"A tour de force . . .
an extremely useful and practical guide to body-centered therapies."
—Jon Kabat-Zinn, author of *Wherever You Go, There You Are*
and *Full Catastrophe Living*

"If you want to heal you must be aware of how you feel. The body is where
the experience is stored and it contains its own inner wisdom. Read this
book and learn how to be in touch with your life."
—Bernie Siegel, M.D., author of *Love, Medicine and Miracles*
and *Assistant to the Creator*

"Mirka Knaster gives us the state of the art in understanding the wisdom
of the body. This book is at once a harvest of the world's best knowings
concerning ways of working with the body, and a superb and sensitive
guide to self-discovery."
—Jean Houston, Director, The Foundation for Mind Research

"Mirka Knaster has written a highly informed book on bodyways that I
strongly recommend to those who seek relief from bodily ills, to those who
wish to know themselves better, and to therapists and teachers of body
therapies. Knaster treats the reader as a valued friend, showing how to
assess one's own needs, how to determine the appropriate type of bodyway,
and how to enhance the experience itself."
—Dolores Krieger, Ph.D., R.N., author of *Accepting Your
Power to Heal: The Personal Practice of Therapeutic Touch*

"Mirka Knaster has a practitioner's passionate commitment to body
work—or 'bodyways,' as she calls them—and a journalist's broad
perspective. Her book is a treasury of interesting and exciting information
on our bodies and keeping them healthy."
—Tiffany Field, Ph.D., Department of Pediatrics,
Touch Research Institute, University of Miami School of Medicine

"Mirka Knaster has performed something just short of a miracle. Like an
experienced tour guide in love with her work, she takes us on a wonderful
safari deep into the most amazing terrain of our own bodies. Hers is not
another boring A to Z book, but a thoroughly engaging and fascinating
exploration into today's alternative body therapies, providing immediate
access for newcomers and old hands alike."
—Jeffrey Maitland, Ph.D., Director of Academic Affairs and Faculty
Chairman, the Rolf Institute; author of *Spacious Body*

# Discovering
## the
# Body's
# Wisdom

## MIRKA KNASTER

BANTAM BOOKS
New York Toronto London Sydney Auckland

DISCOVERING THE BODY'S WISDOM
A Bantam Book/July 1996

The author will donate a portion of her royalties to reforestation projects to replace trees used in the printing of this book.

*Rolfing Movement Integration* by Mary Bond, published by Healing Arts Press, an imprint of Inner Traditions International, Rochester, Vt., U.S.A. Copyright © 1993 by Mary Bond.

*Touching the Mountain: The Self-Breema Handbook, Ancient Exercises for the Modern World* by Jon Schreiber. California Health Publications, 1989. Used by permission of the author.

Excerpt adapted from pages 22–31 of *Relaxercise* by David Zemach-Bersin and Mark Reese. Copyright © 1990 by David Zemach-Bersin and Mark Reese. Reprinted by permission of HarperCollins Publishers, Inc.

Excerpt from *Tao Te Ching* by Stephen Mitchell. Translation copyright © 1988 by Stephen Mitchell. Reprinted by permission of HarperCollins Publishers, Inc.

Adapted from Bartenieff I and Lewis D, *Body Movement: Coping with the Environment.* New York: Gordon and Breach, 1980, pp. 246–247.

The BANTAM NEW AGE BOOKS logo is a registered trademark of Bantam Doubleday Dell Publishing Group, Inc.

INTERIOR ILLUSTRATIONS BY LAURA S. LANIER.

BOOK DESIGN BY GLEN EDELSTEIN.

Library of Congress Cataloging-in-Publication Data

Knaster, Mirka.
Discovering the body's wisdom / Mirka Knaster.
p.    cm.
Includes bibliographical references and index.
ISBN 0-553-37327-7
1. Health.   2. New Age movement.   3. Mind and body.   4. Massage.   5. Exercise.   I. Title.
RA776.5.K57   1996
613—dc20    95-39449
CIP

*Published simultaneously in the United States and Canada*

Bantam Books are published by Bantam Books, a division of Bantam Doubleday Dell Publishing Group, Inc. Its trademark, consisting of the words "Bantam Books" and the portrayal of a rooster, is Registered in U.S. Patent and Trademark Office and in other countries. Marca Registrada. Bantam Books, 1540 Broadway, New York, New York 10036

PRINTED IN THE UNITED STATES OF AMERICA
FG    10 9 8 7 6 5 4

*To my parents, Baruch and Cila Knaster,*
*for the gift of life and all that has made*
*it possible to have the goodness I enjoy today.*

# CONTENTS

INTRODUCTION: THE JOURNEY OF A LIFETIME    xiii

Working with the Body    xiv
What Are Bodyways?    xv
Which Bodyway?    xvi
How to Get the Most Out of This Book    xvii
A Path of Self-Awareness    xx

PART I: DOORWAYS TO THE BODY'S WISDOM

CHAPTER 1: THE BENEFITS OF BODYWAYS
Why People Turn to Bodyways    3
The Power of Embodiment    20

CHAPTER 2: BODY ALIENATION: WHERE WE LOST THE BODY
The Split    23
The Body in the Marketplace    28
Family Influences    32
Education    36
Self-Image and Body Image    38

CHAPTER 3: BODY WISDOM
Matter over Mind    41
Befriending the Body    42
Miracle of the Body    42
Feelings: Emotional and Physical    48
Our Inner Voice    50
Body Perception    52
A Body of Truth    55
Sources of Body Wisdom    57

PART II: GETTING STARTED

CHAPTER 4: CHOOSING AND WORKING WITH A PRACTITIONER
Obstacles to Getting Started    63

The Bodyways Relationship                                    64
Differences Among Practitioners                              71
Where to Look for a Practitioner and What to Look For        72
Your Session                                                 77
Evaluating Your Experience                                   84
Ending the Bodyway Relationship                              90

CHAPTER 5: DECIDING ON A BODYWAY
Not One but Many                                             92
Personality                                                  94
Physical Preferences                                         96
What Are You Looking For?                                    97
Scope of Practice                                           100
Models and Categories: Differences and Similarities         103
Mixing and Matching                                         107
Meandering Like a River                                     109
Developing an Internal Sensor                               110

CHAPTER 6: PSYCHOLOGICAL DIMENSIONS OF
BODYWAYS
The Therapeutic Tradition                                   113
Body Ego                                                    116
Remembering Through the Body                                123
The Practice of Awareness                                   127

PART III: A GUIDE TO BODYWAYS

CHAPTER 7: HOW TO USE THIS GUIDE
What's Included, What's Not, Why Not                        136
Bodyway Entries                                             138

CHAPTER 8: WESTERN STRUCTURE AND FUNCTION:
TRADITIONAL MASSAGE AND CONTEMPORARY
THERAPIES
Comparing Medical Models                                    140
Massage                                                     143
    Swedish Style                                           145
    Contemporary Esalen Style                               149
    On-Site/Seated/Chair Massage                            152
    Pregnancy Massage                                       153
    Infant and Child Massage                                156
    Sports Massage                                          159
    Massage for the Elder Years (Geriatric Massage)         162
    Russian Massage                                         163
The Benjamin System of Muscular Therapy                     164

Bindegewebsmassage                                      165
Lymphatic Massage                                       167
Pfrimmer Deep Muscle Therapy                            169
Lauren Berry Method                                     171
Bowen Technique                                         171
Trigger Point Therapy                                   174
Trager Psychophysical Integration                       178
Craniosacral Therapy                                    181
Ortho-Bionomy                                           184
Body Logic                                              186

CHAPTER 9: STRUCTURAL APPROACHES
Standing Upright                                        188
Rolfing (Structural Integration)                        195
Aston-Patterning                                        202
Hellerwork                                              204
Postural Integration                                    205
Soma Neuromuscular Integration                          206
CORE Bodywork                                           207
Myofascial Release                                      208

CHAPTER 10: FUNCTIONAL APPROACHES
Learning to Move                                        209
The Alexander Technique                                 218
Gerda Alexander Eutony                                  222
Sensory Awareness                                       226
The Mensendieck System                                  230
The Feldenkrais Method                                  232
Hanna Somatic Education                                 238
Body-Mind Centering                                     242

CHAPTER 11: WESTERN MOVEMENT ARTS
Starting from Dance                                     246
Laban-Bartenieff                                        248
The Pilates or Physicalmind Method                      253
Ideokinesis                                             256
Contact Improvisation                                   258
Continuum                                               260
Kinetic Awareness                                       263
Authentic Movement                                      266
Skinner Releasing Technique                             268
Wetzig Coordination Patterns                            271

## CHAPTER 12: EASTERN ENERGY

| | |
|---|---|
| The Life Force | 273 |
| The Chinese Tradition | 274 |
| Invisible Yet Visible: The Body Electric | 279 |
| Chinese Bodyways | 282 |
| Chinese Massage/Acupressure | 282 |
| Chi Nei Tsang | 285 |
| The Japanese Tradition | 288 |
| Anma | 288 |
| Shiatsu | 289 |
| Hoshino Therapy | 294 |
| The Indian Tradition | 295 |
| Ayurveda | 295 |
| Chakras and Kundalini | 297 |

## CHAPTER 13: OTHER ENERGETIC SYSTEMS

| | |
|---|---|
| From Asia to America | 300 |
| Traditional Thai Massage | 301 |
| Breema Bodywork | 304 |
| Lomilomi | 306 |
| Jin Shin Jyutsu | 308 |
| Reflexology (Zone Therapy) | 310 |
| Polarity Therapy | 313 |
| Watsu | 316 |
| Zero Balancing | 318 |
| Therapeutic Touch | 319 |
| Reiki | 324 |

## CHAPTER 14: EASTERN MOVEMENT ARTS

| | |
|---|---|
| Meditation in Movement | 326 |
| The Martial Arts | 328 |
| Chinese Tradition | 330 |
| Chi Kung | 331 |
| T'ai Chi Chuan | 335 |
| Japanese Tradition | 339 |
| Aikido | 339 |
| Karate | 342 |
| Indian Tradition | 344 |
| Yoga | 344 |

## CHAPTER 15: CONVERGENCE SYSTEMS

| | |
|---|---|
| Where Body and Psyche Meet | 352 |
| Rosen Method | 354 |

Rubenfeld Synergy Method 357
Phoenix Rising Yoga Therapy 360
Integrative Yoga Therapy 362
Somatosynthesis 364
SHEN Physio-Emotional Release Therapy 366
Somatic Experiencing 368
Hakomi Integrative Somatics 372
Jin Shin Do 374
Process Acupressure 375
Being In Movement 377

ACKNOWLEDGMENTS 380

APPENDIX: HOW TO DEAL WITH SEXUAL MISCONDUCT 383

REFERENCES 386

INDEX 400

There is a force within
Which gives you life—
    seek that.

In your body
Lies a priceless gem—
    seek that.

O wandering Sufi,
    if you want to find
    the greatest treasure
    don't look outside,
Look inside, and seek that.

        —Rumi

# Introduction:
# The Journey of a Lifetime

People travel the whole wide world looking for novelty and adventure. They want to learn about other cultures, places, peoples, and languages. Yet the greatest territory of all to explore is right where you are—your own body. You don't have to set aside time from work for a long vacation. You don't have to get shots or a visa to go abroad. You don't have to save up a heap of money. And you don't need a special wardrobe or luggage. You just need yourself.

*Discovering the Body's Wisdom* is a passport to begin your journey of exploration and discovery in the most fascinating, miraculous, and meaningful land you'll ever traverse. Through such a voyage, I hope you will come to regard your body not as foreign territory but as home.

Take a moment to check in with your body right now. How comfortable are you? Are you curled up in an easy chair? Sitting at a desk or kitchen table? Standing at a bus stop or in a train station? Lying in bed on your side or propped up against pillows? In this moment, stop to observe how you feel in that position. Does your body tell you, "I feel at ease, supported"? Or does it say, "My shoulders and neck are tight," "My lower back aches," "My right foot hurts"? Are you slouching, hunching over, or pressing your weight down onto one leg and foot instead of standing on both?

Most of us go through the day without being aware of how we are in our bodies and what they are trying to communicate. We tune our bodies out in order to get our jobs done, finish our commutes home, and run our errands before we finally lie down and go to sleep, and we hope to wake up feeling good. Even when our bodies finally get our attention with excruciating sensations that we can't ignore, do we listen as they tell us what they want, what they need? Do we know how to respond other than to shut them up by popping a pill, drinking alcohol, turning on the television, or getting overly busy?

> The human body is not an instrument to be used, but a realm of one's being to be experienced, explored, enriched and, thereby, educated.
>
> —Thomas Hanna

And yet it is possible
for you to find the keys
to your body again . . .
and to find your proper
vitality, health, and
autonomy.

—Thérèse Bertherat

What can you do for the tight neck and shoulders, the aching back, the painful foot? How about the recurring pain from an old running injury or the fact that you tire easily? Are you unable to bend over or turn your head fully right and left? Or maybe you're pain-free, but you sense you can stretch your limits. You're curious how much better you can perform, how much more gracefully you can move, how much more pleasure you can experience, how free and lithe you can feel. Instead of ignoring or anesthetizing your body, consider working with it in a cooperative way.

## WORKING WITH THE BODY

Techniques of working with the body existed long before anyone began to keep records on papyri and clay tablets. As soon as someone noticed that relief came with pressing, rubbing, or moving in a certain way, *bodyways*—the term I've coined to refer to body practices ranging from Acupressure to Zero Balancing®—were born. People have used them for millennia to deal with all kinds of ailments, soothe tensions, boost athletic prowess, gain pleasure, and even deepen spiritual practice. Indigenous cultures in every part of the world have long had specialists who know how to massage. Shamans, *curanderos, balians,* and other native healers generally include it in healing ceremonies. In ancient Egypt, masseurs were special assistants to physicians, surgeons, and veterinarians. In some traditional communities, the skills are still passed from generation to generation. In others, a person may be destined for this role because of an early sign, such as a breech birth. Or a health crisis and near-death experience may precipitate becoming a hands-on healer.[1]

Today, beyond the countless testimonials of successful outcomes, we are better able to measure the results of body practices and explain how and why they are effective. For example, a computer search in *Index Medicus* reveals hundreds of research articles in international journals on massage procedures for humans, and animals as well.[2] The Office of Alternative Medicine (OAM), established in 1992 by the National Institutes of Health (NIH), has awarded grants for further research in various kinds of massage therapy, T'ai Chi Chuan, Therapeutic Touch, Yoga, Chi Kung, and other alternative health-care approaches. In the same year, the Touch Research Institute was founded at the University of Miami School of Medicine as the world's first research center devoted solely to understanding the role of touch therapy in human health and development. Ongoing research studies there continue to prove scientifically what the ancient and indigenous cultures knew instinctively. Wherever possible, I cite research findings that support the use of bodyways.

## WHAT ARE BODYWAYS?

There's a lot of name-calling in the field of body practices. It's not mud-slinging, but a habit of differentiating and labeling. Some practitioners are engaged in *bodywork*.[3] Others consider their approaches *therapy*. Still others say they're neither, but rather *somatic education, movement awareness, structural integration,* or even *emotional integration.*

No system, school, or approach defines the range of body disciplines in the same way. For some, it is manual medicine to fix parts of the body that have been injured, cause pain, or are capable only of limited movement. For others, it is emotional as well as physical work. Some see it not as manipulation but as a neuromuscular learning process. Still others view it as the premier vehicle for experiencing relaxation and pleasure. However, whether they're focused on one aspect of your body or on the unity of your body, mind, emotions, and spirit, all bodyways start from three basic assumptions:

- Something is constricting, restricted, blocked, misused, or out of balance—generally because of excessive muscle tension and habit.
- The body is not set in stone; it is plastic and moldable, repairable and educable—you can always do something.
- The body is *the* place for transformation.

They also all share the same goal of changing a person's life for the better. The change could be the immediate relief of discomfort and distress or the longer-range modification of chronic patterns that results in overall improved function. Where approaches differ is on what needs to be changed and how to change it. Does the practitioner repair and improve your structure to affect function or improve function to modify your structure? Is the goal to cure your symptoms or to educate you—draw out self-knowledge and self-control—through conscious awareness?

To get around all the divisions in the field, I created the term *bodyways.* It broadly incorporates both therapy and education as well as relaxation, while still allowing for each separate category of practice and its distinguishing characteristics. I chose *way* (from the Old English *wegan,* "to move") because it suggests a pathway or process, as in *waterway.*

Think of the many different waterways through which water moves: creeks, streams, rivulets, rivers, channels, brooks, rills, seas, oceans, bays, sounds, and lakes. All of the bodyways involve movement, and often the least effortful way can bring about the most ease. Life is, after all, movement. We are living bodies, always in process. As 70 percent water, we are in constant flux, just like a stream. And just as a stream re-

Apart from inherited shortcomings and damages past remedy, we might say that everyone is potentially in perfect health but does not know how to attain it.

—Franz Wurm

It is as if every discipline of healing, health, and becoming whole that ever was has suddenly been called back into practice all over the earth in order that we might have the richest possible inventory of psychophysical opportunities with which to reinvent ourselves.

—Jean Houston

ceives new water from various sources, so too do we take in new information from a variety of bodyways.

Which bodyway will help you move along is another question.

## WHICH BODYWAY?

In 1973, when I was a graduate student at Stanford University, I bought my first massage book and practiced on a friend. I also showed him the Yoga postures I was doing. At the time, those were two of only a handful of body practices in North America, none of which was widespread, but concentrated mostly in pockets on the East and West coasts. Some of them were popular only among dancers and performers who were interested in body awareness and in taking care of themselves.

There were reasons for these limitations. Medical technology had superseded less-prestigious, time-consuming hands-on work. And massage, if not automatically associated with sex, was often suspect as "touchy-feely" stuff from California, while Yoga was "devil's work" from the Far East. A story in the April 1971 issue of *Newsweek* focused not on healing massage but on thinly disguised houses of prostitution called "massage parlors." Between that year and 1980, the American Massage Therapy Association, the oldest and largest national organization representing the profession, had barely two thousand members. By 1995 that figure jumped to more than twenty-three thousand and is still growing. The state of Florida alone had five thousand licensed massage therapists that year. A study published in *The New England Journal of Medicine* (January 28, 1993) reported that massage was the third most commonly used of sixteen alternative health practices.[4]

More than a hundred body-oriented approaches are now available. I've given up counting because each year new ones spring up like mushrooms after a drenching rain. Other associations, such as the American Oriental Body Therapies Association and Associated Professional Massage Therapists and Allied Health Practitioners International, have been organized to represent the diverse groups of practitioners, now surpassing a hundred thousand. In addition, many health-care professionals such as nurses, doctors, dentists, and psychotherapists have also incorporated some of these practices in their work. According to the American Business Institute, massage was one of the three fastest-growing businesses in 1991. In 1995 there were already more than five hundred massage schools, plus the many other kinds of similar training institutes that exist from Maine to Hawaii and in Canada.

Today more than ever, the field is exploding with both exciting new bodyways and renewed interest in old ones. Increasingly, scientific discoveries in diverse areas of research coupled with the latest explorations in psychology are pushing the frontiers of our knowledge of mind and body and our ability to deal with mind-body conditions. *Discovering the Body's Wisdom* provides a window into these leading-edge therapies, disciplines, and systems that until recently either were not widely accessible or did not yet exist. I could not have written this book ten years ago.

With so much available, how do you decide what you really want or what will truly satisfy your needs? And how do you choose the best practitioner to work with? You can make more informed choices as a consumer-client when you know more about the different bodyways. When you choose well, it can have a transformative effect on your life. But when you don't, it may provide no relief or insight and discourage you from seeking more effective help. Although I can't guarantee that you'll always choose the best bodyway and best practitioner, this book does provide you with the information you need to minimize pitfalls and maximize benefits. And it may help you save money.

## How to Get the Most Out of This Book

*Discovering the Body's Wisdom* is divided into three parts.

Part I discusses causes of body difficulties and what advantages you can derive from working with your body. It also introduces you to the principles that underlie this book: body alienation, or how we lost connection with the body; befriending the body; the miracle of the body; and body wisdom.

Part II describes ways of choosing and interacting with a practitioner as well as deciding on which bodyway approach to work with. It leads you through a process of both evaluating the practitioner and assessing your own attitudes and preferences. I include such issues as ethics, curing and healing, treatment and education, goal and process orientations, and short- and long-term benefits. I also cover scope of practice, "hurts good" versus "hurts bad," mixing and matching, and more. A chapter on psychological dimensions will help you understand why bodyways affect more than your physical structure and presents the practice of awareness as a useful prelude to trying any bodyway.

Part III serves as a guide to the bodyways field itself. Each section examines the foundation of a whole group of practices and how they approach the body. The explanation will enable you to understand how so many differently named disciplines can be both similar and distinct. The description of the bodyway includes its aim, technique(s) used, benefits, a section called "Resources" for more information, and, in some cases, a section called "Experience," which gives you a taste of the practice.

Although it is useful to start the book at the beginning and advance

> It is not only possible but natural for each of us to love our bodies, to find ourselves beautiful—no matter how different, disabled, old, or battle-scared we may be.
>
> —Harriett Goldhor Lerner

> Wisdom is not what comes from reading great books. When it comes to understanding life, experiential learning is the only worthwhile kind, everything else is hearsay.
>
> —Joan Erikson

chapter by chapter to the end, you can proceed in whichever way suits you. If in one section I refer to a concept, system, or person that interests you, you may track the hand symbol ☞ and turn to the appropriate page. And, as circumstances in your life change, you can go back to the book again and again.

If your body sometimes feels like a stranger or enemy to you, Part I offers you the opportunity to investigate where your uncomfortable, even antagonistic relationship comes from, how you can move instead toward friendship with your body, and what that friendship has to offer you. I know very few people who are perfectly at ease in and satisfied with their bodies. However, if you're one of them and want to skip Part I, go ahead.

If you've had little or no experience in working with body practices and practitioners, Part II will guide you step by step in making choices about them. If you're already familiar with the bodyways field, Part II can help you better understand some of the experiences you've had and suggest how to avoid the ineffective or harmful ones. It can also help you understand why you gravitate toward certain body disciplines and away from others. You may be following a habitual pattern, and it might be fruitful to try a different approach.

Throughout the book you will find boxes labeled "Experience." Each experience allows you to explore some aspect of bodyways with questions and/or with physical and visual experiments. You might find it fun and illuminating to do the Experiences with a partner and compare notes. If you would rather listen than read, tape the questions and directions first. These Experiences are yours to do with as you wish; they are suggestions rather than commands to do homework. If any part feels uncomfortable, elicits pain, or otherwise disturbs you, you are free to stop at any point or adjust it to your own needs. You can do all or some as you go through the book. If you don't want to engage in one, you always have the option of trying it on another occasion. You also can return to these Experiences and repeat them, observing the differences in how you respond over time.

If you're a psychotherapist or other health-care professional, *Discovering the Body's Wisdom* can assist you in identifying bodyways that are appropriate for your patients as well as help you work cooperatively with other providers. If you're someone who is contemplating a career change, or if you're a body practitioner who is considering acquiring new skills, the information here can help you choose and get started in a new direction. You may also want to refer your clients to the book so that they can become informed, responsible participants or consumers.

## No Mechanical Prescriptions

Some guides are organized by specific ailments or conditions and the approaches that work best for them. I've chosen not to do this because healing often has less to do with technique per se than with a whole constellation of factors. The process is not a mechanical one, and there is no one right practice for any given difficulty. For example, I know of cases in which people with paralysis were able to move again after sessions of Moshe Feldenkrais's gentle hands-on work called Functional Integration®, Emilie Conrad Da'oud's movement process Continuum, or Thérèse Pfrimmer's deep tissue massage. All of these approaches worked very differently in terms of method and focus, yet each facilitated the same result—greater movement.

If you have back pain, you might find relief, temporary or permanent, with any number of practitioners. That's because your back condition is unique to you—what brought it about, what emotions might be associated with it, how you care for yourself, what kind of work you do and its occupational hazards, how long-standing your difficulty is, what aggravates it, and what eases it. One person may relieve stiffness and soreness by practicing Yoga daily; someone else may resolve a chronic back restriction through a series of Rolfing® sessions or Alexander lessons. Also critical to your healing is the rapport you develop with the practitioner.

Working with the body is not just about alleviating a muscle spasm in your back or some other limitation. It can be the entryway to an education you never got in school, an education that teaches not by rote but by examining and experiencing with your whole being. How many of us ever learned in school how our bodies function and grow, how they communicate to us, and how to take good care of them? Working with the body helps draw out an inner knowledge or intelligence that no amount of reading and memorizing could ever do. As farmer-poet Wendell Berry says, "There's a world of difference . . . between that information to which we now presumably have access by way of computers, libraries, and the rest of it, great stockpiles of data, and the knowledge that people have in their bones by which they do good work and live good lives."[5]

That's why this is not a prescriptive book: You won't be able to look up a symptom and find a quick-fix solution. I'm not a doctor who writes a prescription for a drug to treat a sore throat. Many people are already exasperated with the health-care industry because it looks at them as diseased tissue. It labels them with one disorder or another, sends them to this or that specialist to treat one part of themselves, and gives them the latest magic bullet, which often provides only a temporary cure. Where is the whole person in this scenario?

There is a story told about physicist-turned-somatic educator Moshe Feldenkrais, who abhorred labels and generalizations. Someone once innocently asked him which of his techniques were best for pregnant women. Feldenkrais erupted, "You idiot! There is no such thing as a pregnant

*I learned that knowledge, not yet in my mind, was in my body.*
—Ellen Goldman

*What you do not experience in your whole body will remain merely intellectual information without life or spiritual reality.*
—Gerda Alexander

woman! A fourteen-year-old girl having her first baby is nothing like a thirty-five-year-old woman having her fourth child. What I would do with each is completely different."[6]

Don't be misled by publications that advise which system to use for which body condition. For example, one book recommends Polarity Therapy for eyestrain. It's just not that simple. Eyestrain or headache can be the result of a number of things and, depending upon the circumstances, a variety of bodyways or other measures could help—Acupressure, massage of the head, face, and neck, Craniosacral Therapy, Myofascial Release, Trigger Point Therapy, and so on.

This book is not so much concerned with pathology as with how health and well-being can flourish when given suitable nourishment. Even the nineteenth-century French chemist Louis Pasteur, father of the germ theory, recognized before he died that instead of condemning parasites, bacteria, and viruses as the culprits in disease, it is important to attend to the environment. "The germ is nothing," he said, "the soil is everything."[7]

## A PATH OF SELF-AWARENESS

In many ways, this book reflects my own journey toward befriending my body. In my twenties and thirties, I possessed great stores of energy, stamina, and recuperability. I didn't let anything stop me. I always managed to get around imbalances and weaknesses by being blind to their existence or by plowing ahead with willpower. For example, I had an unconscious habit of overusing the right side of my body in all activities. Instead of developing strength and flexibility equally on both sides, I got tighter on the right side of my back and compensated by stretching harder on the left. My Yoga postures may have looked good, but my body paid the price. The contracted muscles never fully let go and the overstretched tendons and ligaments never had a chance to return to their original length. Instead of doing things with ease, I just worked harder.

During that long struggle, I allowed my mind to hold sway. I pushed my body to do more even when exhausted, constantly found fault with its shape and size, and ignored its messages until it screamed so loudly that I finally had to stop in my tracks and listen. Sometimes that meant barely being able to walk, let alone run, or having to lie in bed even when I needed to keep working to pay the mortgage. Now that I'm gentler and friendlier with my body, I pay attention if it so much as whispers to me, and I don't override its wisdom. The more I've grown to accept and love my body as it is, the more it has become what I'd always wanted it to be. Not surprisingly, it refused to do that when I was trying to whip it into shape.

We cannot escape our physical natures; and a proper pride in oneself as a human being is rooted in the body through which love is given and taken.

—Anthony Storr

I've been exploring my own body through a wide variety of approaches for more than twenty years. Some I have trained in only for myself; others I have practiced professionally and taught to others. During this time I also have done extensive cross-cultural research in body disciplines and healing practices in the United States and abroad, particularly in Asia.

Over the years, my awareness level has changed from focusing on the outside to looking inside. I thought I was aware of my body and was truly living in it because I was engaged in both bodyways and athletic activities. I was, but only to a certain extent. In retrospect, I did Yoga during the early years with the intention of getting the posture picture-perfect right away, even if it meant ignoring an inner voice that counseled, "Less is okay; slowly and gradually are okay." Instead of concerning myself primarily with working near my limits, I felt competitive with other students to look good. With time, I came to understand that making Yoga an exterior rather than interior experience defeats its purpose.

The longer I'm in this field, the more layers I penetrate. It's a lifelong process. I am continually intrigued by new approaches. I keep learning how to recognize which bodyway I need when and for what. And the more I open to my body, the more I open to life outside myself as well.

I can't make you become friends with your body. It's taken me half a lifetime. I *can* share with you what I've learned along the way from the many people who shared with me. By exploring your own body and developing awareness, you too can move into a place of greater ease with yourself and with everything around you.

> The real voyage of discovery consists not in seeking new landscapes but in having new eyes.
>
> —Marcel Proust

## Becoming Your Own Authority

Most of all, I hope that this guide will set you on a course of befriending your body and discovering its wisdom. When you're alienated from your own body, you become a stranger to yourself. You're not aware of the resources you have for making judgments and decisions; instead, you rely on recognized authorities to tell you what to think, believe, and do. Once you have stopped treating your body as an enemy and start to appreciate it as an endless source of knowledge, you can choose over and over on your own. You know and accept what is right for you and reject what doesn't fit.

This book is not about one more person being the authority for your life. No parent, no physician, no teacher, and certainly no writer is the last word on your own body. Don't let any bodyway become yet another standard with power over you. Don't reject one expert, such as an M.D., only to replace him with another, a Rolfer®, for example. *Discovering the Body's Wisdom* is an invitation to become your own authority. If even one of you reading this book reaches that place, then I know that my efforts will have made a difference.

> It is precisely through the veils which authorities have spun for us that our own ears and eyes and nerves must begin to penetrate if our hands are to grasp the world and our hearts to feel it. We must recover our own capacity to taste for ourselves. Then we shall be able to judge also.
>
> —Charles Brooks

# Experience: Your Body Wisdom Journal

Even if you don't keep a daily journal, I highly recommend starting a body wisdom journal. Make it easy: treat yourself to a beautiful bound journal, have your sketch book do double duty, get a looseleaf binder or steno pad. Since I fill a journal every two months, I buy a stack of thick, inexpensive spiral notebooks at a discount store. If you have difficulty writing, record on audiotape. It doesn't matter how you do it; the act of self-examination is what counts.

As you read through *Discovering the Body's Wisdom*, enter your answers to questions and reactions to Experiences in the journal. Keeping a log of your journey will both clarify where you stand in relation to your body and increase your awareness and sensitivity. When you make an inventory, you get to know what you have and what you need.

Journal-keeping will also prepare you for your bodyway sessions and help you evaluate their effects on you, especially if you enter your responses again in six months, a year, two years. Reporting to yourself will be like having a reunion with an old friend. After you've explored one bodyway (or more) for a while, go back and see how much you've changed in attitudes toward your body, feelings of ease and comfort, and behavior patterns. If there's no difference, and if you've given that one a fair chance, perhaps you've not yet found the bodyway that's effective for you, and you need to try something else.

Here are some questions to begin with:

### Physical feelings and energy level

When have I felt the most comfortable or satisfied in my body? Where? With whom? How is my body a place of pleasure and joy?

When have I felt uncomfortable in my body? Where? With whom?

How do I feel right now? Am I relaxed, at ease? Do I feel anxious? Do I hurt all over? Where do I feel pain or tension? Is it always here? How long has that been true? Does it jump from place to place around my body? Do I not feel anything? Am I hot or cold? Have I been sluggish or active lately? Am I tired or energetic? Am I pushing myself? Do I sleep restfully or wake up exhausted? Do I wish I could nap right now? How easy or how difficult is my breathing? Am I constantly short of breath?

### Emotional feelings

Do I like the way I look? What don't I like about myself? Am I calm about the ups and downs in my life, or do I freak out? Am I depressed, angry, anxious, afraid, bored, curious, joyful? Do I swing from one mood to another? Do I cry easily? Is it hard for me to cry? Do I laugh nervously? How often do I smile? How do I feel around other people at home, at work, in school, at social gatherings?

### Dream life

What have I been dreaming about? Have the themes changed, or do the same things keep coming up? Have I resolved anything? Are my dreams giving me messages about my body?

### Habits

Do I eat well, skip meals, grab something on the run? Do I stuff myself when I'm angry, tired, or unhappy? Do I rely on coffee or candy bars to perk me up? What does alcohol do for me, and what does it do against me? What drugs am I using? Am I changing my relationship to any of these: increasing, decreasing, completely eliminating, adding, or substituting?

# PART I

## Doorways to the Body's Wisdom

# CHAPTER 1

# The Benefits of Bodyways

During twenty years of practicing first massage, then Trager® Psychophysical Integration, at Esalen Institute in Big Sur, California, Deane Juhan witnessed one remarkable change after another. It sounds like a scene out of Lourdes, that well-known site of miracles in southwest France:

> I have seen stoops straighten, gnarled deformities become more comfortable and functional, injuries heal more quickly . . . completely. I have seen dozens of imminent surgeries averted, medications reduced or eliminated, eyeglasses upgraded . . . occasionally discarded, chronic pain diminish or disappear, various degenerative conditions slow to a halt or even reverse. And I have heard [people] talk enthusiastically about the positive changes they had experienced at home in their relationship with fellow workers . . . employers . . . friends . . . lovers, spouses, children, parents. And with themselves.[1]

Juhan attributes these changes not to temporary analgesia or the placebo effect but to the cumulative process of getting to know one's body from a fresh perspective. Bodyways can be the means for gaining that new viewpoint.

## WHY PEOPLE TURN TO BODYWAYS

Suffering is a great motivator. Many people first turn to bodyways because the pain of an injury or chronic condition forces them to seek alternatives, often after orthodox treatment—surgery and drugs—fails to give relief or

It is not our lightness of heart but our distress which gives the impetus to seek our inmost truth. Too much medical tranquillizing may actually cheat the more sensitive among us from becoming whole.

—Irene Claremont de Castillejo

Pain is the body's cry for help. You are doing something that the body can't take any longer. The body is very patient. It takes a lot of tension and abuse before it makes pain.

—Marion Rosen

has made them dependent on medication. Practitioners report that frequently clients come to their doorsteps when they have nowhere else to go. In desperation and exasperation, they finally try a bodyway to deal with their arthritis, backache, repetitive stress syndrome, or other occupational strains, to help heal old football or dance injuries, or for recovery after childbirth and automobile accidents. While it may be their last resort, it's also the first step toward a new awareness of being in their body and thus a new relationship to their lives.

Such "last-resort" individuals appeared on a Bill Moyers special on healing broadcast on PBS in the winter of 1993. They were shown learning Mindfulness Meditation and Yoga with Jon Kabat-Zinn at the University of Massachusetts Medical Center. Doctors refer patients to the eight-week Stress Reduction and Relaxation Program for anything from headaches, high blood pressure, and back pain to heart disease, cancer, and AIDS.

One such patient, because of a heart attack, was forced to retire from his own large business, from which he had never taken a vacation in forty years. He was depressed and bewildered. By the end of the program he was healthier and happier, with a sparkle in his eyes and an enthusiasm for living. He went from seeing himself as a heart patient to experiencing himself as a whole person, one who could now express love for his family and affection for others as well. Another man, in his seventies, showed up in a wheelchair. The pain in his feet was so severe he wanted to cut them off. He gradually moved from wheelchair to crutches to cane, and he became a more active and cheerful person. Under other circumstances, neither man would have voluntarily chosen to get involved with his body in the precise and caring way that is taught in the course.[2]

According to Dr. James Lynch, author of *The Broken Heart: The Medical Consequences of Loneliness,* "People most vulnerable to disease are extraordinarily disconnected from their bodies." His research indicates that individuals with the highest blood pressure raise their pressure even more while speaking, but they are less likely to be aware that this is happening. "These were rational thinkers with no bodily awareness," he says. "If I'm speaking to you, and my blood pressure rises by 50 percent, then the dialogue could be killing me."[3]

Many of us have been conditioned to look to authorities rather than to learn for ourselves. The more you develop an accurate picture of your body—from within and from without—and the more you can easily feel the different parts, the more you will know what you need to do to take care of yourself and what you need to tell a health-care practitioner who will collaborate in your healing. Various innovators in the field of bodyways did just that and actually became their own healers. Through acute observation and sensitivity, Elsa Gindler cured herself of tuberculosis, Elisabeth Dicke reversed a circulatory disorder and avoided amputation of her leg, Moshe Feldenkrais healed himself of a knee injury, and F. M. Alexander adjusted his posture and stopped losing his voice. ☞ See their stories, pages 227, 165, 233, and 218. In the process, they all developed effective systems that are popular today.

The other motivation for bodyways comes from a more positive frame of mind, from a natural drive toward healthy or optimal functioning. You feel pretty good, yet you sense that you could expand beyond your present limitations. Maybe you want to gain greater flexibility or improve your posture. You're motivated by curiosity and interest: How can I live to my full capacity as a human being? It's been said over and over that the majority of us operate at a fraction of our potential. However, while that's expressed almost predominantly in terms of the brain, the body's intelligence also remains largely untapped. How can I be more creative? How can I prevent the restrictions and pains that limit my life? How can I age well?

It doesn't matter what your reason is for turning to work with your body. Whether you want to get better or to function better, taking that step will open a whole new world for you and may bring you not only the relief you long for but also knowledge and power you weren't aware you had. That's what fulfilling your potential is all about.

Underlying all the reasons that lead us to bodyways is an instinctive drive toward wholeness. We all also yearn, consciously or unconsciously, to be at peace within the war zone of our own bodies. Countries in the Middle East spend about $60 billion a year buying arms. Imagine how much energy and other valuable resources could be released for better purposes—education, health care, and other social programs—if the Arabs and Israelis shift from enmity to cooperation. The continuation of endless war and misery makes no sense, either in the Middle East or in your own body.

## Sensitivity, Flexibility, and Communication

Bodyways are a useful tool for increasing sensitivity to ourselves. When we become more sensitive, greater communication and flexibility are the result. Instead of trying to silence the body with medication or TV noise, we are willing to receive its messages. When we don't turn a deaf ear, we can avoid greater problems.

Jungian analyst Anita Greene learned the importance of listening the hard way. "Whenever I have denied [my body's] needs or ignored its wisdom," she says, "it has 'spoken': an appendectomy delayed completing a master's degree, a fractured shoulder hindered writing a thesis, a migraine interrupts an overactive life. The message is loud and clear. Disregard the demand of the unconscious for balance and for centered being, and the body pays the price."[4]

And we will be in tune with our bodies only if we truly love and honor them. We can't be in good communication with the enemy.

—Harriet Goldhor Lerner

The aim . . . is to cooperate with the body rather than regard it as a misshapen alien or a rather unreliable but omnipresent companion.

—Jean Houston

# Benefits from Working with the Body

Depending on the kind of bodyways you engage in, the benefits, though they vary, are many, and they may arise directly or indirectly.

- Correction of various disorders and conditions
- Prevention of injury and illness
- Reduction of stress response
- Relief of pain
- Improved posture and functioning; a more upright, lighter-feeling body
- Better balance and coordination
- Reversal of aging symptoms; increased health and longevity
- Greater sensory awareness
- Increased sexual pleasure
- More sensitivity, flexibility, gracefulness; friendlier relations and increased connectedness with self and others
- Definition of personal boundaries
- Access to memories and body wisdom
- Emotional healing; shift from victim role to position of self-autonomy, authority, power
- Groundedness, centeredness
- Fewer inhibitions and repressions; expanded capacity for work and creativity; actualization of potential
- More lucid thinking, enlivened consciousness, and embodied spiritual life
- Wholeness rather than fragmentation; living firsthand from the entire body, not just the head—authentic rather than intellectual responses
- Replacement of old negative habits with new positive patterns—cessation of destructive, anesthetizing lifestyles
- Self-acceptance—recognition of one's uniqueness and beauty as a gift of creation; new self-image, new sense of physical self

*I came to see that my body's tensions and headaches were a protest against the denial of my own self.*

*—Clark Moustakas*

When Jean Shinoda Bolen, M.D., a psychiatrist and author of the best-selling *Goddesses in Everywoman,* was going through a trying midlife transition, she sought bodyways to establish communication with her body and feelings. In *Crossing to Avalon,* she recounts the insight she had one afternoon as she lay on the table for her session.

I became aware that I was holding my left arm in such a way that it shielded my heart, with my left hand in a fist, the position of a shield-carrier. I had been through another difficult week and, as usual, stayed on top of things. However, as I lay there, I became aware not only of how I was holding my arm, but that if I opened and spread my arm like a wing, grief would well up. I also knew in that moment that I needed help to do it. I had too much resistance to opening up; some part of me was invested in keeping the feelings down. . . . I asked my body therapist if she would please move my arm up and off my chest. She did and the tears came.

As I struggled to open up and let the grief out, the physician-observer in me thought of the fairly common disease referred to either as a frozen shoulder or shoulder-hand syndrome. It's an excruciatingly painful condition experienced by some women in midlife. It often lasts as long as a year and then disappears as inexplicably as it came. Without physical therapy, muscle atrophy from disuse may complicate the condition. I think I could have been a candidate for this. The emotional pain I was not allowing myself to feel would then have expressed itself through my body as physical pain.[5]

When bodyways are effective, it is because they help reestablish this internal communication by overcoming our disconnection from our body and our feelings. In turn, we're better able to communicate with others as well. "If you cannot listen to your own heart, then how are you going to get your wife to understand you?" asks Dr. James Lynch.[6] The more knowledge we have of ourselves, the better able we are to state our positions, needs, and desires and to hear what others have to say. When you are sensitive to a friend and engaged in communication, don't you find yourself less rigid and more willing to bend, more creative in coming up with solutions?

*Neurosis consists in being out of touch with one's own feelings and sensory experience; and therapy is the recovery of awareness.*

—Fritz Perls

*Ultimately our knowledge of ourselves will give us more to share with others.*

—Tarthang Tulku

## Relationships

Although it seems strange to imagine that lying on a table to be Rolfed or that moving slowly and carefully in T'ai Chi Chuan could help you in your relationships, it's true. There's no direct correlation, but indirectly many things can happen.

Clyde W. Ford, a chiropractor and the creator of Somatosynthesis, refers to how we relate to others as the dance of bonding and separating. We learn it first through our infant bodies, in response to our parents or other caretakers. How well we can come together with or move apart from others depends on what we experienced as children in terms of intimacy, affection, trust, nurturance, abandonment, and abuse.

Do you lean strongly toward one extreme or the other—always clinging close or forever keeping your distance? Ford calls these two directions the "Lost Satellite" and the "Submerged Self." If you're "lost," you probably have difficulty bonding with others and generally live tight and tense,

When my body
becomes a safer place to
live, I will interact with
you differently . . .
more successfully, more
harmoniously, more
lovingly, because I bring
a body that is living in
less of a resistant field,
or in a nonresistant
field, in relationship
to you.

—Rosie Spiegel

as though your body were a protective shell. If you're "submerged," you're probably constantly trying to bond with others, and you find yourself unable to separate from them. Bodywise, you may tend to be overweight, out of shape, unboundaried, and unaware of large portions of your body.[7]

Bodyways can enable you to become aware of your penchant and also to find a place of balance between the two extremes, an ease in being intimate or distant, according to what's appropriate in a situation. Reclaiming your body—loosening or tightening the boundaries—through bodyways is like diving into the ocean to a sunken ship and finding a lost treasure. When you know where your body begins and ends and how it feels, you gain the power to make choices in life, to seek constructive help, and to create and maintain healthy relationships.

As you learn safe touch and boundaries, you begin to feel at home and safe in your body, and you learn that no one has the right to trespass. It's like having a sign up that says, "Do not enter unless expected or welcome." Once you feel different in your body—for instance, allowing sensations rather than cutting them off—you also behave differently, and thus attract different people and relationships into your life.

A client of Aikidoist and Lomi psychotherapist Richard Strozzi Heckler is a good example. Gerard, as he calls him, was a successful corporate executive but was unsuccessful in maintaining an intimate relationship. For years he blamed women for leaving him, completely unaware of his physical and emotional flatness. His muscles had little tone or definition; his movements were glacierlike; his shoulders were rounded forward and his head drooped over his sunken chest. Working with his body somatically enabled him to finally feel how numb and caved in his chest was.

One winter day, I took a break from writing and walked down the road through the woods. The sun was already melting snow that had been sitting on the trees for days. Pieces would drop off suddenly. I shook the snow out of some of the evergreens because it pained me each time I went by and saw them so bowed by the weight of the wet whiteness clinging to their needles. I wondered whether the rigors of winter would permanently deform them, like the hunchback of Notre Dame, or whether they would gradually realign themselves. They reminded me of people whose bodies are curved by the burden of their lives—their work, their relationships or lack of them, their physical and emotional suffering. I hoped that by shaking the young trees free of snow, I would help jump-start their process of springing back to uprightness. In the same way, I believe the experience of being moved and moving in new ways, even of literally having patterns shook out, patterns formed by the weight of different stresses and traumas in life, can help jump-start our own process, too.

Gerard realized how terrified he was of intimacy: When anyone came too close physically or emotionally, he withdrew by squeezing his throat, chest, and pelvis. Every time he tried to take a deep breath, he'd start choking and coughing. As a boy, he'd nearly drowned while his mother stood by helplessly, afraid to go near him. After that incident, Gerard trusted no woman again. Gradually, as he allowed himself to feel again in his body, he also learned how to stop shutting himself off from relationships with women and business colleagues.[8]

*Knowing others is intelligence; knowing yourself is true wisdom.*

*—Tao Te Ching*

## Inner Knowledge and Freedom

We need to learn to face and effectively deal with all kinds of weather conditions in life. Avoiding and anesthetizing aren't the solution to stormy days. Ultimately, that kind of response requires more energy than does creatively confronting the winds that blow through our lives. Because bodyways can help you know yourself better, they also can enable you to meet and brave what comes. When you know yourself, you're better able to respond instinctively and authentically to each situation, for you can see it clearly for what it is.

This "knowing thyself" is not exactly what the ancient Greek philosopher Socrates had in mind. It's not a knowing from the head. It's not a knowing imparted from a teacher or elder or book. Nor is it a knowing achieved through supplication to a deity. It's a knowing that can come only from within our own bodies, from our own hearts and guts. It's inside-out rather than outside-in. And that's what is crucial to personal freedom—not just freedom from disease and injury, from chronic mental and physical difficulties, but also freedom from habitual restrictions that keep us from becoming all that we were meant to be as human beings. From knowing thyself can come being thyself.

*One cannot understand the rhythms and meanings of the outer world until one has mastered the dialects of the body.*

*—Timothy Leary*

Inside-out knowing is what we need to keep from being seduced by false prophets. After his own devastating experiences in Auschwitz during World War II, the Italian chemist Primo Levi warned that without inner freedom, people can end up faithfully following fascists. "It is better to renounce revealed truths, even if they exalt us by their splendor or if we find them convenient because we can acquire them gratis," he said. "It is better to content oneself with other more modest and less exciting truths, those one acquires painfully, little by little and without shortcuts . . . those that can be verified and demonstrated."[9]

Why else is it imperative to be the authority for our own lives? Aside from avoiding demagogues, we need to eschew opinions that limit our potential. When Raun Kaufman was born autistic, the so-called experts showered his parents with prognoses such as "hopeless," "irreversible," "unreachable," and "incurable." Fortunately for Raun, his parents, Barry

*But he can make no progress with himself unless he becomes very much better acquainted with his own nature.*

*—C. G. Jung*

I am certain that children always know more than they are able to tell, and that makes the big difference between them and adults, who, at best, know only a fraction of what they say. The reason is simply that children know everything with their whole beings, while we know it only with our heads.

—Jacques Lusseyran

and Samahria Kaufman, defied the professional authorities. Even when the doctors scolded them, saying, "Your son has a devastating lifelong condition; he'll never come out of it," the Kaufmans still followed their own counsel. The result is what the medical establishment calls a miracle. Raun, diagnosed also as severely mentally retarded, went on to attend and graduate from high school, enter the university of his choice, make friends, become a member of a debating team, and enjoy life fully.[10] When we don't let someone else be the authority for what we can or cannot do, all kinds of things are possible.

A story I read about a football coach and his team at a New York City high school also demonstrates what can happen when we switch from being influenced by outside authorities—in this case, external images and myths—to relying on information from our own bodies. One semester, the coach decided to have the players take ballet lessons to learn lateral movement and develop strength. In that tough neighborhood, macho males ordinarily would be ostracized for engaging in such "girls' stuff," but these guys got away with it. Much to their surprise, the ballet got them interested and active in social dancing, which they had formerly considered effeminate. After this change, one football player, who had wondered why he was adept on the athletic field but clumsy on the dance floor, realized that his community's ideas of what a man should or *should not* do had turned into a situation of *could not*. Through his body, he learned otherwise: He didn't have to limit what he could do.

## Stimulating Awareness

An addiction serves to numb us so that we are out of touch with what we know and what we feel.

—Anne Wilson Schaef

Most of us in the West are exposed to an unending stream of stimuli—the mechanical noises of vehicles, refrigerators, chain saws, and pneumatic drills; nonstop banter from TV, radio, and boom boxes; the honking of horns and the yelling of people, the barking of dogs and meowing of cats; not to mention the ceaseless chatter in our own heads.

If your sensory circuits are already overloaded, you're probably trying hard to block out what you see, feel, hear, and smell so that you can get through the day. You may be so overstimulated as to be numb, even amnesiac to your own body. You may also be deadened or desensitized because when you felt pain at an earlier time, you withdrew your awareness from that sensitivity and suffering.

By freezing or anesthetizing our bodies, we don't have to feel what hurts. But in doing so, we also keep ourselves from feeling what gives joy. The source of pain is also the source of pleasure. Cut off one and we cut off the other as well. Worst of all, we are no longer aware of how frozen we are. That is the nature of frostbite: Where it has struck, there is no longer any feeling. That means we can't know that the feeling is actually lacking.

The kind of frostbite caused by cutting off your feelings—tension blocks—helped us at one time to stop feelings and impulses that seemed dangerous, painful, prohibited, or unacceptable, but now they're keeping us from feeling altogether.[11]

Working with the body provides a different kind of stimulation, one that eases rather than stresses. Becoming aware of bodily sensations can be an antidote to overstimulation in the modern world and the desensitization it causes. It can be a way to thaw and heal the frostbite. Awakening your body and becoming aware of its insights as well as its sensory delights can be a doorway into a spacious room. It can reintroduce you to the areas you deadened in self-defense. It is also a means to slow down even in the midst of frenetic living, by physically experiencing each moment now instead of speeding along mentally. The body anchors you in the present, the place where time seems full and expanded, rather than short and limited. In that calm you rest, you learn, you change, you heal.

That process can continue to help you to discover who you are and help you to exercise a degree of self-control over your physical and emotional symptoms. By self-control, I mean not rigid suppression but the ability to choose, to respond rather than react. Self-awareness is a prerequisite for this, and it can come from bodyways.

You might wonder why we need to be more aware of our bodies when they seem to run along just fine on their own. We breathe, our hearts

> It is not easy to recognize and choose good nourishment of any kind if the spontaneous and receptive instinctual part of us is numb and neglected.
>
> —Jean Shinoda Bolen

## Experience: Observing Your Breath

Stop for a moment and note how fast, slow, shallow, or deep your breath is. Don't make any effort to change it. Just watch your breath as it enters your nostrils, fills your lungs, and expands your chest. Notice how it makes your abdomen inflate or rise when you breathe in. Then, as you breathe out, feel how your belly deflates and falls and your chest drops back.

Did the air coming into your nostrils feel cold or warm? When the air touched the area above your upper lip as it came out of your nostrils, was it cold or warm? Did you breathe in and out through both nostrils, or in one and out the other? After several breaths, has each breath become easier or more labored? Do you feel calmer or more anxious? Has your heartbeat slowed down or speeded up?

Any emotional response you have will immediately change your breathing pattern. Simply becoming aware of your breathing changes it, but without any active intention or effort to do so. The mere observation of our natural functions is enough to connect us with our body and what it wants to do, given the opportunity. To try this with anger, ☞ see the Experience on page 16.

beat, the food we eat gets digested and eliminated, all apparently without our assistance. However, when we stop to observe even "automatic" functions such as these, the nature of the process changes, generally for the better.

## Avoiding Loss

Another reason to work with the body is to avoid losing what we don't use. "Behind *every* technological innovation . . . is a withered human faculty," says Michael Murphy, cofounder of Esalen Institute. "For every automobile, a little more flabby muscle . . . the more reliance on [technology], the less reliance on the stupendous inheritance [of] . . . our psychosomatic, psychophysical capacities that we don't cultivate . . . our natural birthright."[12]

Part of the purpose in working with the body is to stem the tide of this loss, to awaken these capacities before atrophy sets in. An extreme version of such deterioration is a kind of sensory marasmus. In the 1800s and early 1900s, when infants were left in foundling institutions and not touched, they had no way to activate their sensory-motor systems (the sensing and moving capacities of the muscles through the central nervous system), and they literally wasted away.[13] More recently, such cases have appeared in understaffed Romanian orphanages.

If you've had polio or know someone who has, you understand well this "use it or lose it" principle, for the muscles of the stricken leg, when not exercised, degenerate. This loss of use is true whether or not polio is involved. Stimulation to the neuromuscular system is what helps stem the tide. The input can come from the skillful touch of a practitioner or your own slow movements made with careful attention. You can provide yourself with new feedback through, for example, working with balls in Kinetic Awareness®, with directions from a teacher in person or on tape, as in the Feldenkrais Awareness Through Movement® lessons, or by doing movements such as Yoga asanas. Bodyways furnish new sensory data to break you out of the same old ways and create change. They help form a new template that includes greater flexibility, variety, smoothness, and appropriateness in your movements. As the nervous system resequences muscular activity, it dehabituates old patterns. The result is that you learn to prevent disease, injury, and stress-related illness.

> The prophets preach . . . that pleasure, not will-power and coercion, is how you most deeply transform people.
>
> —Matthew Fox

## Pleasure

You can use bodyways to provide more than relief from discomfort. Through them, you can educate yourself to focus differently on your body—not as a source of pain, but as a source of pleasure and comfort. Take a moment to make a mental list of pleasurable experiences that espe-

## Greater Sexual Pleasure

Joseph Heller, the creator of the structural approach he calls Hellerwork, says that before he worked with his body, he would never have said that he had any problems with sex. He was sexually active and enjoyed it immensely. But when he looks back at that earlier period, he remembers that moving his pelvis demanded effort. His lower back would get tired during sex and sometimes ache. His energy would become depleted, so that after orgasm he wanted only to roll over and go to sleep. And his sensations of pleasure were fairly limited to his genital area.

After a particular body session that focused on his abdominal and pelvic area, Heller's pelvis began to move on its own. His motions during sex happened to him, rather than him having to do them. As a result, the whole act no longer fatigued him, his back stopped aching, and he felt energized afterward. Also, his feelings of pleasure from sex eventually expanded throughout his entire body. As his body became looser, his experience of sex became more fluid.[14]

cially satisfy you. They can be anything: nursing your baby, walking barefoot on the beach, reading a novel in a hot, scented bath, making love with your partner. How frequently do you remember that your body is also a source of delight?

"Every human being possesses an effective internal health maintenance system . . . guided by pleasure," say psychologists Robert Ornstein and David Sobel. "Our senses do more than send alarms about sporadic hazards. They shepherd us to agreeable experiences that increase survival."[15] We learn through pleasure. We heal under such positive conditions. Our brains even come equipped with pleasure substances (endorphins).

In fact, says anthropologist Lionel Tiger, pleasure is not a luxury but an evolutionary entitlement. We need it the way we need vitamins, water, warmth, conviviality, and carbohydrates. Pleasure is what suggested "which behaviors, emotions, social patterns and patterns of taste served us well during our evolutionary history. They were experienced as pleasures and encoded into our formative genetic codes . . . deep in the past, from about 100,000 years ago and beyond."[16]

> It is usually the case that the greater the pleasure the body experiences, the greater the pleasure it is able to give.
>
> —Robert Masters and Jean Houston

### Emotional and Spiritual Development

While psychologists believe that physical changes accompany better emotional and mental functioning, bodyways practitioners believe that better emotional and mental functioning accompanies physical changes. Ida Rolf,

The physical body is the mediator of all our experience. If it seriously malfunctions, everything we perceive is distorted. If it is relaxed and in balance, many of our difficulties fade to insignificance.

—John Mann and Lar Short

the creator of Rolfing, suggested that in certain cases correcting structural deviations could be more effective than psychotherapy. Somatic educators Moshe Feldenkrais and Thomas Hanna asserted that increased movement function leads to improved psychological states. Hanna, a student of Feldenkrais, never discussed psychological difficulties with his clients. Yet, without saying a word, he noticed that once physical restrictions were eliminated, psychological ones followed suit. ☞ See Louise's story, page 239.

Brent Williams, a graduate of the Southern Baptist Theological Seminary in Louisville, Kentucky, observed the same thing in regard to spiritual problems. He switched from his ministry to massage therapy when he realized that when people were depressed and "not feeling right with God," 80 percent of the time there was a physical difficulty behind it rather than a spiritual dilemma. Counseling with words alone left Williams frustrated and his clients still in conflict. But with massage, physical relief led to spiritual relief as well.

Today, more and more individuals are realizing that it is not enough to contemplate, analyze, or reason through emotional or spiritual issues; rather, they must address them directly, in their own bodies. A disciplined body practice can lead to self-confidence and the kind of self-knowledge that emphasizes unity instead of duality. How we are in our bodies alters how we feel about ourselves and life in general.

Feminist writer Gloria Steinem describes what happens during lectures when she asks people to stand and then look at how they place their bodies in space. The women often realize they're standing with their feet together, head slightly forward, arms folded across the chest or hands clasped in front, as though to cover their bodies and take up a minimal amount of room. On the other hand, the men find themselves standing feet apart, head up and back, arms at their sides or one elbow jutting out, thus taking up a maximum amount of space. When Steinem has them exchange their standing styles and see how it feels, they soon realize how quickly their physical posture can influence their state of mind, particularly self-confidence.

"When people in the small-space group expand their stance, they often say they feel odd or exposed at first, then stronger and more confident," Steinem notes. "When those in the big-space group contract their bodies, they often report feeling childlike at first, and then less powerful, even less visible."[17]

Similarly, Promoting Achievement in School Through Sports (PASS), a yearlong course designed for high school students, helps them improve academically by working with what their bodies already know through the physical experience of sports. They discover that they have most of the qualities and skills they need to do well in school. Movement and body concentration exercises in the class leave them more balanced and relaxed, which leads to greater physical power and mental alertness.

# Johnny's Story: Matter or Mind, Bodyways or Psychotherapy?

According to Ida Rolf, the originator of Rolfing and doyenne of the structural body-ways field, some people mistakenly seek help in psychotherapy when what they need to do is become aware of and correct physical aberrations. She uses the story of Johnny as an example.

When Johnny was ten, he roller-skated down a flight of concrete steps, bumping down the last six on his behind. Since there were no broken bones, his mother figured there was no real damage. But a year later, Johnny was no longer able to keep up with his friends in sports or sit cross-legged. His self-image suffered: He began to feel inadequate and insecure. By the time he turned fifteen, his knees were hurting; at sixteen, he grew heavy-hipped. Finally, when he was seventeen, he saw a doctor to find out what "disease" was ruining his knees and impairing his walking.

Eighteen years later, Johnny was trying futilely to unearth and get rid of this "disease" through psychotherapy. Was he insecure because his mother had not given him enough love as a baby? He remembered his father yelling at him, "For God's sake, boy, can't you stand up straight?"

In fact, says Rolf, he couldn't. One leg felt longer because his fall down the stairs had rotated his pelvis, leaving one hipbone forward and slightly higher than the other. The psychiatrist labeled Johnny "insecure." He literally was. Without both legs properly under his body, he couldn't help but feel and act insecure. To compensate, he became withdrawn and timid. To overcome that, he worked out at a gym and built up his muscles. Although he got sturdier, he still felt no more security than before because there was no change at the affected joint.

To Rolf's way of thinking, psychotherapy is not the remedy for Johnny's insecurity because it does not undo the structural deviation of his pelvis. Working with his body—restoring balance in his pelvis—is what would evoke security.[18]

Physical confidence translates into overall personal confidence and thus competence in scholastic work.[19]

Women I know who grew up engaged in sports—some were "tomboys"—refused to restrict themselves to activities and clothing considered appropriate for girls. They became confident women who are not afraid to go and do. From elementary school on, I had to help my father in his business. The experience of lifting boxes and doing other physical tasks instilled in me a sense of strength that I carried forward into my adult life. Other women recognize their strength later in life, through the physical experience of giving birth and then raising children.

The better you feel physically, the easier it is to be happy.
—Martin Rush

Even the most mundane physical tasks can break up mental inhibitions and emotional blocks. Several of my women friends and I have discussed why it is that we clean closets, desks, or the entire house before we get down to the work at hand. We used to call it procrastination, but I've come to understand that the physical activity is truly a warm-up that then gets translated into the mental activity needed for the paperwork. One friend, when her husband died suddenly and left her, a young mother, to raise two sons, found herself thoroughly overhauling the house and rearranging all the furniture. The physical

# Experience: Using Your Body to Change Your Mood

Remember the last time you felt sad, depressed, or aggrieved over some loss. Picture and/or feel how your body was. Were your shoulders rounded and your chest drawn in, as if to protect your heart from more hurt? Did you keep your eyes cast downward? If you were fortunate to have a friend or partner put her or his arm around you, did that touch allow you to expand even just a little bit, to feel less alone in your body? Were you able to take a deeper breath? Did the physical comfort ease some of your emotional tension?

If you're sad or depressed now, straighten your posture, but without forcing anything. Lift and open your chest so that your shoulders unround themselves; pick up your head so it isn't falling forward, then look straight up at the ceiling as you tilt your head back. Whenever I sense I am on the verge of crying in a situation where it's not appropriate, all I do is gaze upward and suddenly the urge for tears is gone. If you find yourself feeling sad while driving a car, lengthen and straighten your spine by pushing down with your buttocks and reaching with the top of your head toward the roof of the car. Instead of slumping over the steering wheel, straighten and lengthen your arms.[20]

To deal with emotions other than sadness, you can try a different exercise. For example, even if you're not angry or anxious right now, you can practice by thinking of and picturing something or someone that really gets you furious or fearful. Get worked up. Really feel it. Then pay attention to how you're breathing. Is your breath short and shallow? Is your heart beating wildly? These are some of the physical sensations that go along with anger or anxiety. Now consciously breathe deeply and slowly: Fully inhale into your abdomen, chest, and back, then gradually let out all the air. Do this until each round of breathing is effortless. Notice that as you have changed physically, you have also calmed down emotionally. Are you still irate or overwrought? You used your body to affect your mind.

act of reorganization helped her get through the grief and begin to arrange a new life for herself.

## *Improvement of Skills*

As awareness increases and relaxation deepens, balance, coordination, and even learning skills can improve. For example, in 1980, Project P.R.E.S. (Physical Response Educational Systems) began a program using Acupressure (Jin Shin Do®) with special-education students in Santa Cruz County, California. Consistently, there has been positive change. As the students relaxed and became more aware, they also became more responsive, sociable, and receptive to learning and affection; difficult behaviors diminished or disappeared. Children saddled with cerebral palsy, mental retardation, or hyperactivity made notable gains in balance, posture, rhythm, and coordination. One teenager finally stopped bumping into things. A young child learned to eat with a spoon, while others learned to catch a ball or ride a skateboard. Although all of the students had language-learning difficulties because of retardation, physical disorders, or emotional disturbances, they made improvements even in communication and cognition. One who had previously only echoed sounds began to speak in three-word sentences. Another increased his attention span. And another jumped almost two grade levels in language development and reading. By the end of six or eight weekly Acupressure sessions, some students experienced as much as three- to five-year growth spurts in academic performance.[21]

The Touch Research Institute, at the University of Miami School of Medicine, conducted a study among working adults and found that a fifteen- to twenty-minute massage (on-site, in their chairs) left them in a state of heightened alertness that improved their job performance. When asked to do math computations, both their speed and accuracy doubled.[22]

In observing children in the British school system, educator Michael Gelb discovered the critical role of posture in academic excellence. He noticed that when young students searched for the right answers to difficult math or reading problems, they would tighten up their bodies and restrict their postures. Once he helped them to become aware of how they sat and demonstrated how they could relax and expand their postures and breathing patterns, the children found that the answers seemed to appear magically, effortlessly.[23] Many bodyways, especially the structural and functional approaches, are useful in promoting better posture; those that emphasize greater awareness and attention are equally helpful. Since poor posture can impinge on the flow of oxygenated blood to the brain, aligning the head and body while sitting or moving can improve thinking and problem-solving.

So, will bodyways make you a brilliant orator or dazzling dancer even though previously you got tongue-tied or stepped on other people's feet? Truly, anything can happen, though no one makes such promises. As you begin to feel different in your body—less inhibited, more balanced and coordinated—you may also have the confidence to get up in front of others to speak or take dance lessons.

## Aging

Can you let your body
become
supple as a newborn
child's?

—Tao Te Ching

Bodyways are also of value as we age. Thomas Hanna declared repeatedly that aging, as we think of it, is a myth: We don't have to become decrepit old men and women. We do this by selecting, often on an unconscious level, attitudes and postures that fit our self-image and rejecting others, restricting ourselves in forming new body patterns and learning. Limitations that we think are due to a lack of suppleness are actually the result of habitually contracted muscles that lead to unbalanced movement. That, in turn, leads to new limitations on muscles, which we avoid using to preclude discomfort or pain. This vicious circle leads to deformation of the skeleton, spinal discs, joints, and so on. The result is premature aging and a reduction of range and variety of bodily movements. Actual age has only a minimal influence on such limitations.

Bodyways practitioners, especially somatic educators, strongly believe and prove through their work that we can learn to restore the ability to move normally or fully at any age. And when we do, it has a markedly rejuvenating effect not only on the mechanics of our bodies but also on our personalities. ☞ See Louise's story, page 239.

We can see bodyways as preventive maintenance as well. Consider painter Georgia O'Keeffe, who attributed nimbleness in her senior years to having been Rolfed earlier. Or Bob Hope, who for decades has traveled everywhere with a personal masseur to work on him daily, and who in his nineties is still working.

## Touch

There is a mysterious
healing power in touch
that is beyond words
and beyond our ideas
about it.

—Aileen Crow

Touch is both a means and an end in bodyways. Touch is something we all need—for comfort, pleasure, sensory-motor stimulation, even life itself. Studies indicate how decisive touch is to an infant's survival and an adult's well-being. For example, when separated from their mothers, rat pups go into shock; without touch, all their systems shut down and stop producing an enzyme crucial to the development of major organs. Earlier I mentioned what happens to human infants left untouched in foundling institutions—a kind of sensory marasmus.

Conversely, more recent research reveals that a daily massage enables prematurely born infants to catch up in their growth and development. It can also keep them from contracting pneumonia. Pharmacologist Saul Schanberg and other scientists at Duke University are researching a complex chain of gene interactions to clarify the link among touch, protein synthesis, and cell regulation. To conserve energy in survival mode—when lack of touch means absence of the mother—a baby's developmental proteins, such as growth hormones prolactin and insulin, will stop working. Elsewhere, in earlier laboratory experiments with animals, deprivation of tactile and movement stimulation led to abnormal social and emotional behavior—aggression, fearfulness, violence, and sexual abnormality—and brain damage.[24]

The need to touch and be touched does not diminish with age. The late Virginia Satir, a member of the American Orthopsychiatric Association, used to say, "You need four hugs a day for survival, eight for maintenance, and twelve for growth." Anthropologist Ashley Montagu suggests that among the elderly the quality of tactile support before and during an illness greatly influences its course and outcome, perhaps making the difference between life and death.[25] According to ophthalmologic surgeon Stephen Turner, having their hand held during a cataract operation reassures and relaxes his patients.[26]

Touch helps define body boundaries and body image. If you grew up thinking that you were large and heavy or small and weak, the more you sense your body through touch, the more you'll know how it really is now, rather than how you still imagine it to be based on worn-out beliefs and misconceptions. If you feel like a Hercules or an Amazon, touch may help you establish contact with your gentleness and vulnerableness. If you've always felt fragile, it might help you identify strength in your body. Unless you know your body—feel it, sense it, rather than deny it—you can't go beyond the still picture you have of yourself. You're frozen in a snapshot rather than moving in a film.

If you bring a despised body to bodyways, don't be surprised if your image changes for the better and shame about your body decreases. Someone working with you nonjudgmentally allows you too to stop judging, to accept your own body instead of being repulsed by it. That acceptance also allows a wider range of experiences to come in. As you feel different in your body, you may change how you treat yourself—perhaps you'll dance or hike through a beautiful woods, cook yourself wonderful meals, or make a new friend.

If in the past touch was a painful, even abusive, shameful, unloving, or uncaring experience, bodyways provide an opportunity to have an opposite encounter and to learn that touch can be safe, loving, and healing. It also gives you the chance to know the difference between the two, so you can make healthy decisions about what kind of touch you allow.

Touch facilitates awareness. "Touching hands are not like pharma-

Touching is nourishment.

—Gay Luce

Hands are the heart's landscape.

—Pope John Paul II

Often the hands will solve a mystery that the intellect has struggled with in vain.

—C. G. Jung

ceuticals or scalpels," says Trager practitioner Deane Juhan. "They are like flashlights in a darkened room."[27] Where we are touched is where our attention goes and, in so doing, provides information we were not aware of. For example, you may not realize you're tense or sore until you're touched in your calf, neck, shoulder, or lower back. You get new information about your body. That new information allows and encourages new choices. Similarly, you may not be aware of where your body feels good and comfortable until you're touched there and you feel the pleasure of it.

When touch leads to ease in the body, it opens a whole new way of being and living. Instead of fighting discomfort and pain and contracting around it, we have the energy to embrace pleasure and comfort, to open to what's around us.

### Access to Memories and Overcoming Trauma

Like a sponge filled with water, anywhere the flesh is pressed, wrung, even touched lightly, a memory may flow out in a stream.

—Clarissa Pinkola Estés

Working with the body through touch rather than words (verbal therapy) can help access what can't come through in language, especially a preverbal experience. Although anything that engages our senses can trigger a memory—a door banging shut, the light of dawn, the stench of rotting garbage, the sweet creaminess of cheesecake—touch seems especially evocative when the original incident powerfully affected the body. When that part of the body is touched again under certain conditions, a past experience is touched, too, and a "body memory" surfaces. It's as though the body's tissues remember a particular event or series of them. Uncovering that memory through touch enables you then to work with hidden material that talking alone couldn't find. ☞ See box on body memory, page 83.

Particularly in cases of abuse, body therapists can, in conjunction with psychotherapy, assist you in reclaiming parts of your body "lost" to trauma through dissociation and repression. They can facilitate your overcoming feelings of disgust and shame and self-violence so you can develop a friendly and compassionate relationship with your body. They also can help you to experience your body as a source of strength and groundedness and to know pleasure through nonsexual touch. Eventually this can lead to reconstructing a sense of trust that makes genuine caring connections with people possible again.

## THE POWER OF EMBODIMENT

The key to unique individuals is: They keep their power.

—Bernie Siegel

Bodyways help us get to know our own bodies—to know where we live, how we feel, act, and sense. That kind of knowledge brings power. How often have we heard, "What you don't know won't hurt you"? It's not true. What we don't know *does* hurt us. What we don't know limits us and deprives us of autonomy over our own lives. When we do know, we can make appropriate choices, we can respond effectively, and we are better able to take care of ourselves.

Historically, it has been in the interest of the powers that be—church hierarchy, royalty, industry, dictatorship—that we not know through our bodies. It serves them to have us rely on an intermediary—priest, general, teacher—and stand apart from ourselves, to view our bodies as a thing to labor or kill with. ☞ See "The Split," page 23. To connect with our bodies is to learn to trust ourselves, and from that comes power.

To connect with our bodies makes it possible to move as easily, grace-fully, and instinctively as an animal. If we don't meddle in the natural development of a kitten, it grows up walking lightly and stretching long without being trained to. The foremost teachers in somatic education and movement arts believe that, like a kitten, we start out knowing how to move well, but somewhere along the way we get interfered with, through certain restrictive forms of parenting and education and/or through injuries. Bodyways can help us learn anew natural movement and physical grace, effortless being in the body. That means becoming more coordi-nated, flexible, and appropriately responsive or "intelligent." This kind of integration makes us better able to resist depression and disease and to attend to and repair ourselves in times of stress or injury.

Bodyways are also a way to become embodied. For all of our dieting and fitness crazes, in Western culture an "unembodied" way of being is the norm—psychologist Sidney Jourard called it "a kind of normalized mad-ness."[28] Being unembodied is what makes it possible for people to endure the boredom, stress, and violence of a conventional, status-quo-maintaining lifestyle. Or we anesthetize the body with alcohol, sedatives, or food when we haven't successfully repressed our feared vitality. Maybe that vitality was punished because our early experiences of sexual play, sounds, or

> There are many pathways that reconnect the personal to the political, the spiritual, and the sexual. There are no authorities, hierarchies, or gurus. Empowerment comes from within, from the connection to the life force.
>
> —Elinor Gadon

## Baby Elsi's Story

When newborn Elsi came home with her mother from the hospital, her grand-mother insisted she learn to sleep through the night without disturbing the family. She was left alone at the far end of the house so that no one would hear her cry. By the sixth night, Elsi no longer cried. But everyone soon saw that the child had little sense of her own body. She never seemed to know if she was hungry, cold, or tired. Others had to tell her when to eat, when to go to bed, and when to put on warm clothes. She had learned to deny her instinctual bodily needs, and now she no longer knew how to respond to them unless told.[29]

People should be inspired to have confidence in their innate wisdom, in their basic creativity, and their fundamental goodness. The choice of how to live their life is their creation.

—Barbara Dilley

If you can stand whole in your physical body, there is nowhere on earth you cannot stand whole in your being.

—Arisika Razak

movements that are a normal part of growing up disturbed the adults around us.

We repress the experience of our bodies to protect ourselves from threatening pleasure and pain. For example, it's natural for a baby to explore its body, including the genital area, but if parents have certain set ideas—"Don't touch there"—because of their own unresolved sexual issues, then that child will learn to inhibit this natural tendency for pleasure. Somatics professor Don Johnson recalls growing up in a family in which sensual knowledge was associated with sin. As a small child, he went to sleep at night afraid that he would end up burning in hell for all eternity if he even once let down his guard against following his own physical impulses. He remembers being warned, "If you touch your penis with pleasure, or enjoy looking at your naked body in a mirror, you're committing a mortal sin, worthy of eternal damnation."[30]

We also become disembodied when others take over the function of detecting our own bodily states and estimating our strengths, weaknesses, needs, or desires. How often have you continued to take a medication after it has ceased being effective only because the doctor kept prescribing it for you, not because of what you felt in your own body? You can use bodyways to help you get back in contact with your own body so that *you*, not someone else, knows when and how much to eat, sleep, drink, exercise, work, play, and so on.

And the more at home you are in your body, the more competent you will feel. Knowing your personal boundaries, respecting your body, and being in touch with its wisdom and power can all contribute toward freeing yourself from feeling overpowered by others—as a victim or potential victim. When we are truly embodied—living fully from within our bodies—that feeling gives us a presence that's empowering.

CHAPTER 2

# Body Alienation:

# Where We Lost the Body

It is ironic that a culture so obsessed with the appearance and functioning of the body—consider the billions of dollars and the amount of media attention devoted to food, fitness, fashion, and sex—is simultaneously so ignorant of and divorced from it. The irreverent, iconoclastic Episcopalian priest cum Zen student Alan Watts put it this way: "The commonly accepted notion that Americans are materialists is pure bunk. A materialist is one who loves material, a person devoted to the enjoyment of the physical and immediate present. By this definition, most Americans are abstractionists. They *hate* material, and convert it as swiftly as possible into mountains of junk and clouds of poisonous gas."[1]

The words *material* and *matter* come from the Latin *mater,* "mother." The lack of respect for matter is akin to a long-standing disrespect for woman, nature, and body. Events that began thousands of years ago gave rise to this attitude.

## THE SPLIT

Most of us have punished, abused, hated, or ignored our bodies at some time, if not regularly. It seems a given in Western civilization, though it was not always that way, and it's not true around the world. Where does this difficult relationship come from? Why do we obsess over or neglect our bodies instead of relate to them as sacred friends or equal partners? Why do we impose our power on the body the way the media impose dictates on us? The origins of how we feel and live in our bodies are many and varied. They come from the actual experiences we've had and from underlying attitudes and beliefs that prevail in our families, cultures, and educational systems.

Few of us have lost our minds, but most of us have long ago lost our bodies.

—Ken Wilber

## Goddess Civilization

In reexamining the past, archeologists have found evidence of a civilization in which body, mind, and spirit were one—the body itself was considered sacred. Feminist historians and theologians harken back to a Goddess-centered culture that flourished in Europe during the Stone Age. It was a time when the female body was appreciated and worshiped for its voluptuousness and fecundity. Then, at the end of the fifth millennium B.C.E., marauding tribes descended on this society and imposed a male-dominator patriarchal system. European civilization shifted from a model of partnership and cooperation to one of conquest and domination. Gradually men took control as patriarchs at home, autocrats of the state, fathers of the church, and giants of industry.[2]

"The wisdom of woman, gained through her identification with her body, with the Goddess, and with the earth, was no longer revered, but ridiculed and rejected," says psychotherapist Judith Duerk. "Once honored as prophetess and seer, woman was now scorned. Her instincts and intuition, through which she perceived the elemental energies in the cycles of nature and her knowledge of healing, were rebuked and humiliated."[3]

The new way of life was based on what's designated as "the masculine principle"—a valuing of mind over matter, intellect over senses, logos over eros, head over heart, spirit over body, and man over nature. The split was clear. All that was identified with woman—nature, body, matter, earth—was devalued and brought under control. Men sought ascension to a spiritual realm and separation from the uncontrollable, necessary urges of the "disgusting" body, the messiness of earthly birth and death, and the chaotic powers of nature.

## Religious Dualism

While the Goddess-centered culture considered the body sacred and not separate from earth and spirit, later religions established a dualistic doctrine. In many of his books, former Dominican priest Matthew Fox talks about the devastation wrought by Christianity when it uses original sin as its starting point and builds itself exclusively around sin and redemption. It teaches distrust of our bodily existence. "The fall/redemption tradition considers the soul to be an interior dimension to our bodies, held in check by the cage that our bodies are," says Fox.[4]

Derogatory labeling of the body has included everything from "the dark prison," "the living death," and "the sense-endowed corpse" to "the grave thou bearest about with thee" and "a dung heap." In 1752 English writer Samuel Johnson continued the condemnation when he said, "Thy body is all vice, and thy mind is all virtue."[5]

This duality doesn't make sense, says farmer-poet Wendell Berry. "You cannot devalue the body and value the soul—or value anything else. The isolation of the body sets it into direct conflict with everything else in Creation. Nothing could be more absurd than to despise the body and yet yearn for its resurrection."[6]

The doctrine of original sin plays into the hands of politicians, empire-builders, slave masters, and patriarchal society in general by dividing and conquering. It pits our thoughts against our feelings, our bodies against our spirits, and people against the earth, animals, and nature. Philo, a first-century philosopher in Alexandria, said: "We must keep down our feelings just as we keep down the lower classes." When we suppress or repress the body, we can oppress the body politic.[7]

## The Mechanical Enlightenment

As the centuries passed, nothing undid this duality. In the 1600s, European scientists and philosophers—Bacon, Kepler, Galileo, Newton, Descartes—perhaps more than any other group, deepened the split to such an extreme that it still informs our thinking today. The Italian astronomer and physicist Galileo believed that everything, including the natural world, could be reduced to measurable particles of matter. Thus human understanding would come not through qualitative and subjective criteria but only through quantitative measurement and mathematical analysis. That which could not be known in mechanical terms was not important.

New discoveries about the solar system, gravity, physics, and analytic geometry reinforced Enlightenment thinking that all of nature worked like a machine, particularly the clock. Even animals came to be considered clockwork beast machines or "soulless automata." For the German philosopher and mathematician Gottfried Wilhelm Leibniz, "Living bodies are even in the smallest of their parts machines *ad infinitum*."[8]

Then French philosopher and mathematician René Descartes delivered the crowning touch: He divided human life into mind and body. *Cogito ergo sum* ("I think, therefore I am") gave supremacy to the mind. Although human beings had a machinelike body, they also possessed an immortal soul, based on reason, but the two did not make a unified whole. The human body went from being sacred, created in the image of God, to being a finely functioning machine whose parts can be replaced but which in time will wear down and out.

## The Industrial Revolution

Promoting man as machine did not end with the Enlightenment. Beginning in eighteenth-century England, the Industrial Revolution fur-

Almost all civilized peoples have been brought up to think of themselves as ghosts in machines . . . as souls or spirits in alien bodies, as skin-encapsulated egos, or as psychic chauffeurs in mechanical vehicles of flesh and bone.

—Alan Watts

Describing everything in mechanical terms undermines our capacity for experiencing wonder, awe, reverence, spontaneity, and mystery in relationship to nature, other people, and even in relationship to ourself.

—James W. Jones

Cartesianism tells us that we are schizoid creatures, one-half of which is little more than a mechanical rig for getting us about in the world.

—Maxine Sheets-Johnstone

thered alienation from the body. Rather than save humans from the drudgery of labor, as it purported to do, industrialization made them another cog in the machine. By 1918 a U.S. public health publication reported: "From the standpoint of industrial physiology, the worker is looked upon as bringing to the general physical equipment of the factory his own bodily machine, the most intricate of all machines used in the plant. This machine must be understood . . . watched, used . . . so as to obtain from it the most profit."[9] The Industrial Revolution took the workers' bodies and made them possessions of the bosses.

To the extent that the body failed to be machinelike, it lacked value. When performance artist and theater director Leonard Pitt was growing up in Detroit in the 1940s and 1950s, he felt puny and inconsequential next to a new car off the assembly line. To him, the billowing smokestack seemed to say, "Turn your body into a machine, and then you're worth something!"[10]

## Cultural Evolution

Our intellectual and scientific "establishment" is, in general, still spellbound by the myth that human intelligence and feeling are a fluke of chance in an entirely mechanical and stupid universe—as if figs would grow on thistles or grapes on thorns.

—Alan Watts

The Cartesian legacy left us relying not on our own living, sense-making bodies, but on what modern science tells us about our bodies with regard to food, sex, stress, and health. We became top-heavy with mind, brain, language, and consciousness, instead of equally weighted with touch, kinesthesia, and feelings. This shift away from the body and the immediate experience of our senses and toward the intellect is an aspect of what we call cultural "progress."

It's not that intellectualizing is wrong, but without emotional meaning or feeling, a concept doesn't truly convey a message. "Primitive man had concepts," said psychoanalysts Arthur Burton and Robert Kantor, "but they were more immediately related to his personal world of experience, and in this experience his body played a uniquely mediating part." When a culture evolves into more complex social forms and abstractions, it also diminishes and devalues the immediacy of personal experience. Burton and Kantor went on to say, "The prevalent cry of alienation and 'loss of meaning' today is just that quality of culture which denies the body and ignores the integrative aspects of its impulses."[11]

## Cycles of Heresy and Orthodoxy

All the while that Western civilization has been evolving toward more intellectual forms, it has also struggled through cycles of heresy and orthodoxy. Heretical or countercultural movements, such as the pre- and early Christian cult of Gnosticism, believe that spirituality is an inner or personal experience, not an intellectual doctrine, and value the bodily life as sacred in itself. (*Gnosis* is Greek for "direct internal or visceral knowledge," in contrast to rational-analytic knowing.) Orthodox movements co-opt the heretical ones, become the political power in charge, and mediate experience for others. As French writer Charles Péguy put it: "Everything begins in mysticism and ends in politics."[12] Rather than see and experience the sacred in the here and now, the orthodoxy defers to a heavenly afterlife. "Orthodoxy, in other words, opts for map instead of territory, for the travelogue instead of the trip," says philosopher and social critic Morris Berman.[13]

In some respects, the present flourishing of bodyways is a resurgence of heresy in its best sense. Instead of striving for vertical ascension, we're learning to live in the horizontal here and now. The emphasis on centering or grounding in the martial arts and movement awareness leads to a greater appreciation of the lower body's strength and importance. Reaching with your head has its limitations when you need to plant your feet on the ground, when you want to stand tall yet stable, like a tree or mountain. Instead of having others mediate your experience, you have it yourself, in your own body.

It is also heretical to accept and trust the body we have, rather than condemn it as a repository of sin, as the Christian orthodoxy would have us believe. We have the opportunity to let go of equating bodily ills with moral turpitude. In such misguided thinking, we consider our bodies' imbalances, crookedness, and tensions as somehow a sign of spiritual degeneration. Yet in the Old Testament story of Job we read that a "perfect and upright" man who loved his God suffered unendurable losses, including having his healthy body disfigured by painful disease.

Not much has changed since Job's time. Some New Age beliefs foster a similar guilt, that we are to be ashamed if we don't succeed in overcoming an illness, that maybe we don't love ourselves enough, aren't trusting enough of ourselves and others, or have some deep-seated fear we're not in touch with. Larry Dossey, a physician of internal medicine and author of books on the relationship between physical health and spiritual awareness, points out the dangers of this kind of thinking. One of his healthiest patients prided herself on "taking full responsibility" for her health and for "consciously creating [her] own reality" 100 percent. Even when she experienced major signs of appendicitis, she didn't go to see Dossey until she wound up in the emergency room in the middle of the night. When he asked her why, she responded, sobbing, "I felt like a complete failure!"[14]

"In nature the occurrence of disease is considered a part of the natural order, not a sign of ethical, moral, or spiritual weakness," says Dossey. "Sickly saints and healthy sinners show us that there is no invariable, linear, one-to-one relationship between one's level of spiritual attainment and the degree of one's physical health."[15]

Our grandfathers often felt that they had spirits striving to free themselves of fleshly bonds. Are we not flesh, perhaps, striving to free ourselves of intellectual bonds?

—Charles Brooks

The typical middle-class American carries around a huge load of habitual unreflective guilt about the body.

—Richard Smoley

# Experience: How Did You Become Disembodied?

Aside from the centuries-old legacy of duality that we've inherited, there are many reasons why we become disembodied. Stop to consider what they might be in your life:

Religious inculcation. What did the religion(s) of your family teach you about the body? Is it something to be ashamed of or joyfully celebrated? Is your body a blessing or a curse? Are some parts of your body acceptable but others not even mentionable? Is the spirit high and good but the body low and bad?

Abuse and violence. Were you physically abused? Sexually abused? Did it make you hate your body as the scene of the crime and want to escape it? Did you numb your whole body or certain areas to the pain in order to survive, cope, and adjust? Did a rape or beating make you dissociate from and leave your body? Did you come away with the belief that the body is a source of pain and powerlessness rather than pleasure and power?

Social mores. When you were growing up, did your family touch affectionately or have little to no physical contact? Was masturbation disapproved of or allowed? In your social group, were outward displays of closeness considered improper manners or expected behavior? Were people proud of their physicality, or did they try to hide their bodies? Did they hold themselves stiff or swing their hips? Was sex considered natural and pleasurable or something to be despised yet endured? Were menstruation, pregnancy, and childbirth rued as women's curse or considered a celebration of life?

Trauma. Were you ever in a serious car accident? Have you been mugged, raped, kidnapped, or robbed? Did you undergo a terrifying surgery? Were you in a war? Were the experiences so painful and frightening that feeling became unbearable? Do you still flinch and avoid certain things?

Guilt. Did you ever inflict hurt on someone else, even unintentionally? Did you ever kill a person or animal, even accidentally? Did you ever hit someone younger, smaller, or less powerful? Do you wish you could vacate the body that committed the damage?

## THE BODY IN THE MARKETPLACE

I am not a mechanism, an assembly of various sections.

—D. H. Lawrence

At the end of the twentieth century, we are still struggling to swim out of the eddy of alienation that Western civilization has been caught in for centuries. We're not only a human motor but also a collection of parts, commodities sold or used to sell other products. Turn to any TV channel or open any popular magazine. The media display bodies, especially the semi-clad female body, to market everything from cars to chain saws. We've even become marketable merchandise ourselves. Wombs are rented for growing babies, and body parts and materials—organs, blood tissue, genes, eggs, semen—are manipulated, engineered, patented, and put up for sale in a worldwide market. Andrew Kimbrell calls it "the human body shop."[16]

There are whole industries—plastic surgery, cosmetics, dieting, fashion, pornography, and fitness—that continue to disconnect us from our bodies. They constantly barrage us with ideal images that most of us can't attain; yet they never tell us that those images are often illusions created by a camera and computer after hours of collaborative effort by a large team. For example, instead of seeing pictures of themselves in magazines, women see girls made up to look older. While the average North American woman is thirty-six years old, stands just under five feet four inches tall, and weighs 144.2 pounds, the standard demanded by modeling agencies is a long-necked, long-legged, broad-shouldered woman in her teens or twenties who measures between five feet eight inches and six feet in height and between thirty-four and thirty-five inches for bust and hips, with a narrow waist. After looking through forty thousand photographs, one agency came up with only four "ideal" women they could book! [17]

During the last few decades, the disparity between the average and the ideal woman has increased in a steady trend toward greater slimness. In 1954 the reigning Miss America stood five feet eight inches tall and weighed 132 pounds; by 1980 the average contestant was down to 117 pounds. In 1970 the average model weighed 8 percent less than the average woman; twenty years later, she weighed 23 percent less, yet overall women have increased in weight.[18]

Men and women alike have grown dissatisfied with specific body areas, height, weight, and overall looks. As a result, we spend more on the industries that pander to that dissatisfaction than on social services or education. From 1989 to 1990 alone, Americans increased their expenditures on dieting from $29 billion to $33 billion. "Aesthetic" surgeries rose 61 percent from 1980 to 1990, according to the American Society of Plastic and Reconstructive Surgeons. Given these statistics, by the turn of the century we could be spending $77 billion—close to the entire gross national product of Belgium—on changing our bodies.[19]

In trying to measure up to what we think will attract others, do we ever stop to consider that we don't really know what is attractive about ourselves and that magazines, movies, and other media influence us into becoming such harsh self-critics? To investigate this, psychologist Thomas Cash and graduate student Lora Jacobi at Old Dominion University in Virginia posed a series of questions to sixty-six male and sixty-nine female students, all white. For example, they asked, "What would you change about your body if you could? What physical traits do you find most attrac-

The body is like an earth . . . as vulnerable to overbuilding, being carved into parcels, cut off, overmined, and shorn of its power as any landscape.

—Clarissa Pinkola Estés

When the body is treated as a purely material possession, our humanness is diminished.

—Maxine Sheets-Johnstone

The human body is a beautiful work of art. Women damage their spirits immeasurably by being at war with their physical selves.

—Nancy Neff

Each of us in this culture, this twisted, inchoate culture, has to choose between battles: One battle is against the cultural ideal, and the other is against ourselves. I've chosen to stop fighting myself.

—Sallie Tisdale

The quest for the perfect body is, like most wars, a costly one—emotionally and physically, to say nothing of financially. It leaves most of us feeling frustrated, ashamed, and defeated.

—Judith Rodin

A culture of domination like ours says to people: There is nothing in you that is of value, everything of value is outside you and must be acquired.

—bell hooks

tive? What traits do you think members of the opposite sex look for in you? What is the ideal body type?" Although most men thought women wanted a tall, muscular, blue-eyed guy and women thought men lusted after a busty, blue-eyed blonde, both sexes were wrong. Instead they preferred fit but moderately sized people. Yet most of these students were not satisfied with their own eye or hair color, height, build, or figure.[20]

This dissatisfaction is futile, for we are born with a particular genetic inheritance that includes a basic structural body type, chemical balances and imbalances, metabolism, and nutritional needs. Some of us have a light build with slight muscular development; others support a stocky, rounded build with a tendency to gain weight; yet others are husky and muscular. We might be longer in the legs, wider in the shoulders, heavier on top or bottom, or evenly proportioned. We may have congenital bone or joint deformities that affect how we carry ourselves or other predispositions, diseases, or illnesses that set off a chain of aftereffects in the body.

We can't change the anatomy and physiology we are born with, yet we do everything possible to conform to the latest ideal. In the process, we pay an even bigger price than the financial cost: We betray or deny who we truly are and what we feel. And if we don't fulfill the ideal, we often hate ourselves because we define ourselves and our self-worth by the way our bodies look, as though our shape and size were a true reflection of who we are.

When we're taught to hate our bodies, we're also taught to disconnect from them. The visual media have become so powerful that they can both determine our sense of reality and override our physical experiences: Thin is normal and everything else is an aberration. Women have become so alienated from their bodies that in one survey, 75 percent of the participants considered themselves overweight even though 45 percent of them were actually underweight.

It seems preposterous to me now, but when I was a teenager in the 1960s, we wore panty girdles so that nothing would jiggle and our clothes would glide smoothly over hips and buttocks. I remember wearing a red wool sheath to a party at a "friend's" house. At one point she came up to me and said, "Your stomach is sticking out; you really should be wearing a girdle." I already was! Long after that episode, I was still so self-conscious of my abdomen that I tried to keep it flat by sucking it in and holding my breath. Then one day, when I was in my thirties, my friend Rocco said, "Why do women hate their bellies? To me, it's the most beautiful part of a woman's body." I took in what he said, but it was a few more years before I overcame my estrangement from that distinctly feminine part of myself, the fertile part that generates new life.

If it's not the abdomen, the breasts may be the object of hatred.

# Experience: Cultural Ideals

Every culture and every era have different ideals of physical beauty, particularly for women. Traditionally in India and in the Arab world, plump is desirable, whereas thin is highly unattractive because it reflects undernourishment and poverty as well as possible infertility. Skinny women are not considered marriageable. In America in the 1920s the slender, flat, unrounded body of the flapper was all the rage, but in the 1940s and 1950s shapely, "stacked" women like Jane Russell were sought after. From the 1960s on, an obsession with losing weight—"You can't be too thin"—has reigned.

What did you experience while growing up? Was there an ideal look that you strove for? For women, was it "in" to be flat-chested and lean like Twiggy or to be curvaceous and buxom like Marilyn Monroe? If you were a tall girl among short boys, did you slouch to diminish your height? For men, was being skinny an embarrassment? Were you more popular if you could flex your jock muscles or your brain muscles?

How much hatred toward your body did you absorb because of ethnic prejudices? Did you try to lighten or darken your skin? Did you make your straight hair curly or your curly hair straight? Did you bleach your black hair blond or dye your brown hair red? Did you have your nose made smaller? Did you have the epicanthic folds of your eyes cut to take the "slant" out? Do you wear blue or green contact lenses over your brown eyes?

Think back: Were you really "too" anything in the earlier years of your life—too short, too fat, too big, too tall, too small? If you have pictures of yourself from childhood, pull them out and take a good look. What do you see? Did you have a cowlick that was impossible to smooth down? Did your ears stick out? Was any of that really so terrible?

Or did you experience what others could only long for—the perfect look? What did that feel like? Were you afraid you were popular only because of your good figure or great physique, that nobody cared how smart you were, only about how good you looked?

Today: Can you look at the child you were and love yourself just as you were?

---

Feminist writer Gloria Steinem tells the story of a woman who was so ashamed of hers that she scheduled breast reduction. Then, a week before her operation, she suddenly remembered the painful bindings her grandmother had subjected her to as a girl to keep her safe from boys at school. Fortunately, the woman realized she didn't need to have her breasts cut to be healed. "How many people try to change the part of the body that is only trying to help them remember?" asks Steinem.[21]

We've come to measure our social worth so much by appearance

## Experience: How Do You Treat Your Body?

There's nothing wrong with being fit—I strive for it myself—but how do you try to get fit? Be honest in answering the questions. If it helps, close your eyes and picture yourself working out, and remember what it feels like. Or ask yourself these questions the next time you exercise.

Are you aggressive toward your body, showing it you have power and control? Do you override its messages even when it tells you to slow down or stop to recuperate? Do you ruthlessly exploit it and run it like a machine? Do you treat it as Cinderella's stepmother and stepsisters treated her, making it the scapegoat for your problems? Even though you're being physical, are you actually alienated from your body? What is the real reason you pump iron?

Consider also how you dress. Are you comfortable in your clothes, or do they deny your body's needs? How tight is the waist of your pants, skirt, or dress? How restrictive is the belt you're wearing? Can you take a full breath even when sitting down? Do your stylish shoes pinch your toes and make you worry about getting bunions? Is your tie knotted so tightly it's cutting off the blood circulation to your brain? Do you present the "right" appearance but wrong your body?

---

that we've even allowed it to become a new moral imperative: An attractive, fit, healthy body—the "lean, mean machine"—equals a healthy soul. Yet something is askew. "Body preoccupation has become a societal mania," says psychologist Judith Rodin. "We've become a nation of appearance junkies and fitness zealots . . . driven to think, talk, strategize, and worry about our bodies with the same fanatical devotion we applied to putting a man on the moon. Abroad, we strive for global peace. At home, we have declared war on our bodies."[22]

### FAMILY INFLUENCES

*What if,* when you were a toddler, you had been toilet-trained when you were ready and had never been shamed about natural elimination?

*What if* you had been applauded every time you got up and managed to walk by yourself?

*What if* you had not been yanked up or made fun of when you fell down?

*What if* your mother hadn't slapped you for exploring your genitals when you were a baby and toddler?

*What if* you had been comforted and helped to get back on your bicycle when you fell off and hurt yourself instead of being pooh-poohed for your tears?

*What if* you had been allowed to have your feelings instead of being told, "Boys don't cry" or "That's nothing to cry about"?

*What if* no one had teased you when you put on weight as a teenager while hormones raged through your body?

*What if* you had not been forced to sit still and uncomfortable at a desk all day but had been allowed to learn while also moving your body?

*What if things had been different*—you were accepted just as you were, you were praised each time you showed competence, you were comforted with understanding as you went through strong bodily changes, your feelings and ideas were acknowledged and considered instead of dismissed? Might you have developed a relationship of friendship with your body rather than alienation?

Clyde Ford, a chiropractor and the creator of Somatosynthesis, calls the body our "earliest classroom." According to the late Swiss child psychologist Jean Piaget, during the first two years of life our thinking takes place through the body, for we have little or no language yet. Before we ever speak or understand words, we go through a sensory-motor stage of learning. We come to know the world around us by grasping, squeezing, crawling, shaking, bouncing, turning, falling, twisting, and tasting with our bodies.

What we learn forms the foundation of our emotional life beyond childhood. Take how we're handled. If our needs are disregarded, eventually we shut down to them, too. If we're mistreated, we learn to mistreat ourselves. If we're protected and lovingly cared for, we learn we're worthy of kind attention. From what we see and hear, we learn effective or destructive ways of being in our bodies. Our parents or other caretakers are our first models for relating to the body.

But sometimes our families invade every aspect of our development, leaving us little room to respond naturally. If they encourage or force us to sit, stand, or walk before we're ready, we may wind up with muscular tensions that affect our movements and distort our postures. If, for the convenience of their schedule, we must stop playing or wake up before we're finished sleeping, we may learn that there is no internal rhythm to follow. We lose a sense of harmony with ourselves and our environment. We begin to confuse and doubt our own capacities for judging with our body sense and trusting it. ☞ See Baby Elsi's story, page 21.

One day when Charlotte Selver, the doyenne of Sensory Awareness, was visiting some friends, she observed how a parent can interfere with a child's innate way of being in the body:

And is there not shame at the core of all one learns as one learns propriety? The terrain of forbidden acts. Hungers, expressions, evidence of flesh permeating an atmosphere of denial. Shame commingling with skin, cells, bone, even breath.

—Susan Griffin

To like myself means to be, literally, shameless, to be wanton in the pleasures of being inside a body . . . the way I'd felt as a child, before the world had interfered.

—Sallie Tisdale

Among the guests there was a couple with their daughter, a little girl of eight, a thoughtful and very graceful child. While we were talking the little girl played in the garden, and I had the pleasure of watching her through the window. Then she came upstairs and sat down, one leg hanging down, the other one on the couch. The mother: "But Helen—how do you sit? Take your leg off the couch. A girl never should sit like that!" The little girl took her leg down, causing her skirt to fly above her knees. The mother: "Helen—pull your skirt down! One can see everything!" The child blushed, looked down and pulled her skirt down, but asked, "Why, what is wrong?" The mother looked at her in shock and said, "One does not do that!" By this time the atmosphere in the room was completely uncomfortable. The little girl not only had her legs down, but had them pressed against each other. Her shoulders had gone up and she held her arms tight against her little body. This went on until she could not stand it any longer; she suddenly stretched herself and yawned heartily. Again a storm of indignation from her mother. By now—this all lasted about ten minutes—the child had changed completely. Her gracefulness had turned into awkwardness; all her motions were stilled, her little body was tense; she hardly seemed to be alive any more.[23]

Like Helen, many of us learned to inhibit ourselves—our feelings, our movements. We learned to hold back our fear and terror, our anger and rage, by tightening our muscles, keeping ourselves from crying or screaming, in order not to lose connection with a parent or other caretaker, in order to win approval, acceptance, or love, or in order to survive. In his memoir *Shot in the Heart,* Mikal Gilmore recalls such advice from his brother Gary Gilmore, the murderer notorious for successfully challenging Utah authorities to execute him by firing squad in 1977:

> You have to learn to be hard . . . to take things and feel nothing about them. No pain, no anger, nothing. And you have to realize, if anybody wants to beat you up . . . you have to let them. . . . Lay there and let them do it. It is the only way you will survive [in our family]. . . . Promise me you'll be a man.[24]

As we stopped listening to our bodies, we gradually stopped knowing *how* to listen. How many of us, then, wound up like Mr. James Duffy, the bank cashier in James Joyce's *Dubliners,* who "lived at a little distance from his body"? And how many of us developed such physical discomforts as TMJ, headaches, ulcers, back pain, or asthma because we learned to shut down feeling? Did we gain self-confidence only by losing physical presence through

# Experience: Family Models of the Body

**What kind of models did you grow up with? Did members of your family practice poor health habits? Did they take good care of themselves? Did they complain of pains and limitations? Were they sick a lot? Did they work their bodies hard? Did they know when to rest? Did they abuse each other physically? Were they restrained or exuberant? Did they attend to their bodily needs behind closed doors, as though they were shameful? Did they allow themselves physical pleasures? Did you try to stand tall like your daddy, the soldier? Or did you hunch over the way he did after a hard day's work? What kind of body messages did you get?**

anorexia and bulimia? Did we tune out sensations because we didn't want to know that something is really wrong? Do we blindly hope that if we ignore and forget it, it'll just go away—that if we don't feel it, it's not there?

In "forgetting" what we feel, we may come to accept how others see us. If someone tells us we're clumsy, even though we're not, we may adapt ourselves to fit that image. And as a clumsy person, we become prone to accidents, reinforcing the image. We may also unconsciously imitate those around us. Psychotherapists Gay Hendricks and Kathlyn Hendricks tell of a father and three sons who came to share a particular posture: head jutting forward and chest caving in. The boys assumed this was genetic until they discovered that the youngest son was adopted at the age of four. In photographs of him before then, he showed no inclination toward this stance. It slowly appeared in elementary school and became pronounced by high school.[25]

In his autobiographical work *Lovesong,* former civil rights activist Julius Lester describes the body relationship he had with his parents. Here's what the arrival of his elderly parents for a visit evoked in him. After you read it, try to imagine what such a visit would elicit from you.

> I put my arms around [my father] and hug him. He chuckles nervously, pleased, and pats me on the back. We are not accustomed to touching, he and I, she and I, he and she. It is as if their bodies are forbidden to them, as if their bodies have been sanctioned only for work, as were the bodies of their parents and slave grandparents, and if their bodies were to know joy it could only be through the smooth wood of a hoe handle, the upraised ends of a plow, in arms extending above the head to pin damp clothes to a line. I want to hold him closely enough so I can feel the clods of earth in a cotton field, his grief for those bodies of his youth whose souls went to God with the burn

*People have lost their bodies and want them back.*

—Alexander Lowen

marks of a lyncher's rope. But I dare not. I want to hold her thin body and touch apple blossoms and the fuzz of the peaches she pulled from the trees in the orchard, the loneliness and fear in long, waist-length black hair and skin as luminous as the new moon. . . . But I dare not.[26]

Remember, our bodies are our earliest classroom. From our first days of life, physical learning forms the template of our emotional lives, governs our relationship patterns, and provides resources and challenges. In working with our bodies now, we have an opportunity to discover what was taught well and relearn lessons given poorly. "Touch, movement, and body awareness are the teaching tools we can use," says Clyde Ford.[27] Bodyways provide them.

## EDUCATION

*Ironically, we are all too often educated out of rather than in to an awareness of the body.*

—Jean Houston

While writing this book, I audited a class for my own interest at the university in my area. Twenty years after completing graduate school, I was shocked to find that nothing had changed physically. I cramped myself into an uncomfortable little seat with a small area to write on. Set in rows, these chairs did not allow me to face anyone, only to see the back of heads. There was no way to interact with those behind or to the side of me, unless I uncomfortably twisted my body one way or the other. There was no fresh air in the room, and fluorescent lights hung overhead. The atmosphere was physically deadening. If it hadn't been for the fact that the subject was stimulating and the professor dynamic, I think I would have fallen asleep.

According to some critics of the American educational system, this kind of structure does not teach us what is fundamental to basic self-knowledge—awareness of our bodies. It does not teach us to make effective and efficient use of our bodies so that we don't hurt ourselves. It does not teach us how movement, sensing, thinking, and feeling are all interrelated in the interaction of our minds and bodies. As a result, we don't even know the true range of our potential and how to use it productively.

*A child who enters school today faces a twelve- to twenty-year apprenticeship in alienation. He learns to manipulate a world of words and numbers, but he does not learn to experience the real world.*

—Rudolf Arnheim

Dancer Elaine Summers, originator of Kinetic Awareness, believes our confinement to school desks for long periods as children is a major cause of the physical difficulties we have as adults. We had to and still have to adapt to chairs, which contributes to muscular imbalance and joint inflexibility, compared to cultures in which people squat. And in order to sit still we had to block out sensations from our bodies. "Movement is restful," says Summers, "holding a position is not."[28] The result is too often a slumped position that distorts and contracts the back.

Having to sit still at a desk is not the only way we develop painful body conditions. In her medical practice, Christiane Northrup regularly sees women with constipation and urinary disorders and an inability to move their bowels in public rest rooms. As children, they had to follow regulations in school (and perhaps at home) about when they could go to the bathroom. These rules damaged their capacity to know when their bodies need to perform normal functions.[29]

How many of us became alienated from our bodies after spending hours all week confined to our desks? Did we learn what things are by words, which abstractly label them, rather than by our senses, which concretely explore them? Were we able to use and heighten the power of our bodies' senses, especially kinesthesia, rather than erode them through using our senses less and less? A woman I met at an Alexander workshop

## Experience: Check Out Your Posture

What relationship did you develop with your body at school? Were you forced to sit still at a desk for hours on end to concentrate on mental tasks at the expense of your body's cries for movement? Did you slump forward, your back rounded, your shoulders hunched? Did you continue that poor posture at home while doing homework? Stop and check how you sit at a desk or table now. Do you revert to your classroom posture?

When you hear the command "Stand straight" or "Correct your posture," do you flash back to a teacher's or parent's orders? How does your body respond to those words? Check yourself. Have you sucked in your belly and thrust out your chest? Are your shoulders tight and close to your ears? Are your arms stiff by your sides? Are you holding your breath? Is your neck rigid? Maintaining this so-called good posture, walk around the room. Do you feel like a wooden soldier? Are you able to take in with your eyes all that's around you, or do you see only what's directly in front of you? Notice your thinking. How clear are you when you're so contracted?

Now try a different posture. Stand with your attention focused on the center of your body, about two inches below your navel, deep within your pelvis. Instead of holding your breath, inhale deeply into this place and drop your shoulders. Keep your knees soft rather than locked so that you have a stable but flexible base of support. Relax your arms. In this posture, walk around the room again. Notice the range of your vision: Are you able to see up and down, right and left, or are you still staring only straight ahead? Do you feel fluid or rigid? How does a shift to a belly-centered posture affect you overall? How are your perception and thinking now?

remembers how, as an eighth grader in New Jersey, she was forced to take an etiquette class in which she learned to sit straight with her knees pressed together and ankles crossed, to get up from a chair with a book on her head, and ultimately to hate her body because it wouldn't conform to the ideal being taught in the class.

## SELF-IMAGE AND BODY IMAGE

Our sense of self—our image of who we are—is first and foremost an image formed through our body.

—Clyde Ford

We're not born with an ego, according to developmental psychologists. In the beginning of our lives, we're not aware of ourselves as separate or of the world as distinct from us. There is no differentiation. But gradually our egos begin to emerge. Since body boundaries mark off our existence from the surrounding environment, our first sense of identity is in our bodies. Our selves are somatic, corporeal, fleshy, bodily selves—body egos.

Thus, self-image is essentially body image, for we know who we are through our bodies—as we physically feel them and as we visualize them. It has to do with how our bodies are oriented in space and time, with the contours of our bodies, and with our kinesthetic sensations and visual perceptions.

However, body image or self-image is not only what we see when we look at ourselves and how we sense and control our body parts. It is also mental, emotional, and historical—how we feel and think about our appearance and how all our experiences, both pleasurable and painful, full of praise or criticism, shaped us. Our perception of our bodies is based on all of these—physical sensations, ideas, emotions, projections, instructions, and expectations.

If you ask Western people where "I" exists, many point to their foreheads. If you asked [anthropologist] Margaret Mead that question, she responded matter-of-factly, "Why, all over me, of course."

—Jean Houston

Each of us acts in accordance with this self-image. We eat, walk, sit, speak, think, and love in our own particular ways. We identify with this image, even though it doesn't necessarily coincide with what our physical bodies actually are. For example, if we somehow absorbed a message that the body is inferior or bad, that sensual needs are wrong, that we should not explore and know and enjoy our bodies, then this would have led to a negative self-image. We probably wound up embarrassed or ashamed about what we do with our bodies. We wouldn't even have had the experience of touching ourselves to form a rudimentary tactile map of our own bodies. For these and other reasons, our bodies become a suspicious mystery we don't trust. We don't have an accurate picture of them: Some parts are missing, while others are indistinct or even distorted. In turn, a negative or poor body image can have such dire consequences as depression, eating disorders, low self-esteem, inhibited sexuality, and fearfulness.

Instead of forming our self-images through our own physiology and perceptions, we collect them through a variety of social filters—from our families, communities, ethnic groups, and religions. We form them from what is required and expected of us as we grow up. We may wind up with images of ourselves as coordinated or ungainly, tall or short, homely or pretty, all in comparison to what was around us. Using other people's ideas, we *think* rather than *perceive* our self-image or body image. Our body image also develops gaps, distortions, and vagueness through disuse and misuse of the body. For example, sexual anxieties may cause the genitals to become faint or even disappear from the body image.

It took me years to match my physical body and body image. I always thought I was taller and larger because even before I finished elementary school, my parents were already shorter than I was. When I was a teenager, for some reason people assumed I was at least five feet seven inches tall, yet I was only five feet five inches. It was not until my twenties, when I had a boyfriend who was a foot taller, that I realized I was of only average height and weight. However, for many years afterward, I still thought I needed a bigger size in clothes, until a couple of petite friends insisted I try on their outfits. Much to my surprise, everything fit.

Over time, my self-image changed to be more accurate. But I know that many other women still think, incorrectly, that they're bigger than they are. In a study conducted at the University of South Florida, more than 95 percent of the women (without eating disorders) who participated overestimated their body sizes, in most cases as one-fourth larger than they actually were. Nearly 50 percent estimated at least one of four body parts to be 50 percent larger than it was.[30]

To change the self-image we developed gradually as children, we need to feel differently in our bodies. We need to know ourselves through

Everyone's body is the invention of somebody. The question is, who invented my way of being incarnate? My mother? My spouse? My coach? Me?
—Sidney M. Jourard

## Experience: How at Ease Are You with Your Body Image?

Are you comfortable with how you look? Are you excessively self-conscious? Do you constantly compare yourself with others? Are you obsessed with the size of certain parts of your body? Do you call them "thunder thighs," "big butt," "saddlebags," or "balloon belly"? What are you ashamed of? Do you wish a genie would grant your wish to change your body? If so, how?

Do you check on how you feel inside, or do you look in the mirror a lot? Do you see yourself differently each time you look? Does the slightest change in your body size—for example, your abdomen swelling after a meal or before menstruation—terrorize you into immediately starting a diet or increasing your exercise regimen?

The founder of Hasidic mysticism once said, "Since the dawn of creation no two human beings have been born alike. All are unique. And it is the task of each adult to further his uniqueness. And it is the failure to work on this task that has held back the coming of the messiah."

—Lawrence LeShan

self-touch and the touch of others. We need to feel our feelings, sense our sensations. Slowly, as we plant new seeds, we begin to harvest a different bounty from the garden of our bodies. As our bodies change, our images change, coming from deep inside us, not from thinking, willing, or reasoning. Gaps are filled in. Vagueness becomes clarity. Distortions turn into regularities. Low self-esteem turns into self-confidence. And, as psychologist Rita Freedman says, body loathing transforms into bodylove.

In bodyways, the goal is to fully feel all of the body and recognize its entire movement potential. That allows us to function unimpeded and to avoid injuries. Even if you have no aches and pains that bring you to bodyways, certainly coming to know, as completely as possible, who you are in your body is a worthwhile aim. It leads to being your own person. "The privilege of a lifetime is being who you are," rather than imitating someone else, said mythologist Joseph Campbell.[31] Even if that someone else is Mother Teresa, when you're not being yourself, you're headed down the wrong road.

# CHAPTER 3

# Body Wisdom

Despite the crucial role of the body in every aspect of our lives, we have overemphasized the mind, as though the body were nothing more than nuisance baggage to drag around or a pedestal existing solely for the purpose of holding and showing off the head. Think of the marble and bronze heads of Roman emperors on pedestals that you've seen in museums or art books. The entire essence of who they were is stored entirely in the topmost part of their bodies. In fact, when we say "body," aren't we referring to all that's dangling below the neck, without including the head?

*There is deep wisdom within our very flesh, if we can only come to our senses and feel it.*

*—Elizabeth A. Behnke*

## MATTER OVER MIND

The expression "mind over matter" is probably the best example in the English language of how much we put the mind first. Indeed, science has proved this maxim to be true—our mental intentions can overcome pain and send a disease into remission. We also know that prolonged depression and repressed anger eventually can take their toll in physical illness, even death.

Yet "matter over mind" is just as valid. How we feel in our body—whether we're fighting pain or gravity or reveling in pleasure—is as influential in how we think and feel as the other way around. All of our thoughts and feelings are simultaneously physical sensations. Thinking is inseparable from electrical and chemical activity in the brain and nervous system and from accompanying muscle tensions and movements.[1]

In considering the body to have an equal influence, we are finally "giving the body its due," says Maxine Sheets-Johnstone, an independent scholar, professor, and former dance artist. We are challenging the culturally em-

*No matter how closely we look, it is difficult to find a mental act that can take place without the support of some physical function.*

*—Moshe Feldenkrais*

The quite ordinary body of quite ordinary experience holds the key to lightening its own miseries, provided one stops to listen to it and gives it its due.

—Maxine Sheets-Johnstone

bedded ways we deride or ignore the body's role in our humanness—in knowing and making sense of the world, in learning, creativity, self-understanding, and interpersonal relations.[2]

"Life is so generous a giver," said Fra Giovanni in the sixteenth century, "but we, judging the gifts by their covering, cast them away as ugly or heavy or hard." Giving the body its due is a gesture toward inviting in the outcast, the feared, the misunderstood, the hidden. "Remove the covering and you will find beneath it living splendor, woven of love, by wisdom with power," he concluded.

## BEFRIENDING THE BODY

How often do you berate your own body? Do you get angry at it when it breaks down, when you get sick, when you're in pain, when it doesn't look or feel the way you want it to? Do you turn information about your body against yourself? Do you feel guilty because of its needs and desires?

Would you blame a tree because it's bent over rather than standing straight, has a growth on its trunk, or is infected with a fungus? Would you chastise it because it requires rain and sunshine? If a friend were in pain, would you censure her by saying, "You're such a bad person, you deserve to hurt" or "You're so stupid [or ugly or disgusting]"? Yet we talk to our own bodies in such hateful terms.

What we reject in ourselves is usually what we most need to befriend. Once we accept it and respond with compassion, it can heal or blossom. When Helen Keller finally accepted her deafness and blindness rather than cursing them, she was able to make a significant life for herself and contribute to society. When Eleanor Roosevelt stopped comparing her own looks to those of her beautiful mother and valued what she did have, she became internationally loved and respected for her goodness.

What we need to learn is how to be an accepting, kind, and understanding friend to our own bodies, as we are with our dear friends. When we establish an amicable relationship with our bodies, they are sure to respond in kind—with comfort, pleasure, energy, strength, flexibility, ease . . . *and* wisdom.

Why not fall in love with the body you've been sleeping with all your life?

—Stewart Emery

## MIRACLE OF THE BODY

If you're interested in transforming your life, a shift in attitude will take you a long way. Instead of looking at the body as an imperfection or pathology to be fixed or cured, accept it as a gift. According to Confucianism, a philosophy-religion indigenous to China since the sixth century B.C.E., the

# Experience: Honoring and Loving Your Body

Instead of spending time, energy, and money on trying to remake yourself into the ideal the media exhort everyone to aspire to, here are three things you can do to honor and love the uniqueness of your own body.

1. Draw a line down the middle of a piece of paper to make two columns, or fold it in half lengthwise. On one side list twenty things you appreciate about your body: a long neck, strong shoulders, thick hair, good digestion, a wide pelvis that makes giving birth easier, powerful hands, full breasts that feed your baby, clear vision, fine coordination, graceful fingers, and so on. If you can't come up with twenty, list ten. If that's still too many, then write down five. And if you have trouble even with five, two will do, but you must have at least two. Once you've done that, in the other column enter only one thing you don't like about your body. Look at your list. Can you allow yourself to treasure more than you condemn?

2. If you have difficulty generating such a list, begin by making a positive statement about your body, even if it feels outlandish—for example, "I love my belly." Then write down every critical statement that comes up to counter it until you've exhausted all the negative voices. Once you've gotten them out, repeat the positive statement and try to add others to it.

3. Whether you're sitting up or lying down, close your eyes and scan your body from top to bottom or vice versa. Is there a part you quickly go past? Is it something that you've rejected and kept out of your whole body image? Is there an area you don't feel, perhaps don't even know you've rejected? Is there an aspect of your body you dislike and denigrate with such words as revolting or hideous? Focus your attention on that area. Does it have a particular quality, color, sound, image, temperature, texture, density, pressure, or other sensation? Now, with each inhalation, draw energy into your heart from whatever sacred source you believe in; on each exhalation, breathe out love from your heart to the area you reject or don't feel. Repeat this breathing until you notice something. Do you feel a softening, a release of compassion for yourself? Has the color, quality, picture, or sensation changed?

body is the ultimate gift we receive from our ancestors. Instead of obsessing over how thick your thighs are or how small your breasts are, how long your nose is, or how big your ears are, you can direct your attention to the

It is difficult to dislike your body or a specific part of your body and still like yourself.

—Linda Tschirhart Sanford and Mary Ellen Donovan

miracle of being here as a human body and consider the wonder, wildness, magic, and beauty of it, as poet Gary Snyder does:

> Our bodies are wild. The involuntary quick turn of the head at a shout, the vertigo at looking off a precipice, the heart-in-the-throat in a moment of danger, the catch of the breath, the quiet moments relaxing, staring, reflecting—are universal responses of the mammal body. . . . The body does not require the intercession of some conscious intellect to make it breathe, to keep the heart beating. It is to a great extent self-regulating: it is a life of its own.[3]

Indeed, as one of the psalms says, we are "fearfully and wonderfully made."

• The eye, about the size of a Ping-Pong ball, weighs only a quarter of an ounce. The muscles operating its lenses move up to a hundred thousand times a day so that we can focus on all the varied objects that attract our attention. We would have to walk fifty miles every day just to give our leg muscles the equivalent amount of exercise. Each optic nerve is composed of about 1.25 million individual fibers.

• In the nine ounces of red marrow in our bones, red blood cells are created at the rate of approximately two million every second to replace an equal number destroyed.

• The brain has ten million nerve cells and each has a potential twenty-five thousand interconnections with other nerve cells.

• The nose can detect up to ten thousand different odors, yet our sense of smell, located in the upper part of the nasal cavity, is no more than two patches of membrane containing several million receptors.

• The inner lining of the stomach is a mucous membrane into which are set up to thirty-five million tiny glands that secrete gastric juice to break down proteins and carbohydrates.

• In the three hundred million air sacs (alveoli) of the lungs, carbon dioxide is exchanged for oxygen in one third to three quarters of a second, depending on whether we're at rest or engaged in exercise.

• The kidneys filter five hundred gallons of blood daily.

• The heart, no bigger than a fist, pumps blood day and night through a network of blood vessels calculated to be sixty thousand miles long. When a person is at rest, the heart pumps at sixty-six gallons an hour. Over a lifetime of seventy years, that amounts to nearly sixty million gallons of blood. When a world-class athlete is at

All the scriptures and spiritual teachings which have been passed from generation to generation have revealed, in one way or another, that it is an honor to be a human being—to have this body—even though there are times when the suffering and difficulties are great.

—Stephen R. Schwartz

the height of exertion, the rate increases sixfold. Remarkably, the heart carries out this feat with no more power than that of two tiny electric motors of the size found in many toys. It beats a hundred thousand times a day without rest our entire lives.

• The liver alone, sometimes referred to as the body's chemical factory, is able to perform more than five hundred different functions, including the production of more than a thousand enzymes essential for good digestion and healthy metabolism.

And how beautifully the body is organized. Each part of a cell—the average human body consists of about fifty trillion cells—and each cell as a whole performs a special function. Each tissue, in turn, is specialized to accomplish characteristic tasks. Each organ and each system are experts in particular operations for the benefit of the body as a whole. Everything is intricately integrated. Whenever something happens in one part of the body to disturb the existing condition, other parts compensate to restore the original condition—they adjust to maintain a steady state, or homeostasis.

Suppose you're standing on a street corner talking to someone you happened to meet. Suddenly you look at your watch and realize you'll be late getting back to the office or picking up your child if you don't hurry. Your whole body shifts gears to enable you to run down the street and into your office building or to the parking lot. You breathe more rapidly, your heart beats faster, your blood pressure rises, all in order to bring more oxygen to your muscles so you can run. When you arrive, you're probably warm and perspiring, which is your body's response to all the heat generated by your muscles. If that heat were not dissipated, it would cause the albumin—a protein that occurs in our blood and muscles—to become stiff, just like the white of a hard-boiled egg. Once you stop, your breathing and heartbeat will slow and your blood pressure will drop down again.

If you've ever been in an accident or otherwise seriously hurt yourself, consider the miracle of healing and recovery: how you didn't bleed to death even though a part of your body was open, how bones rejoined and wounds closed up, how you were able to walk again, how your eyes went from swollen and purple to normal size and color. Within split seconds, chemicals sent out a warning signal and cells lined up like an army to defend against invading bacteria and viruses that threatened your life.

Like musicians playing in an orchestra, our muscles contract in concert and lift our bones so we can stand up, walk, dance, jump, or speak. Just lifting one leg forward requires more than forty muscles tugging in unison, "like deckhands hauling out a boom." Our first steps in the morning call on two hundred pulling muscles. Even opening our mouths to greet someone

*Your body is a three-million-year-old healer. Over three million years of evolution on this planet it has developed many ways to protect and heal itself. . . . You have all the knowledge, tools, materials, and energy necessary to keep yourself healthy.*

*—Mike Samuels and Hal Bennett*

with a hello means intricately coordinating the muscles of the lips, jaw, tongue, palate, pharynx, larynx, and respiratory system, which in total contract more than five hundred times per second.[4]

Consider also the body's plasticity, its continual and lifelong changes. Although we start life complete with a genetic blueprint, all of our days are filled with changes. We are not "a frozen anatomical structure, but literally a river of intelligence and information and energy that's constantly renewing itself," says medical doctor and best-selling author Deepak Chopra.[5] Every second of our lives we are remaking ourselves more effortlessly and spontaneously than we change our clothes. For example, in less than one year, we replace about 98 percent of all the atoms in our bodies:

- a new liver every six weeks
- a new skeleton every three months
- a new stomach lining every five days
- a new skin once a month

And the raw material of DNA, which, as Chopra points out, "holds memories of millions of years of evolutionary time," comes and goes every six weeks.[6] Knowing this, recognizing this miracle in your own body, maybe you too will ask the question novelist Janet Burroway posed to herself.

> My question is: Why—when, even after a half-century, and even after its ability to reproduce itself is past, a body not particularly well looked after will demonstrate its enthusiasm for survival . . . will speed good about the veins, pump blood and antibodies, set itself to coagulation, osmosis, cleansing, and creation, will mend so thoroughly that mobility and convenience are restored that could not be had from half a ton of technology—why, I say, should I ever have bitterly blamed it for such trifles as I have blamed it for: for having too much flesh in this spot, too little muscle in that, for producing this wrinkle, that sag, that gray hair, or this texture? Dear body! My dear body! It has gone about its incessant business with very little thanks.[7]

## Intelligence in the Body

We don't tend to associate intelligence with our bodies. We don't think that it is with our bodies that we discern, understand, and know. Yet, as Thomas Edison said, "Great ideas originate in the muscles."

Take a moment to consider Edison's words. How often have you had a breakthrough in your thinking while moving your body? A lot of my ideas in writing this book, including the term *bodyways*, came as my mus-

*The human body is vapor materialized by sunshine mixed with the life of the stars.*

—Paracelsus

*Think with the whole body.*

—Taisen Deshimaru

cles moved me back and forth across a pool or through the woods, or while standing at the sink washing dishes. It was daily walks that inspired Russian composer Tchaikovsky to create many of his symphonies. It was on a stroll that inventor Edwin Land came up with the concept that led to his discovery of the Polaroid camera. Somehow movement serves to remove the silt that blocks creative waters from flowing freely. Even Albert Einstein, one of the most brilliant scientists of our century, said, "My primary process of perceiving is muscular and visual." Or, as writer Laura Riding penned to the young daughter of friends:

> When the sun shines, when the wind blows, when you breathe or see things or walk or sit down or sleep—this is doing. Your whole body is doing. The body part of everything is doing. . . . You must feel this doing, this body part of you, before you can begin to think.[8]

It is also through our bodies that we sense the rightness of a situation or detect danger. Like a radar system, our body wisdom lets us know when we're going too fast and need to slow down, or when we need to be vigorous and in motion. Our bodies signal what to do as long as we don't override the messages with abstract goals and ideas and the latest faddish information in the name of health, success, morality, beauty, or spirituality. For example, as a vegetarian for two decades, I couldn't imagine changing my diet, for it had worked so well for me. But after I turned forty, my hormones turned up the volume to make sure I heard that it was time to incorporate more protein and fat. Instead of sticking with something that was no longer suitable, I added eggs and fish, and my body thanked me for them. In a similar way, Jungian analyst and author Jean Shinoda Bolen dramatically changed her diet. Upon returning to California from a month-long pilgrimage to sacred sites in Europe, she found herself standing in front of the meat section at the market and hearing her body say, "No, thank you." Her habit of eating a small New York steak for breakfast every morning suddenly vanished. And with it also went her pleasure in drinking champagne.[9] For both of us, no willpower was involved. We merely followed what our bodies wanted.

But on another occasion I didn't heed my body's voice, and I paid for it. A week before my first marathon, I went on my last training run in an area that a friend insisted was fairly level. In fact, it was very hilly, but since I'd driven all the way over there, I pushed to do my quota anyway—foolishly. While I managed to finish my run that day, I never made it to the Napa Valley Marathon. I had hurt my left knee straining up and down those hills. To protect me from greater damage, my knee made it clear I would not participate in the race.

This attitude [that consciousness is limited to reasoning] devalues the intelligence of the senses, the "thought of the heart," the thinking hand and eye, and the thoughtfulness of the moving body.

—Shaun McNiff

Only by being inwardly attentive can we learn to tell what we should take in, who feels safe to be with, where we want to be, what is true for us.

—Jean Shinoda Bolen

Our own body is the
best health system we
have—if we know how
to listen to it.

—Christiane Northrup

Learning to listen
to ourselves is a way
of learning to love
ourselves.

—Joan Borysenko

The body's life is the
life of sensations and
emotions. The body
feels real hunger, real
thirst, real joy in the
sun or snow, real plea-
sure in the smell of
roses or the look of a
lilac bush, real anger,
real sorrow, real tender-
ness, real warmth, real
passion, real hate, real
grief. All the emotions
belong to the body and
are only recognized by
the mind.

—D. H. Lawrence

In this regard, body wisdom acts like a smoke detector. We may be "asleep"—as we often are in waking consciousness—and not sense fire, that is, a problem. But the slightest sign—a feeling of discomfort or uneasiness, a stiffness, the flare-up of an old injury, or a sudden headache—will set off the alarm and wake us up to what we need to do. Body wisdom always strives to ensure our survival. The nose detects bad smells to help us avoid eating spoiled food; the digestive system responds acidically when we eat food that doesn't agree with us; an ulcer forms to signal that something's deeply wrong and needs attention; at the first sign of threatening intruders, the immune system sends forth white blood cells to keep harmful bacteria and viruses from damaging our health with disease and infection. That instinct for self-preservation is also built into primitive nonconscious structures in our nervous system that are able to perceive certain events as potentially dangerous to our survival and mobilize us to respond effectively—to flee or fight. But if we don't or can't respond instinctively, we may wind up with a disorder or even endanger our lives.

In some extreme cases, the loss of built-in body intelligence can eventually lead to death. Many years ago I had a young massage client who had developed diabetic retinopathy, which blinded her; she also developed necrosis (localized death of living tissue) in her lower legs and feet. Because she could no longer see or feel in her feet, she didn't know that she had stepped on a heating vent in the floor and burned herself. She never recovered from the subsequent infection and died in her early twenties.

We're outfitted with all the apparatus we need: neurotransmitters, sensory receptors, homeostatic adjusters, detoxification units, chemical regulators, and so on. Intelligence suffuses every cell in the body—in all of its enzymes, genes, hormones, antibodies, and nerves—regulating essential functions with perfect know-how. Even seeking pleasure and avoiding pain are part of the body's design for survival and well-being. ☞ See "Pleasure," page 12. Everything will continue to work precisely and exquisitely as long as we can listen and take care.

## FEELINGS: EMOTIONAL AND PHYSICAL

We have no emotional feelings unless we also have physical ones. It is through our bodies that we know love—that we receive it and give it—and other emotions. Bodily gestures and facial expressions convey what we're feeling without one word. Even when we do speak, our bodies often contradict our words. We may say we're not interested in someone, but the blush on our face and the quickening of our heartbeat belie our attractions. We may claim we're not nervous, but our palms are wet with anxiety. We may not admit we're bothered, but our shoulders are contracted up to our

# Experience: Where Do You Feel Anger, Fear, Grief, Love?

How do you know when you're comfortable, in pain, bored, or terrified? How do you know when you trust or don't trust someone? How do you know when you're happy, sad, pleased, disappointed, or neutral? Remember the last time you laughed so hard that you cried and the last time you cried your heart out. Even though in both situations tears came out of your eyes, didn't you know the difference? Did you know that from thinking about it or from feeling it in your body?

The next time you're angry, frustrated, peaceful, scared, or in grief, ask yourself: Where in my body do I experience this feeling/emotion? What are the specific sensations of this feeling/emotion?

---

ears with anger. We may deny we're sad and lonely, yet our chin is down and our chest caved in.

How are the emotional and the physical connected? In the third week of our lives as an embryo, three sheets of cells are present. One of these primitive or germ layers, the ectoderm, gradually gives rise to the skin, brain, and nervous system. This means that from the same group of cells we develop the structures that allow us to feel physical sensations—sensory receptors—*and* those through which we experience emotions. "Depending on how you look at it," says Deane Juhan, a Trager practitioner and instructor, "the skin is the outer surface of the brain, or the brain is the deepest layer of the skin."[10] They function as a single unit.

Scientific research in the field of psychoneuroimmunology is proving that the "brain" and its functions are actually located all over the body. Candace Pert, formerly of the National Institutes of Health, and other brain researchers have found receptor sites for neuropeptides (brain chemicals) not only in the brain, nervous system, and immune system but also throughout the body.

When we are aware of physical changes taking place in our bodies, then we also know what emotions we're feeling. Specific body sensations act as protective signals or convey emotional meanings. Alicia Appleman-Jurman experienced this dramatically during World War II. In her autobiography she recounts how she lived with constant fear as a Jewish girl hiding from the Nazis and their collaborators in Poland. Her body gave her signals she knew she could trust more than anyone's words: "I felt a cold hand lodged inside me, twisting my insides whenever danger was present."[11]

The body is a multilingual being. It speaks through its color and its temperature, the flush of recognition, the glow of love, the ash of pain, the heat of arousal, the coldness of nonconviction. . . . It speaks through the leaping of the heart, the falling of the spirits, the pit at the center, and rising hope.

—Clarissa Pinkola Estés

We have neglected
our emotional reality,
and the source of
our self-nourishment:
our bodies.

—Stanley Keleman

Through trial and error, clinical psychologist Harriet Goldhor Lerner has learned how to recognize and heed physical sensations as warnings of emotions. This enables her to respond consciously rather than react unconsciously. When she feels "an anxious, uncentered sort of intensity," it's a red light to "stop, think twice" before rushing into obnoxious confrontations that damage relationships. She's able to distinguish this feeling from a "fire-in-the-soul passion" that energizes and adds zest to her work and friendships.[12]

## OUR INNER VOICE

Listen to what you
know through your
body.

—Frances Payne Adler

When we become more aware that we have inside us resources for knowing and evaluating, then we begin to listen to the "still, small voice" we find there. That voice enables us to develop an inner source of confidence, which has repercussions in our self-concepts, self-esteem, morality, and behavior, as well as in our relationships, health, and creativity.

A woman named Inez discovered this for herself. "There is a part of me that I didn't even know I had until recently—instinct, intuition, whatever," she says. The "whatever" she's talking about is body wisdom. "It helps me and protects me. It's perceptive and astute. I just listen to the inside of me and I know what to do. . . . I can only know with my gut. I've got it tuned to a point where I think and feel all at the same time and I know what is right. My gut is my best friend—the one thing in the world that won't let me down or lie to me or back away from me."[13]

"Gut knowing" sometimes makes such unusual appearances that we don't immediately recognize or accept it. Jean Houston, director of the Foundation for Mind Research and author of human-potential books, tells a story of one such perplexing manifestation of body wisdom. When she was twenty-three years old, she lay utterly fatigued from what the doctor diagnosed as influenza. In the middle of the night her temperature would soar, even up to 105 degrees, and hallucinations would commence. In one, a group of garden club matrons in flowered hats kept insisting that Houston wake her mother, that she had to have the blood test that's given to alcoholics. Since she rarely drank, she feverishly whined at the women to leave her alone. When the ladies wouldn't let up, she finally called out to her mother, who agreed to phone the laboratory in the morning. The blood tests uncovered Houston's raging case of hepatitis, not the flu. With a new and appropriate course of treatment, she duly recovered. This experience convinced Houston that her collective body wisdom had insinuated its way into her consciousness through the whimsically decked out ladies bearing vital information. In an altered state induced by the high fever, she was able to receive a message her conscious mind was not aware of.[14]

# Experience: A Guided Journey to Body Wisdom

You might want someone to read you these directions or record them yourself to play back.

Sit comfortably or lie down. Close your eyes. Begin to relax your body from your toes to the top of your head by taking nice deep breaths and letting the air out in an easy, slow manner. As you inhale, feel your abdomen and chest expand. As you exhale, feel yourself letting go of tension. Take several breaths to experience these sensations of fullness and emptiness. Then, after a deep in-breath, focus on your feet and as you exhale imagine that breath going straight to your feet. Like a gentle tropical breeze, it caresses and softens what it touches. Using the breath in the same way, move up until you've covered every part of your body. If, when you get to the head, you're not yet fully relaxed, repeat the whole sequence, starting with the feet again.

Once you're relaxed, imagine that you're on a mountain, ready to descend. You notice a path. Take it as it winds around and down, around and down. Be careful as you go, so as not to slip or trip over rocks and roots. Take as much time as you need to find your way down the mountain.

When you reach the bottom, the path becomes a trail through the woods around the mountain. You haven't gone far when you notice a big rock outcropping. As you get closer, you see that it is a cave in the mountain you've just walked down. Enter the cave. There's no need to be afraid of anything in there. There's plenty of air, so you can keep breathing easily and remain relaxed. You can see your way because there are candles lit along the cave walls. Their light leads you to a being seated at the back of the cave. You sit down in front of that wise being and politely bow to show your respect. Picture her (him, it) clearly, for this is Body Wisdom, who knows everything important about you. Body Wisdom has access to countless bits of information about your body—its health and its needs.

Be respectful, but don't be shy. This is your opportunity to learn what could help you. Seated in front of Body Wisdom, ask general or specific questions about yourself. Wait patiently for whatever answers come. They may be in words or images, or you might feel them as sensations in your body. Just stay relaxed and receptive so you can pay attention to the messages that come. Take as much time and ask as many questions as you need to.

When you have gotten all that you can use at this time, bow again with thanks and take leave of Body Wisdom. Walk out of the cave and through the woods until you come to a clearing. Then gradually wiggle your toes and fingers, stretch long but easy, and slowly open your eyes. It's now up to you to implement the information that has been imparted for your sake.

Whatever I wanted to express in its truest meaning must emerge from within me and pass through an inner form. It cannot come from outside but must emerge from within.

—Meister Eckhart

Sometimes gut messages are not about health but about creativity. Through experience, British classical scholar and poet Alfred E. Housman learned to recognize such physical notes in regard to his work. When he shaved in the morning, he carefully watched his thoughts, for if a line of poetry strayed into them, suddenly his skin would bristle to the extent that his razor would stop working. He'd also get a shiver down his spine and a constriction of his throat; his eyes would tear, and he would have the sensation of a spear going through the pit of his stomach.[15]

## BODY PERCEPTION

Psychologist Sidney Jourard called the body's wisdom *somatic perception.*[16] Others have called it *vivacious perception* or *life-to-life communication.* Hippies called it *picking up the vibes.* It's the capacity we all have for "seeing" or testing the world with our bodies. When we're awake to it, we're intelligent: that is, we know when, what, and how much to eat, exercise, rest, interact with others, or be alone; we know when something is beneficial or destructive to us. When we're numb to this kind of body wisdom, we become stupid (from the Latin *stupere,* "to be benumbed")—we make unintelligent decisions and act carelessly.

He who feels it, knows it more.

—Bob Marley

This mode of perceiving is similar to the old-time miners' practice of carrying a canary into the mine. If the air was not fit and the bird died, the miners knew the atmosphere would soon kill them too. "One's entire body functions like a canary in a coal mine," Jourard said.[17] How else would we know when a person is truly angry or deeply sad while hiding behind a false smile?

In response to the energies around us, our bodies vibrate at various rates and amplitudes, informing us of what's going on. For instance, an African !Kung San can sense the approach of animals at a great distance or the location of water not by what he sees in the landscape but by consulting the feel of his body. When naturalist Terry Tempest Williams traveled in the Serengeti savanna, she observed that her Masai guide had not abandoned this native intelligence. "Samuel felt the presence of animals long before he saw them," she writes in *An Unspoken Hunger.* "I saw him penetrate the stillness with his senses."[18] Similarly, Polynesian men have learned to navigate not so much by the location of stars but by exquisite body sensitivity to the subtlest swells in the ocean. The wayfinder sits cross-legged and nearly naked on the bottom of a canoe and, by the feeling in his testicles, reads the shape of a swell in order to tell the direction and strength of the current beneath it.[19]

I shut my eyes in order to see.

—Paul Gauguin

The French writer Jacques Lusseyran recognized this ability in himself after he was blinded in a school accident at the age of eight:

This tendency of objects to project themselves beyond their physical limits produced sensations as definite as sight or hearing. . . . How should I explain the way objects approached me when I was the one walking in their direction? Was I breathing them in or hearing them? . . . Did I see them? It seemed not. And yet as I came closer, their mass was modified, often to the point of defining real contours, assuming a real shape in space, acquiring distinctive color, just as it happens where there is sight.

As I walked along a country road bordered by trees, I could point to each one of the trees by the road, even if they were not spaced at regular intervals. I knew whether the trees were straight and tall, carrying their branches as a body carries its head, or gathered into thickets and partly covering the ground around them. . . . Trees and rocks came to me and printed their shape upon me like fingers leaving their impression in wax.[20]

My whole body
is covered with eyes:
Behold it!
Be without fear!
I see all around.

—Eskimo poem

Consider how many functions the skin, the body's largest organ, performs. Take a quarter and place it on your forearm. Try to imagine what's in that small patch of skin under the coin:

- more than three million cells
- a hundred sweat glands
- twelve feet of nerves and hundreds of nerve endings
- three feet of blood vessels
- three feet of lymph vessels

It is a remarkable organ: waterproof in both directions (keeping water in and out); germproof (protecting underlying tissues from infection); protective against the sun's UV rays; productive (turns ergosterol into vitamin D when exposed to sunlight); flexible and supple (stretching when we move, then springing back); long-lasting (instead of wearing out, it repairs itself when damaged and always replaces itself); regulatory (maintains body temperature through sweat glands); repository (stores sodium chloride and glucose); and tactile (has a sense of touch). It is our most important sense organ. Containing hundreds of thousands of sensory receptors, which are responsive to touch, pressure, pain, and temperature changes, the skin is a constant source of information about our environment.

Within me even the most metaphysical problem takes on a warm physical body which smells of sea, soil, and human sweat. The Word, in order to touch me, must become warm flesh. Only then do I understand—when I can smell, see, and touch.

—Nikos Kazantzakis

What Lusseyran experienced was validated in experiments conducted by Georg von Békésy, 1961 Nobel prize winner in medicine. Because the size and inaccessibility of the human inner ear proved an obstacle, he worked with the skin, which also is a vibration-sensitive membrane equipped with an extensive system of nerve fibers. Experiments by Paul Bach-y-Rita showed that with some training through vibratory pressure on their skin, people who were blind from birth could visually image and deaf individuals could "hear" the sound of the human voice. Research by a French writer and Academy member, Jules Romains, demonstrated the existence of visual perception outside the retina, in certain nerve centers of the skin, particularly in the hands, the forehead, the nape of the neck, and the chest.[21]

Allan Gurganus, author of *The Oldest Living Confederate Widow Tells All,* uses his body to help him in his writing. He calls it "the ultimate testing ground" of what works or doesn't work on the page. He knows when he's hot on the trail of a story by the physical sensations he feels. When he's working well, he perspires so freely that he sweats his way through the fiction. And since he has to use something so abstract as the twenty-six letters of the English alphabet "to bear all the human investigations and all the aspirations and appetites that we have and that have ever existed in human history," again he lets his body be the test of how well he's put those letters together. He reads his stories aloud dozens of times until he gets "a kind of rhythmic synchronicity" with the readers' biological chemistry and somehow pulls them rhythmically into the fiction, creating "a kind of heartbeat on the page." What Gurganus has learned from this process is: "By trusting my body and making it my active collaborator, Hammerstein to my Rodgers, I have a kind of company in the isolation of working."[22]

Somatic perception is vital not only to the survival of seafaring navigators and tribal hunters but also to us "modern" human beings. If we can't discern how our relationships with others affect us, if we can't judge how our physical habits influence our well-being, then we're doomed to suffer the breakdowns, physical and psychological, that result from not changing our lifestyle. If we're operating on automatic pilot—that is, "stupidly"—we are not sensitive to how we're being influenced by what we eat, where we live, the way we work, and our actions, thoughts, and emotions. When we're not aware of these connections, we also remain baffled why we're sick, tense, in chronic pain, or depressed.

Our body is a source of truth.

—Albert Pesso

This wisdom or ability to listen to your body and respond appropriately to it is also essential in collaborating with health-care professionals. Only you know what your symptoms feel like and how you are responding to treatment. "Learning to listen to your own body is vital to improving your health and the quality of your life," says Jon Kabat-Zinn, founder and director of the Stress Reduction Clinic at the University of Massachusetts Medical Center.[23]

## A Body of Truth

If honesty is a quality you prize, then relying on your body's wisdom can keep you honest—with yourself and with others.

That's what psychologist Harriet Goldhor Lerner learned when she was trying to decide whether to marry an old friend. Although he scored well on her checklist of qualifications, she was ambivalent. Finally one day, unable to tolerate the situation any longer, she decided to make a full emotional commitment and marry. She fell asleep relieved, but awoke the next morning nearly paralyzed. Lying heavy and immobilized in bed, overcome by depression, she knew she could never marry this man.[24]

Similarly, a friend of Lerner says that her body keeps her honest even if her head wants her to get away with things: "When I don't tell the truth, I feel it in my body. So I don't get off the phone, for example, by making excuses, like someone's at the door or I'm late for an appointment. Telling a big lie, like faking sexual pleasure, would make me physically sick."[25]

As Lerner learned, body wisdom comes through feeling and sensation, not through thinking and figuring out. While we're making a list of pros and cons to help us decide which way to go, we probably already know the answer in our gut but are not ready to hear it. Eugene Gendlin, a psychology professor and the originator of a process called Focusing, calls this inner feeling the "felt sense." He describes it as "not a mental experience but a physical one . . . a bodily awareness of a situation or person or event. . . . Think of it as a taste . . . or a great musical chord that makes you feel a powerful impact, a big round unclear feeling. . . . A felt sense doesn't come to you in the form of thoughts or words or other separate units, but as a single (though often puzzling and very complex) bodily feeling."[26]

I've often had such whole-body feelings telling me which direction to take. One time I tried to convince myself to take a well-paying position as publicity director for an arts and cultural center in the making. It would have helped tremendously at a time when living as a freelance writer was precarious at best. Finally I said yes after calculating the advantages. But when I visited what was to be my new office, a feeling of darkness and uneasiness came over my body that I couldn't ignore or dispel. That night I had a dream that clearly revealed to me I had my own path to walk and it didn't include that job. As hard as it was to give up the financial security I longed for then and to disappoint the person who had gotten me the position, I had to withdraw. More than a year later, I talked to the woman who did take on the work; the job had proven to be worse than demanding.

When you allow this natural sense to function—too often it's socialized out of us so that we will conform to society's rules and regulations—you also begin to pick up in your own body the truth of what's going on in

If you're an alive body, no one can tell you how to experience the world. And no one can tell you what truth is, because you experience it for yourself.

—Stanley Keleman

Stress: the feeling you get when your gut says "No" and your mouth says, "Yes, I'd be glad to."

—Dick Francis

When you get into the body, it keeps you true.

—Jennifer Reich

Your health is bound to be affected if, day by day, you say the opposite of what you feel, if you grovel before what you dislike and rejoice at what brings you nothing but misfortune. Our nervous system isn't just a fiction, it's part of our physical body, and our soul exists in space and is inside us, like the teeth in our mouth. It can't forever be violated with impunity.

—Boris Pasternak

others. The more you know your own body, the better able you are to read other bodies and distinguish between your feelings and theirs; you can determine when you're perceiving and when you're projecting. This was true for a student of Robert Frager, the founding president of the Institute of Transpersonal Psychology in Palo Alto, California. She would often tell him, "I don't know what is going on with a certain client, but my stomach felt funny when he brought up this topic." As she learned to trust her stomach, she became "an extraordinarily effective therapist" who was sensitive to the slightest nuances in her clients even when she couldn't rationally understand what was happening.[27]

If you are not sure whom to trust, even when everything appears perfect, then your body will tell you something doesn't feel right. An incident in my own life comes to mind. After some years of living on Maui, I decided to build a cottage. I interviewed several candidates for the task. One man came carrying a book on *feng shui,* the Chinese ancient art of placement. As we stood in the driveway, he held the book up and said all the politically correct things, but my body wouldn't trust his words. No matter how much I tried to be open, my body kept withdrawing from him. I never did invite him inside to discuss any details, even though I already believed in the principles of *feng shui.* On the other hand, when another prospective builder came to the house, my body said I could go beyond appearances and trust him, though something about his looks reminded me of men I had been warned away from as a girl. He didn't try to dazzle me with popular books and ideas, yet he proved to be immensely creative, knowledgeable, trustworthy, and competent. He did such an excellent job that even the building inspectors praised his work.

# Experience: Feeling a Lie or the Truth in Your Body

Try to remember how you felt the last time you told a lie. Did you lower your head and look down? What sensations did you have? And what did they provoke you to do? Did you get busy to avoid what you were feeling? Did a tightness in your throat, chest, or belly make you grab for some food? What does your body do now in response to that memory?

Now remember how you felt the last time you told the truth. What sensations do you notice in your body as you review the memory? Is there a warm feeling, a fullness, a lightness?

If you have difficulty remembering an incident, try this. Alone, say out loud an outrageous lie and see how your body responds. Notice sensations. Then say a deep-down truth. Again, notice how you feel in your body.

## SOURCES OF BODY WISDOM

Where does body wisdom come from? What gives us access to it?

How we know what we know is a complex, even mysterious process that we don't fully understand. However, everything in the body and mind plays a role in a total communication system. Our brain receives messages about changes in the external environment from sensory receptors in the eyes, nose, ears, and skin, and within our bodies from receptors in the muscles and joints. These signals travel along sensory nerves to tell the brain what is happening. In turn, the brain decodes and translates them into adjustments of the internal environment, which register as heat, cold, pressure, pain, and movement. These signals go out along motor nerves, which have connections to every muscle. As tiny electrical impulses arrive, a muscle contracts. That message then returns to the brain for yet another adjustment, and another message is sent out—it's a constant feedback process.

We know through all our senses, but vision is emphasized the most in Western culture, even though touch is the sense that involves the entire body and the one we can't survive without. Every tactile experience we have brings in a flow of information. Measuring more than twenty square feet if laid out flat (for an average adult), the skin is the body's largest organ and its most constantly active source of sensations. Replete with sensory receptors, the skin is our outward connection to the central nervous system within. What we feel through touching or being touched is as important to our thinking as reasoning and language.

### *Proprioception and Kinesthesia*

In a sitting position, close your eyes, then reach with your hand to touch your left knee. Or extend both arms out to the side at shoulder height, then bring the tips of your index fingers together. If you can't make the contact, then something is amiss with your proprioception.

Everyone is familiar with five of our senses—sight, smell, hearing, taste, and touch. But we also know through various inner senses that make up our proprioceptive system (*proprioception* literally means "own reception"). Through that system we receive stimuli that are produced within our own bodies rather than smells, sounds, and light that come from outside. When we sense ourselves from within, we know when to eat or drink or when to stop eating or drinking, when to cool off or warm up, when to urinate or defecate, and so on. Our internal or visceral organs feed us the information—for example, we sense fullness, hollowness, stretching, contraction, pressure.

Our sense organs of balance and position play the greatest role in how we move. *Kinesthesia,* from the Greek, means "perception of movement."

What you cannot find in your body you will not find anywhere else.

—Asian proverb

We have five senses in which we glory and which we recognise and celebrate, senses that constitute the sensible world for us. But there are other senses—secret senses, sixth senses, if you will—equally vital, but unrecognised, and unlauded . . . unconscious, automatic.

—Oliver Sacks

The body knows to protect itself because the body thinks faster than the mind.

—David Woodberry

Kinesthetic receptors are sensory receptors that inform the brain of what kind of movement is going on in different parts of the body: that our legs are moving and how far and fast, that our heads are turned, that our arms are behind our backs, that we are lifting, pulling, or pushing, and that we are keeping our balance. For example, special structures inside skeletal muscles communicate muscle length, letting us know how the muscles are moving. Golgi bodies (cell organelles) in tendons detect muscle force and the pull on tendons. Joint receptors monitor compression in our joints. Hair cells called maculae and cristae in the inner ear monitor equilibrium; this labyrinthine or vestibular feedback lets us know our position in space. ☞ See illustration of inner ear, page 214. Bodily movement and tensions stimulate all of these sense organs.

Without kinesthesia, the various muscle groups needed in walking would never cooperate. The muscles would send our legs in one direction and our torso in another. We wouldn't be able to control our movements and would probably stagger around, jerk about, and fall down often. Proprioception gives us coordination in time and space and monitors every movement. It's what enables excellent typists as well as accomplished musicians to place their fingers exactly and with the right amount of pressure without looking. It makes it possible for us to adjust our muscular efforts to the particular task at hand. Otherwise, when you bend to pick up a package, you wind up tensing more muscles than the job requires. Or you don't tense adequately and wind up unprepared for the weight. In either case,

## Experience: Proprioception

Although bodyways will help you to know yourself better, you can start that process on your own before you ever make an appointment. Stand relaxed with your eyes closed in front of a mirror (if possible, a set of mirrors that reflect your sides and back as well). What do you sense about how your feet are planted on the floor? Are they pointed straight ahead? Is one turned more left or right, out or in? Do you feel more weight on one leg and foot than the other? Are your knees relaxed or hyperextended? Do you feel level across your shoulders and hips, or is one side higher and the other lower? Do you feel the weight of your body more forward or leaning back? Are you balanced on the balls and toes of your feet or on your heels?

Now open your eyes and look in the mirror(s). Check yourself visually against what you felt with your proprioceptive senses. How much do you already know about how you live in your body? How much did you learn?

you're likely to hurt yourself. That's why this proprioceptive sense is what certain bodyways—Sensory Awareness, the Alexander Technique, Gerda Alexander Eutony™, Kinetic Awareness®, the Feldenkrais Method®, Hanna Somatic Education®, and others—address. They strive to reawaken and expand this inborn capacity.[28]

When this muscle sense is combined with touch, we are able to judge the texture, weight, and shape of objects even if we're blindfolded. This ability is called *stereognosis* or *solid knowledge*. In fact, for the blind French resistance fighter Jacques Lusseyran, this was a truer way of knowing something than by vision alone:

> Our eyes run over the surfaces of things. All they require are a few scattered points, since they can bridge the gap in a flash. They "half-see" much more than they see, and they never weigh. . . . They are satisfied with appearances, and for them the world glows and slides by, but lacks substance. . . .
>
> [Objects] are alive, even the stones. What is more, they vibrate and tremble. . . . Touching the tomatoes in the garden, and really touching them, touching the walls of the house, the materials of the curtains or a clod of earth is surely seeing them as fully as eyes can see. But it is more than seeing them, it is tuning in on them and allowing the current they hold to connect with one's own, like electricity. To put it differently, this means an end of living in front of things and a beginning of living with them. . . . This is love.[29]

Bodily perception gives each of us privileged access to information about our own bodies that no one else has about us nor we about them. It partly explains why we say "my own body." If we lose this self-sensing, the body becomes blind and deaf to itself. Neurologist Oliver Sacks tells the story of a twenty-seven-year-old mother and computer programmer who suddenly lost her sense of proprioception. From top to toe, she couldn't feel her body and thus felt disembodied or unreal. Unable to be certain of her existential basis—her very body—she also lost her fundamental identity, or body ego. She had to relearn how to function by vision, not by feel, and lived in a realm of "nothingness."[30]

## Energy Sense

Another source of body wisdom is what some people call the "energy sense." We perceive not only what is palpable physically, but also that which is invisible—the electromagnetic field surrounding everything. ☞ See "Energy," page 273. We sense this energy as subtle vibrations emanating from others—almost like sound waves lapping at the shore of our bodies.

Deep within us there is a natural intelligence operating that houses a multitude of information.

—Richard K. Heckler

This is the wisdom:
If we bless our bodies,
they will bless us.

—Gloria Steinem

In order to be
maximally sensitive to
another person, one
must be maximally
sensitive to oneself.

—Thomas Hanna

Jungian analyst Joanne Wieland-Burston says that when we learn to use our bodies as an extremely sensitive seismograph, capable of registering the slightest instabilities, we have a valuable tool we can consult. What it communicates about our state of being—whether unpleasant sensations or those of pleasure, relaxation, and enjoyment—enables us to make decisions appropriate to the point of view the body-seismograph is expressing. That communication allows for a new order to emerge from the chaos of our physical symptoms. That sensitivity also allows us to feel what is transpiring with other people, animals, and plants, too.[31]

Whether you call this inner knowing *body wisdom, bodily intelligence,* or *body perception* makes no difference. You could just as easily say, "My guts tell me . . ." or "I know it in my bones." What matters is that you recognize that you have this knowing and learn to use it.

# PART II

# Getting Started

# Choosing and Working with a Practitioner

Whether you're new to bodyways or you've already experienced one form and are curious about others, you may have some reservations. Perhaps a friend or relative had a negative experience, or you read about a bodyway that did not appeal to you. Many people also have more intimate personal concerns.

## OBSTACLES TO GETTING STARTED

Do any of the following sound familiar?
- I'll have to take all my clothes off.
- I feel exposed and vulnerable when I'm naked.
- The therapist will be disgusted and gasp when she sees my body.
- Why bother? My body has always hurt.
- It'll mess up my hair and makeup.
- The practitioner will ask me personal questions.
- I can't afford it.
- I don't have the time.
- I'll get so relaxed I won't be able to function.
- I'll get turned on and embarrass myself.
- What if the therapist makes sexual advances?
- My condition is genetic, so no one can help me.
- What if I hate it?
- I'm uncomfortable having anybody but my husband/wife touch me.
- I'm afraid awful memories will come up.

> We are all bodies—sensing, moving creatures, wonderfully simple, wonderfully complex. . . . In the flesh, down to and into our bones, we are all bodies.
>
> —Maxine Sheets-Johnstone

- I'll find out I'm a total mess.
- I'll get addicted to it.
- What if it's painful?

In addition, you may notice such negative feelings as hatred of your own body, unworthiness, and unlovableness. Or you may have learned early in life that to go for any kind of help means there's something wrong with you, that you're weak and dependent on others or not in control. You may also feel shame and failure when your body doesn't function as you wish.

Instead, consider that getting assistance is what can spark change. Incident after incident in my own life taught me that getting help is an act of strength, an acknowledgment of my humanness, and that none of us is truly independent. That myth is an especially strong illusion in the American "can do" ethic; it plays off the romantic image of the lone cowboy. Just as every organ and system depends on every other in our body, so we as whole beings are interdependent.

One last point about fears. Some people don't like to be touched, period. It doesn't matter whether the person who does the touching is mother or stranger. There are various reasons why you might shy away from touch. Maybe you were abused and are terrified of having your personal space violated again. Maybe you have a skin condition you're embarrassed to let anyone see or a nervous system that is truly ultrasensitive. If you resist the idea of being touched, you can still try a bodyway that teaches movement awareness or that works only on the energy field surrounding your body.

> *The deeper we live the life of our bodies, the deeper is the upwelling of love.*
>
> *—Stanley Keleman*

## Can You Do It Yourself?

When it comes to the body, books, videos, and friends go only so far. Certainly you and your partner or other family members and friends can achieve a fair level of mastery by learning from a book or video and practicing on each other. I wouldn't have participated in the video "Massage for Health," with Shari Belafonte, if I didn't think it would help a lot of people to get started. But if you want truly professional work, go to a professionally trained practitioner.

## THE BODYWAYS RELATIONSHIP

Your relationship with a body practitioner may be similar to the one you have with teachers, health-care professionals, or psychotherapists, yet it is almost always more physically intimate. Touch is often involved, in some cases, so is partial or full nudity.

Trust is crucial to this relationship—trust in the practitioner's professional competence, confidentiality, commitment, sincerity, and ethics. You want to be able to form an alliance or collaboration with that person so that your concerns, not his or her needs, are the focus of the work. Look for an interactive rather than strictly hierarchical relationship; the latter is often typical of doctor-patient or teacher-student relationships, in which someone else is considered the authority and gives orders, and you take them.

As in any relationship, it's important to be clear about what you expect and what you need. Remember that this is a relationship of exchange—the body therapist provides you with services in return for an agreed-upon payment. It is an economic as well as therapeutic relationship. It is also a professional relationship, with certain boundaries. You're not paying someone to be your friend, mother or father, sister or brother, aunt or uncle, or grandparent. Check your expectations to make sure they are appropriate. At the same time, body practitioners should also be conscious of their expectations and needs in doing the work. As a client, you're not there to be a friend, child, or parent, either.

If you're seeking help at a time of distress—you're hurting physically and/or emotionally—you may be scared and confused. You may hope someone will "fix" or "cure" you. While the wand-waving godmother is fine for fairy tales, she is not likely to figure in your real life, and it's dangerous to ascribe that role to therapists. More important, you have your own inner resources to activate and engage so that you can participate in the healing process. Look for someone who is interested in partnership, in a back-and-forth exchange of perceptions. The relationship between you and a practitioner works best as a two-way process, not a one-way intervention. Ideally, the practitioner is able to both follow and guide you.

Many centuries ago, Hippocrates, the father of Western medicine, said, "It's more important to know what kind of patient has a disease than what kind of disease a patient has." Aileen Crow, a New York therapist, teacher, and performance coach, adds, "Following each person's unique process (and one's own) without imposing even the most impressive program on it, is a more relevant technique and a more difficult skill to acquire."[1]

Certainly you want a professional's expertise. In fact, skillful guidance is especially important when "people don't always know what they want or even what there is to want, let alone how to ask for anything . . . [and] may need educating about the possibilities that exist," says Crow.[2] But you don't want to become wholly dependent on that person, particularly if he or she reinforces helplessness and inadequacy.

Be wary of practitioner-saviors who claim possession of secret knowledge and promise you they're the answer to your prayers. It's better to trust someone who says, "Let's see if, in working together, we can chart a course

Nothing is more exciting than knowing that our bodies and our feelings are a clear, open pathway toward our destinies.

—Christiane Northrup

Doctors are cast in roles of authority in our culture, but I see I am not an authority on anything as much as the ability to take moment by moment leaps of trust in my self and in life. This authority is in all of us.

—Jemille Cox-Hardy

in the direction you're interested in moving." The world's greatest massage therapist cannot relax your muscles unless you let go from within. The most excellent Alexander teacher will not improve your posture unless you're willing and able to focus your attention on how you move. Your body therapist serves best as a hands-on consultant, facilitator, intermediary, agent, or catalyst, providing the input your body needs to reorganize itself—to relieve a spasm, unsway your back, or balance your energy. What you do in the session is just as important as what the therapist does.

## Your Role

Whichever body practice you decide to use, your experience will be greatly enhanced by three things on your part: receptivity, participation, and commitment.

**Receptivity.** It helps to approach your session believing that change or relief is possible. That doesn't mean having expectations that a magical solution will suddenly present itself. It does mean going in without negative thoughts such as "I'll always feel like this, so what's the use?" or "I'll never get over this, it's hopeless." If you're convinced no one can help you, no one can. Also, if you believe feeling good and experiencing pleasure in your body is a sin, then you'll be reluctant to truly enjoy the session and fully partake of its benefits. Jeffrey Maitland, the Rolf Institute's director of academic affairs, says, "Without some fundamental decision that [you're] going to get better, even if you have Buddha, Krishna, and Christ helping you, it wouldn't work."[3]

**Participation.** You're not a car, nor an item of clothing. The bodyways practitioner is not a mechanic or dry cleaner. Bodyways are not about dropping your body off for an hour, then coming back to pick it up all done. The more you are involved, the more you pay attention, the more you make connections between what you do in your body and what you feel, the more you link what you do in a session and what you do in the rest of your life, the more the work will have lasting results. Otherwise, it becomes a case of bringing your car in to have the clutch replaced over and over again because you're not even aware that you continuously keep your foot on it.

**Commitment.** Pain is a great motivator, but once it's gone, do you return to old habits instead of following through on suggestions the body practitioner makes? Are you willing to do what it takes to keep the pain from recurring?

## Understanding Client-Therapist Psychodynamics

Even if your body therapist or educator is not a trained psychotherapist, there are certain psychodynamics that can occur in a bodyways relationship

What we are learning today is that one of the keys to good health is a state of heightened awareness.

—George Leonard

simply because of its therapeutic nature. Transference, countertransference, and projection are common.

## Projection

We all have the tendency to project onto others what we're feeling. Maybe we woke up tired and feeling as though we're coming down with the flu. When we greet our coworkers first thing in the morning, we might say, "Did you have a bad night? Are you feeling okay?" Or we may not be able to accept our emotions—anger, sadness, sexual desire—if we are afraid of them or find them unacceptable. Instead, we might think that someone else is in a rage or is sexually attracted to us.

I remember two women clients who projected their own discomfort with their bodies. One had had a mastectomy and assumed I would find her scarred chest repulsive. I didn't. In fact, I appreciated the opportunity to work with her. Another woman, much heavier than she wanted to be, was certain I'd freak out when I saw her body and would run screaming out of the room. She too learned to take back the projection and realize I wasn't feeling or thinking what she was.

*The infinite ways we are taught that we do not belong to ourselves may amount to a total erosion of connection with and love for our bodies and what they stand for.*

*—Harriet Goldhor Lerner*

## Transference

Transference is different from projection in that you transfer certain emotions and reactions from earlier in your life onto the therapist or bodyways practitioner. The way he dresses, smells, or talks may remind you, negatively or positively, of someone important to you from the past. In one session, you might think the person is the best and most understanding therapist ever or even a miracle worker. In another session, if you're disappointed by something, you might find the same therapist insensitive, stupid, or ineffective. In either case, consciously or unconsciously, you hold the other person responsible for how you feel. Your mood is dependent on what that individual says or does. A skillful therapist will know how to use the transference to break through old patterns and find new ways of perceiving and responding. If this arises with body practitioners and they are not equipped to handle it, they should be prepared to refer you to a psychotherapist who is trained to do so.

## Countertransference

Therapists or body practitioners may also have strong negative or positive reactions to you, the client, based on their past. When this occurs, the dynamic is countertransference. Ideally, therapists are trained to recognize this in themselves and to be responsible for then consulting with a colleague to avoid disrupting or damaging the professional relationship with you.

Boundaries

Being in touch with our bodies, or more accurately, being our bodies, is how we know what is true.

—Harriet Goldhor Lerner

Issues of confidentiality, safety, boundaries, and trust also come into play in a therapeutic relationship. Boundaries are both a dividing line and a point of meeting. If you look at the shoreline as a division between land and sea, you realize it's also the place where water meets land. That boundary changes according to tides. People build their houses accordingly to protect them from being destroyed. The same principle holds true here. Professional boundaries are set up for the safety and protection especially of the client but also of the therapist or body practitioner. While we tend to think of therapists as taking advantage of clients' vulnerability—and certainly the media have reported such cases—it also happens that some clients are flirtatious and seductive, even vengeful if rejected.

As a consumer of bodyways, you have a right to respectful, safe, considerate treatment that is free from physical, sexual, or emotional abuse. If the treatment crosses the boundary of appropriateness, you can stop the session and refuse any further work. Don't let anyone pressure you to continue. Feel free to discuss what happened with friends or other practitioners and to report the unethical behavior if necessary. If the situation becomes too uncomfortable and the practitioner oversteps professional boundaries into a sexual relationship, there are steps you can take to help yourself. ☞ See Appendix: "How to Deal with Sexual Misconduct," page 383.

## Ethical Considerations

Whether someone is a medical doctor, bodyways practitioner, or psychotherapist, the most basic ethic to follow is the Hippocratic oath: "First, do no harm." Unfortunately, as the media have revealed, professionals have breached this rule again and again.[4]

Vulnerability and trust are built into the relationship between doctor and patient, therapist and client, or teacher and student. Because the person with more power in the relationship can take advantage of this situation, licensed professions have adopted codes of professional ethics. Unlike the law and medicine, body disciplines are not uniformly regulated. There is no code that covers everyone. Unlicensed or uncertified practitioners are not accountable to professional or state ethics committees or licensing boards. However, the field is still guided by ethical principles. There are certain standards you can judge by.

The majority of body practitioners conduct their work ethically. By discussing ethical issues, I am not trying to make you distrust the profession wholesale. Rather, I'm recommending that you be an informed consumer and keep your eyes open.

# Too Much Intimacy?

**You have a right to question any action that seems invasive or sexual. If you are at all uneasy about how the therapist is behaving, but have difficulty articulating it, consider these questions:**

- **Do you feel more like a confidante than a client with this bodyways practitioner? When you go for your session, are you getting professional treatment, or are you paying the therapist only to wind up hearing all about his personal, even sexual anxieties? Is the session taking care of his needs or yours? Do you find yourself comforting him?**
- **Does she make sexual jokes or references that are unrelated to the treatment?**
- **If you hug at the end of a session, do you find him holding on longer than a good-bye warrants?**
- **Do you find yourself sexually aroused by her? Do you sense she is aroused, too? Do you fantasize about a sexual relationship with her?**
- **Are you trying to attract him? Do you dress a special way when you know you'll see him?**
- **Does she invite you to social events? Have you invited her?**
- **Do you get together for drinks or recreational drugs?**
- **Does he pry too deeply into your personal life?**
- **Do you try to bump into her in town to have more contact?**
- **Are you financially involved with him other than paying for services?**
- **Is she an active listener, acknowledging your feelings and experiences, or does she go beyond the scope of her practice and try to be a psychotherapist too?**
- **Does he suggest certain kinds of intimate touching, even a sexual relationship, as therapeutic for your condition?**

The central ethical principle of any therapy is concern for the welfare of clients. That means therapists should

- not suggest or try to engage you in anything immoral, illegal, or harmful.
- not discriminate against you because of gender, age, weight, religion, sexual orientation, national or ethnic origin, profession, and so on.
- not offer services outside of their scope of practice or area of competence. For example, a massage therapist without adjunct training in psychotherapy should stick to massage and make referrals to a licensed counselor. If someone is trained in massage, but not in Trager Psychophysical Integration, the business card should not cite Trager.
- not offer services when they're incapacitated by illness, life crisis, personal difficulties, alcohol, or drugs. These factors make the

practitioner ineffective or compromise your health and well-being.
• not impose their values but respect your right to your values and choices.
• assume responsibility for their work with you.
• respect your privacy and confidentiality.
• refer you to other professionals when appropriate, rather than keep you as an exclusive client.
• prevent the complications of dual or multiple relationships (when you have overlapping roles—social, sexual, financial—with different expectations and responses) by avoiding sexual involvement and financial entanglements and by not socializing unless you've established clear boundaries about payment, sexual intimacy, and confidentiality.

These guidelines may seem stringent, but I'd rather err in this direction. It's like working with a piece of elastic. Even the tightest piece can be stretched, but once overstretched, it becomes too loose to be useful. Here are two experiences where I had to draw the line.

Years after he had been my client, a psychotherapist told me he was perplexed by the fact that I had maintained distance and not become friends with him. At the time, I lived in such a conservative community that the licensing procedure for practicing massage was through the police: You had to wear a photo ID card, and your place of work was subject to their unannounced drop-ins, presumably to make sure you weren't engaged in prostitution. In order to keep my practice as circumspect as possible, I did not encourage friendship or dating with my male clients. I also didn't trust this man; he seemed far too nosy about me. And, as a licensed counselor, he should have known better. By keeping things strictly business, I avoided complications and established a respected reputation.

As a client, I also experienced someone not drawing the line. Many years ago, when I tried the services of a Shiatsu practitioner, I wound up the recipient of unexpected and inappropriate touch. Under the misguided illusion that it was what women wanted, the man tried to roughly stimulate my breasts. He even insinuated that, of course, I really liked this, didn't I? I lay there immobile, curious to see what he would do. When I didn't respond, he stopped. I am sorry now that I didn't confront or report him. It had never happened to me before, and I was so shocked that I didn't know what to say at the time. Afterward, however, I did warn other women not to go to him.

Once you have tasted inner relaxation, your body will be your truest guide.

—Tarthang Tulku

## Differences Among Practitioners

Even within the same body therapy or discipline, practitioners have a wide range of backgrounds, perspectives, and skills. Some also are or were philosophy professors, engineers, computer programmers, musicians, physicists, dancers, nurses, or ministers. They vary greatly in their bodyway approaches and manners. They may bring science, aesthetics, love of nature, or a spiritual practice to the work. Just as no two potters work exactly the same way with clay, no two people practice a bodyway identically, even though they may have trained with the same teachers at the same time. The method they practice is filtered through their bodies and personalities.

Each of us learns and then teaches through the sensory modes we have particular gifts in or feel most comfortable with. Some have the ability to "see" inside the body through touch or "see" what the lungs or diaphragm are doing by hearing the quality of your voice. If you have difficulty with particular practitioners, it may be that you're operating in different modes of knowing or perceiving. They may try to direct you visually, while you sense better through your muscles.

Other variations in how people practice include whether their approach is holistic or symptom-oriented, and whether the sole goal is relaxation or activation. This can be applied to any system because it depends on the way practitioners work. Do they just try to mash out the knot in your shoulder? Do they inquire about the kind of work you do and then help you alter your movements during work postures to prevent tense shoulders? Do they consider what connections might exist between a recurring knee injury and your shoulders? ☞ See "Scope of Practice: A Triple-Lens Look," page 100.

Some practitioners specialize, while others have an eclectic practice. Some are purists, while others synthesize. There are people who work exclusively as an Alexander teacher, Feldenkrais instructor, Rolfer, or T'ai Chi Chuan master. Others have a variety of skills at their disposal that enable them to address different conditions multimodally. Neither way is more valid than the other. This temperamental difference characterizes other professions as well. Some people are predisposed to be archeologists who dig deeper and deeper at the same site for decades, while others study one culture after another, finding the common ground among them.

There are advantages and disadvantages to both ways. When you have a bag of tricks to pull from, surely one of them will work; however, you might not be an expert in any of them. On the other hand, a Rolfer may know Structural Integration exquisitely but tend to see every condition and person strictly through the lens of Rolfing. There's an expression:

Intelligence is present everywhere in our bodies . . . [and] our own inner intelligence is far superior to any we can try to substitute from the outside.

—Deepak Chopra

*Any technique can become a static one-size-fits-all prescription that doesn't exactly fit anyone.*

*—Aileen Crow*

If the only tool you have is a hammer, everything looks like a nail. Some people work with a variety of techniques and skills because they may have found it difficult to earn a living at only one. They don't want to limit their earning potential by being categorized. Also, it often happens that in the process of their own healing journeys, body practitioners may have moved on from one system to another.

Today, the trend in the bodyways field is to address the fact that emotional issues may arise during the course of working with a client. Some bodyways schools have already incorporated a certain amount of psychological education in their programs; others require that students pursue adjunct training. Working practitioners who come face-to-face with clients' emotions, though they did not solicit them, have sought additional instruction on their own or have made themselves familiar with psychotherapists to whom they can refer clients. Similarly, various bodyways have gone beyond a strictly hands-on approach and added lessons in movement as well. If a bodyway does not include a movement component, you can ask for a referral or select a movement art to work with after reading that section in Part III. For an example of how one body therapy became a multisystem approach, ☞ see Ilana Rubenfeld's story, page 357.

## WHERE TO LOOK FOR A PRACTITIONER AND WHAT TO LOOK FOR

Once you decide which bodyways you want to try ☞ see "Deciding on a Bodyway," page 92, how do you go about finding someone to work with? Just as you wouldn't get a bid from only one contractor to build your house, shop around for a body practitioner unless you live in an area where your choices are severely limited. In that case, it is still wise to inquire about that person.

Aside from looking in the telephone directory, you can get referrals through several channels:

**For a better sense of where the practitioner stands, don't hesitate to ask:**
- **Have you completed training in each of the modalities on your business card? Beware of practitioners who list many approaches on their cards after only a brief introduction to them.**
- **If you are an exclusive practitioner, are you open to other systems and how they might complement yours? Are you willing to refer me to them? Beware of individuals who rigidly advocate only their way.**

- Friends, coworkers, neighbors, classmates, and family.

- Other health-care professionals, especially chiropractors and naturopaths, who may have body therapists as staff.

- Health clubs and fitness centers.

- Health-food stores.

- Body therapy schools and institutes. These usually can provide a list of their graduates. They also have intern programs through which you can try a session for a moderate fee or sometimes for free if students need to accumulate practice hours for completion of training. But remember, these students cannot give you the kind of experience you get from an accomplished practitioner.

- The American Massage Therapy Association, American Oriental Bodywork Therapy Association, and other organizations. See "Resources" for organizations with nationwide and international directories.

- Holistic health centers. Some hold open houses at which you can meet practitioners.

- Health fairs and expos. These often include body therapists who give free or low-cost samples of their work.

- Magazines. Various health and specialty periodicals, such as *Natural Health, Yoga Journal,* or *Massage Magazine,* have ads from individual practitioners or sometimes offer directories. Articles may be written by or about bodyways professionals.

## *Getting Your Feet Wet*

If finances are tight and you're hesitant to commit money before you know this is really what you want to delve into, be creative. There are several ways you can test the water before jumping in.

- Attend a lecture or demonstration at health fairs or holistic health centers.

- Participate in a class or workshop given by practitioners to get a sense of what they know, how they communicate, and how you feel around them.

- Try a reduced-price first session and other special discounts.

- Volunteer to be demonstrated on at a massage school or other training institute.

> We can begin to heal our lives at the deepest levels when we begin to value our bodies and honor their messages instead of feeling victimized by them.
>
> —Christiane Northrup

> If we had a culture that nurtured intelligence implicit in blood and bone from infancy on, we wouldn't need remedial efforts, and there's no telling how far we might advance.
>
> —Gloria Steinem

• Ask for an introductory mini-session.

• Interview the practitioner. Would you buy a car without asking certain important questions of the salesperson? How much more important, then, to ask when entrusting your body to a stranger. Sometimes you can tell just from speaking over the phone whether you feel compatible enough to try working with someone.

## Compatibility Is Key

Ideally you want someone who's well trained, has lots of experience, and is simpatico—personable yet professional, warm yet respectful. According to Jack Engler, Ph.D., a member of the clinical faculty at Harvard Medical School, and Daniel Goleman, Ph.D., former senior editor of *Psychology Today,* "research is showing more and more clearly that certain interpersonal, social, and emotional factors are prominent ingredients of *all* types of therapy, and . . . that how well you and your therapist work together . . . is the single most important determinant of a satisfactory outcome."[5] Success depends on the personal chemistry between the two of you and an atmosphere of mutual trust.

## Competence

Although the overall quality of the healing relationship is considered the most important predictor of a good outcome, don't discount skills. It is especially important that they be appropriate to your needs. Before you experience someone's work, you can't determine how effective it is, except by favorable reports from other clients, but you can start out with a provisional assessment.

## Ask Yourself:

- **Do I feel more comfortable with a woman or a man? Do I think a woman won't be strong enough? Does the thought of a man touching me make me anxious? Do I feel safer with a woman? Will she understand me better and be more sensitive?**
- **Would I prefer to work with someone I already know, or am I more comfortable with a stranger who's not connected to my family or circle of friends?**
- **Does the person's sexual orientation affect how at ease I am?**
- **Does it matter what ethnic group the practitioner belongs to?**
- **Do I care whether the person is my age, older, or younger?**
- **Is the individual's spiritual path or religion important to me?**

Bodyways practitioners come in all shapes and sizes with respect to training and experience. Even within each body discipline, the extent of training can vary greatly, from a few casual classes to a rigorous four-year program. It is up to you to inquire. Be wary of individuals who take a weekend workshop and decide to hang out a shingle based on that one experience.

Depending on the particular training, not everyone who is certified or licensed is necessarily highly competent or sincere: Requirements may or may not be stringent, and some individuals may be better test-takers than practitioners. Some people are just plain gifted, with or without framed certificates and licenses on the wall. Those who have trained with masters in foreign countries may be adept teachers or therapists yet lack documentation because apprenticeship is a different kind of educational tradition.

A diploma is not necessarily a guarantee of skill or honesty. Some practitioners have all kinds of framed documents, yet may not do the work well. I went to one who had a respectable array of such papers, but when I asked her to use one of the techniques she supposedly had trained in, she admitted it was her weakest point. She tried, but I could tell she was fumbling, and finally I said, "Never mind, just do what you can." Remember, this is a professional relationship. It's one thing to get a back rub from a friend, but when you pay professional fees, you should expect professional services.

If the practitioner doesn't have a brochure that outlines the services provided, training and experience, appointment policies, fee structure, recourse policy if you're not satisfied, and details of what happens in a session, then ask the questions yourself. If you really want to be thorough, you can check on the person through the local licensing board, especially if you're concerned about sexual issues.

Here are some questions to ask:

- How did the practitioner get his training in this bodyway? Try to find out if the person read a book, attended a weekend workshop, or participated in an extensive program, some of which take hundreds of hours or even several years.

- Is the practitioner licensed? That depends on your state. ☞ See box on licensing and certification, page 76. Is she certified nationally or by a particular training institute?

- What do the letters after the practitioner's name stand for? Such abbreviations don't always mean legitimacy. Don't be afraid to ask whether they were obtained by fulfilling requirements or granted as honorary or mail-order degrees. I knew an instructor who put *N.D.*

# Licensing and Certification

There is no national law or licensing procedure that uniformly covers the entire field of bodyways across the country. Institutes and schools certify their students. States license practitioners. For example, only nineteen states have state boards administering massage practice laws: Arkansas, Connecticut, Delaware, Florida, Hawaii, Iowa, Louisiana, Maine, Nebraska, New Hampshire, New Mexico, New York, North Dakota, Ohio, Oregon, Rhode Island, Texas, Utah, and Washington. The other thirty-one have various kinds of regulations, ordinances, and statutes according to county, city, town, township, or village, of which there are thousands, so you have to ask locally at the offices of the city attorney, mayor, or county commissioner.

The National Certification Board for Therapeutic Massage and Bodywork (NCBTMB) was established in 1992 as an independent certification board and accredited in 1993 by the National Organization for Competency Assurance (NOCA), a public-protection, standards-setting organization in accord with U.S. Department of Education guidelines. In order to be eligible for national certification, practitioners must have completed at least five hundred hours of training in massage and/or other body disciplines, such as Trager, Rolfing, Polarity Therapy, Shiatsu, Neuromuscular Therapy, or Reflexology, before taking a written examination. Training must include a specified number of hours of anatomy and physiology, theory and practice, and ethics. Once certified by NCBTMB, practitioners maintain that status for four years, during which time they are required to obtain fifty additional continuing-education units. NCBTMB also holds practitioners to a code of ethics and has a disciplinary procedure for processing grievances filed against them. For a list of nationally certified practitioners in your area, contact NCBTMB, 1735 N. Lynn St., Suite 950, Arlington, VA 22209, (703) 524-2000, fax (703) 524-2303, or (800) 296-0664.

after his name and allowed himself to be called Dr. So-and-so. The only school of naturopathy he'd attended was by mail.

• How long has the practitioner been engaged in this work?

• Is the person professionally affiliated (holding membership in a national association, state chapter, or training institute, or a staff position in a clinic, agency, or school)?

• Would any of the practitioner's clients be willing to share their experiences with you? However, keep in mind that what worked for the client you talk with may not suit you. Ultimately, you're the only one who can tell if the shoe fits.

## YOUR SESSION

When you call or meet a practitioner and are considering making an appointment, it's also up to you to be forthcoming. State who referred you or how you found out about the person and explain why you're calling without giving your whole life story. For example:

- "I run [bike, surf, play tennis] and I heard that massage will help me do it better [longer, faster]" or "Yoga will help me stay flexible."

- "I'm a dancer who gets injured frequently and can't afford the downtime."

- "I'm under a lot of stress."

- "I fell and hurt my hip; I'm recovering from surgery."

- "I'm divorced [or widowed], live alone, and read somewhere that touch is as vital as food and helps with depression."

- "I'm a secretary who comes home every day with knots in my neck and shoulders" or "I'm a truck driver and sit for ten hours a day."

*The body, too, calls out for compassion; it doesn't want to be treated the way the polluters treat the rivers and the skies.*
*—Sy Safransky*

## *How to Avoid Misunderstandings*

To avoid misunderstandings and worries that keep you from relaxing during a session, clearly agree on the following before your first session:

- What approach(es) does the practitioner take? What is it best for? How is it limited? Does she specialize in a particular group—athletes, pregnant women, the elderly—or in particular conditions, such as TMJ, headaches, back pain? If you want to relax with an oil massage on a table, be sure you're not going for a clothed Shiatsu session on the floor.

- Where do you meet for appointments? In a private office or at home? In a clinical setting with other professionals? Is there a sauna or whirlpool there, and is it included in the session? Can you shower before or afterward if necessary?

- How long does a session last? Is extra time included for a client assessment? What happens if you arrive late or cancel? Are emergency appointments possible?

- How much does a session cost? Is there a sliding scale? Is payment by cash, check, or credit card? Could the service be covered by health insurance? If so, do you need the referral of a medical doctor? Do you pay after the session, or are you billed? Are there discounts for paying

## A Note on Cost and Time

The cost of a bodyway session varies widely, depending on the particular system as well as what the practitioner's expertise level and reputation can command. It also reflects location. Services in big cities, such as Los Angeles and New York City, tend to cost more than in small towns. Time is a factor, too. A session can run anywhere from fifteen minutes for an on-site seated, clothed massage at your desk to an hour of Shiatsu or a two-hour T'ai Chi Chuan class. One practitioner may work a strict fifty-minute session, while another goes for one and a half hours. Fees run the gamut as well. If you take a private class in Yoga, you'll pay a lot more than if you take a group class. Because of the great variations, I do not discuss length of a session or class, nor do I quote fees. It is up to you as a consumer to discuss this with the practitioner ahead of time.

in advance for several sessions? Is a shorter or longer session a different price? If house calls are possible, is the fee the same?

• If it's a series, how many sessions are in it? Do you have to do the entire series? What happens if you need to drop out at a certain point? How much time should elapse between sessions?

*My belief is in the blood and flesh as being wiser than the intellect.*

—D. H. Lawrence

If the practitioner doesn't automatically volunteer information and you're someone who needs to know as many details as possible before acting, inquire about the following as well:

• Do I wear my clothes or do I get undressed—fully or partially?

• Will I be lying on a table or floor pad, sitting in a chair or on a stool, or moving around?

• Will I be touched or not?

• Will I keep my eyes open or closed?

• Will you use a lubricant—oil, cream, or lotion—or nothing at all?

• Will I remain motionless—passively receiving—or do I actively participate, and how?

• Will I be asked to use imagery or visualization?

• Will you play music? What kind?

## Reasonable Expectations

Once you go for your session, it's reasonable to expect that the practitioner's environment and approach will be both professional and safe, that she or he will treat you with respect, inform you adequately, listen to you carefully without criticism, accept you without judging, neither flatter nor criticize your body, and not touch your genitals.

Especially if you're new to the experience, it's important that the practitioner educate you about it and also let you know that it's okay if you need to cry, yawn, burp, or fart (bodyways are about movement, and things start moving in your body). The same is true should you need to sit up if you're lying down, sit down if you're standing up, get up to go to the bathroom, or drink some water.

Unless you say you are comfortable having your breasts touched (if you're a woman) or your nipples touched (if you're a man), it is not appropriate for a practitioner to assume that it is okay. There is nothing inherently wrong with touching this part of the body, but some people fear being aroused. Don't let a body therapist demean you for not being open if you don't want your breasts or nipples massaged. It's your right to limit or extend

The body is many worlds in one.

—Tom Monte

## Before a Session

1. It is important to check with your physician to make sure you don't have a condition that could be aggravated by certain kinds of bodyways. For example, vigorous leg massage is not advised for someone with severe varicose veins or phlebitis because it could dislodge a blood clot, increasing the risk of stroke. ☞ See "Contraindications," page 149. Most practitioners take a health history and make an assessment based on the information you present before determining a course of action. This is not the same as making a medical diagnosis, which is the identification of a disease from its signs and symptoms. If they don't ask, let them know about any sore or sensitive areas, recent injuries, or chronic conditions.

2. Whenever possible, schedule your session two to three hours after a meal so that you won't be uncomfortable if you lie on your stomach or have your abdomen worked on.

3. Generally, it's best to remove jewelry and glasses so they won't get in the way of the therapist's work and also won't pinch you. You'll also be more comfortable without your contact lenses.

4. If you are allergic to certain oils, lotions, creams, herbs, or scents, be sure to let practitioners know ahead of time in order to have them work with the most neutral substance. You can also do a patch test to see whether or not you have a reaction.

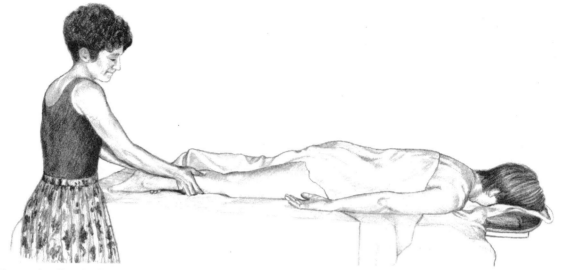

Appropriate Draping During a Massage Session

the area of contact on your body. You can also expect the practitioner to leave the room while you're undressing or dressing, and then to drape you with a sheet or towels, uncovering each section where he or she will work.

Ultimately, it's your prerogative to decide whether and how much clothing to remove, to determine how much physical pressure is acceptable to you, to choose whether or not you want to talk or listen to music, and to *stop a session if you're uncomfortable at any time, for any reason*. If you experience pain, are ticklish in certain spots, or find the amount of pressure unpleasant, speak up. It's also reasonable for the practitioner to expect that you will cooperate by giving information relevant to the treatment or education that will be provided—present physical health, medical history, past experiences in bodyways.

## Hurts Good vs. Hurts Bad

Bodyways don't have to hurt in order for you to get your money's worth. On the contrary, that could work against your benefiting from the session. One of the body's defense mechanisms against pain is to tense and hold the breath, so you can easily defeat the very purpose of the work if you just lie there and grit your teeth.

Which of the following best describes your attitude?

- If it hurts, then something is wrong.

- Unless it hurts, it doesn't do any good.

- If it feels good, it must be right.

During my cross-cultural research in Asia, everyone I met believed that if a massage was not intense—the harder the better—it probably wasn't affording any benefit. Sometimes it was so hard that I had to steel myself against the painful sensations. One man in Java pressed deeper and deeper into my calves until I could no longer bear it and cried out, much to his delight. This, among other experiences, made me finally realize that it was really of no value for me to push beyond the edge of endurance. I did not want to experience a massage as a matter of survival or competition. I did not want someone to invade and force me. And it was not that I'd become too "soft." Rather, I had learned to have a new relationship with myself and with others, one in which I know and respect my own threshold and assert that others respect it, too.

None of the above attitudes is right or wrong, only limited. What hurts is subjective and relative. It depends on your pain threshold, the context of the touch, and the intention behind it. If a person grabs your arm angrily to harm you, it won't feel the same as a body therapist's work on your arm even though the amount or depth of pressure is the same. The first will probably hurt, while the latter probably feels therapeutic. The deep pressure a body therapist applies may feel like pressure to you, while to someone else it's pain. Not only do you have an individual threshold of pain, but you also carry fears and experiences from the past. If you don't tense your arm as the practitioner bears down but receive it openly, you're less apt to feel pain and more apt to sense it as pressure.

The body is more likely to respond positively when you approach it not with the intention of making it wince but with the idea that you can give it pleasure. However, that doesn't mean categorically that if it feels good, it must be right. A lot of things can feel good but harm rather than heal you—certain drugs, for example. And in some cases the extra pressure may release a trigger point and the pain with it. A practitioner will often direct you to focus on your inhalations and exhalations to help you get through the intensity.

Even in exercise, moderation is what's finally recommended. The mottoes used to be "go for the burn" and "no pain, no gain." Now it's acknowledged that the middle path is generally the best way. Sometimes the feeling may be more intense, but if you are always hurting and having to grit your teeth during a bodyway session, then something is wrong.

Gentle work can be more powerful than harsh handling, and a light force often accomplishes more than a heavy one. A biological law supports this thinking. The Arndt-Schulz Law, named for the two German doctors who first described it in 1899, states that light stimuli enhance the function of biological systems, while heavy ones arrest it. After years of critical comments on how brutal their work felt, Rolfers found a milder way to get the

> The gentlest thing in the world overcomes the hardest thing in the world. That which has no substance enters where there is no space.
>
> —Tao Te Ching

same results. Don Johnson, who trained with Ida Rolf herself, criticized her for promoting the belief that everyone needs to conform to her ideal of posture and spinal alignment. He believes that somatic therapists may produce painful experiences if they adhere to an idealistic model.

> If I worked on your foot, for example, with the idea that I know before entering your connective tissue where your ankle belongs, I will tend to force the ankle toward the "norm." But the direction in which I've chosen to move the foot may be in conflict with the organism's innate sense of rightness, and the conflict produces pain, often interpreted as resistance on the part of the client. [Thus] the client's experience of pain may signal, not his or her resistance to change, but a conflict between his or her bodily wisdom and the goals of the therapist.[6]

Only you can determine the difference between what hurts good and what hurts bad in your own body. Experiment with what feels appropriate in each individual situation. Play with your own limits, but don't let anyone force you to go beyond them.

### What If You Become Aroused?

Life without feeling isn't worth living.

—Alexander Lowen

The fact is, humans are sexual beings. Sexual feelings are part of being alive and vital. There's nothing wrong with them per se, but we may have learned from our family, culture, or religion to avoid this aspect of ourselves. If sexual feelings come up in you or the practitioner, what's *not okay* is acting on them or expecting the other person to interact with you sexually. Touching with sexual intent falls outside the bounds of professional practice.

In a culture that is not known for easy and frequent touching, we may not have the opportunity to touch another adult except in the context of sexual relations. Nudity, touch, intimacy, and sex tend to get all bunched together. Given this confusion, it should come as no surprise that you might get aroused during a session, regardless of the therapist's behavior. Caring, skilled touch can wake up the whole body. For some people, the first bodyways session often is a powerful sensory and emotional experience. It's not unusual for it to lead to a dreamlike state in which fantasies and fears might emerge.

If you're afraid you'll be aroused during a session, you can address it with the practitioner beforehand. The body therapist can let you know it's not uncommon for a woman's nipples or a man's penis to become erect and that it's nothing to be embarrassed about. Most of the time the arousal will subside. Only in a few cases, when sexual inquiries accompanied a man's erection, did I find it necessary to clearly inform the client that I was

# If a Memory Arises

You may notice an assortment of memories and emotions come up during and after a bodyway session—even days after, as your body continues to release. Note them. Accept them. You don't necessarily have to do anything about them right then, except to observe as you would watch a landscape you drive through. If your body practitioner is trained to deal with psychological issues that arise with certain memories, you can work with her or him. Otherwise, if you don't already have a psychotherapist, ask for a referral. If you've opened up a Pandora's box—incidents of abuse, terror, pain—you probably need professional help.

Whether you work with those memories depends on several things: Do you feel ready or reluctant? Do you feel safe and supported—do you have inner and outer resources—for a process of change? Will you take the time to integrate the experience into your conscious awareness? If not, maybe you need to let the memory lie quiescent and even skip bodyways for now. Don't let anyone force you to go beyond where you're prepared to be.

For a fuller discussion of body memory, see ☞ "Remembering Through the Body," page 123.

strictly a massage therapist, and the issue never came up a second time with that person. In a professional relationship, the therapist is ultimately responsible for maintaining appropriate interaction, no matter what the client initiates.

A final note about sexual issues in bodyways. As a consumer, you may find it confusing that your session can take place in a number of different environments, each one having its own connotation or atmosphere. Some are more casual, others more clinical—anything from a spare bedroom in someone's home to a chiropractor's office or a hotel or cruise-ship spa. No matter where you receive your session, you should be able to count on the fact that you will not be taken advantage of sexually.

## What If Your Session Triggers Memories?

Today, bodyways practitioners report more and more incidents of "body memory" occurring with their clients. Like Jungian analyst Anita Greene, they know that "certain images and memories, both positive and negative, are so imprisoned in body tissue that they may never appear . . . until released through touch."[7]

## EVALUATING YOUR EXPERIENCE

*When anyone is in the healing process they are re-connecting with lost or misplaced parts of themselves, connecting with new parts of themselves, making connections between past and present and dreaming the connection to their future.*

—Jude Franko

Once you've gone through the process of finding a bodyways practitioner and had your session, take a few minutes to reflect on the experience. Some of these questions may sound simplistic, even silly, but in the charged atmosphere of intimate contact and the vulnerability inherent in the session, even small details can loom large.

- Was it easy to explain why you came? Were you comfortable talking about yourself?

- Did you feel the person was attuned to you, genuinely engaged, and interested in you? Was he distracted, running to the phone during your session?

- Did you feel her sincere concern? Were you just another client to be dealt with and quickly ushered in and out?

- Did he treat you with courtesy and respect? Was he patronizing and condescending?

- Did you feel heard? Did the therapist disregard what you said and do what she wanted to? Was she sensitive to your body and pace, rather than imposing an agenda, or did she expect you to match hers instead? For example, my Rolfer always took into account how my body and psyche were responding. Sometimes he'd break up a session, let's say number eight in the series of ten, into two parts instead of trying to do all of it at once. He also varied the interval between sessions rather than following a strict schedule. He didn't make me fit his style, but instead fit his style to me every time we met.

- Did the therapist clearly answer your questions or brush you off with, "You know what I mean"? Did he try to impress you with quick and clever interpretations of you and your body in incomprehensible and meaningless jargon?

- Was the therapist sensitive to your vulnerability, even embarrassment?

- Did you feel judged and criticized, or did you feel accepted?

- Was the person cloyingly sympathetic, overly solicitous, and too eager to please, or was he the opposite extreme, aloof and cold, or somewhere between the two?

Only you know whom you feel compatible and comfortable with, so it helps to be clear about your likes and dislikes. Based on your encounter, think about what you prefer. Here are some possibilities:

• Someone who goes about her work quietly, keeps chatter to a minimum, engages you in dialogue, or runs a monologue the whole time? For my friend Bill, silence is best. "It's a nonconversational experience," he says. "The communication is in the touching."

• Someone who is friendly, yet businesslike, or completely informal. What about the person who gets nosy beyond what's necessary in the session? Does he talk more about his aches and pains than yours? Does he gossip about other clients, referring to them by name? Is he flirtatious?

• Someone who has a sense of humor, who tends to be exclusively serious, or able to be purposeful yet light?

• Someone who is more parental and authoritative, or someone who is more of a peer, exploring with you instead of having all the answers?

There are practical considerations as well.

• Was the bodyways practitioner on time for your appointment?

• Did the person work in his bedroom or living room or in a separate, specifically designated room? Or did the session take place in an office? Was the environment an inviting balance between austerity and clutter? Or was it distracting and unpleasant because of noise, filth, or bad smells? Were lights glaring in your eyes? Did you have easy access to a bathroom? Did you have privacy for undressing and dressing? Was there a place to hang your clothes?

• Did you feel comfortable there, safe? Did the person use professional equipment or a bed? Was the table or floor padded enough? Were the sheets clean? Did the therapist wash her hands before touching you? Were you warm enough? Was there a face cradle so you wouldn't have to kink your neck, and was it adjusted to your comfort level? Did she use pillows, bolsters, rolled-up towels, or other props to ease strain at certain joints? Did she take these and other precautions if you are pregnant or elderly? If it was difficult for you to get on and off the table or floor, did she offer assistance? Did she check to see how you were doing during the session? Did you feel it was okay to express your discomfort or needs? Were you given choices in terms of lighting, temperature, music, oil or lotion, and so on?

If you were in a class, consider the above questions as they relate to the environment and attention given in instruction.

> For the body knows what it is about but we in the Western world have very largely lost our living connections with these knowings.
>
> —Jean Houston

## When a Session Doesn't Work

If your session doesn't go well, don't automatically assume that there's something wrong with you, that it's your fault. For example, a practitioner may ask you to visualize a knot in your shoulder as a symbol of the tension and pain you feel there. If you don't see a knot with your inner eye, that doesn't mean you're responding incorrectly. You may be perceiving it differently. Perhaps you can *feel* a knot untying, even though you can't see it. The more skilled therapists are, the more versatile they can be instead of trying to force you unsuccessfully to "get it" in their mode.

On the other hand, consider how important timing is. Did you come at a time when even a genie couldn't make you relax? Did you squeeze the appointment between business meetings that kept you from putting your full attention on your session?

It's also possible that the approach you tried is not the one you need. Before a race, don't get a relaxing massage that makes you sleepy, but do get one that primes your muscles and awakens your nervous system. If your body aches after you've just run a marathon, skip structural work and get a massage that flushes from your tissues the waste products that accumulate from metabolism. That will help speed your recovery from such an intense workout. Or try the Trager Approach to loosen and free all the tightness from enduring 26.2 miles.

If your session leaves you less than satisfied, you might want to try working with this practitioner again after communicating your complaints or try the same bodyway approach with a different therapist. If it works better with another person, fine. Remember, you want the professional to be your ally. If you have the same reaction with this person too, this may not be the kind of work you need right now.

## Resistance

Don't let anyone bully you by saying you're resistant. *Resistance* is one of those shaming or guilt-inducing terms that has no place in a respectful practitioner's vocabulary. If, in fact, there is resistance, so what? Maybe it's a message that you're not ready for this brand of bodyway yet or that it's not suitable for the condition you're dealing with. If you try to overcome resistance willfully, you may not learn anything anyway, so why bother?

"Clients need to be told that they have a choice about going with the directions, suggestions or manipulations of the body therapist, or not," says Aileen Crow, who combines the Alexander Technique, Authentic Movement, and other approaches in her practice. "They need to know that they can choose to reject the therapist's ideas, and use them as stimuli toward finding out what they themselves want to do. When a client resists a . . .

> Too much technique dulls the mind. Too much creativity makes the body flabby.
>
> —Merce Cunningham

# After a Session

Don't be surprised if sometimes you actually feel worse before you feel better. There are several reasons why this happens. Many bodyways help stimulate the circulation of blood and lymph. As things begin to move through your body, toxins that have accumulated in the tissues (anything from the metabolic by-products of exercise to all kinds of pollutants, whether from the environment, food, drugs, tobacco, or alcohol) may be released into the bloodstream. You may feel slightly dizzy, nauseated, even mildly sick. As your body tries to clear itself and achieve equilibrium, you may need to relieve your bladder or bowels. You may even experience some soreness, not unlike what you feel after a hard workout. This is usually lactic and carbonic acid being worked out of the muscles. The charley-horse feeling should subside within a day or two.

It's also possible that your body has compensated with certain postural changes, and even though you're more structurally balanced, you feel out of kilter standing and walking. In addition, sometimes as your more superficial muscles relax, deeper tensions rise to the surface. I remember massaging a woman who said she was enjoying the experience but had a headache by the end of the session.

What helps after your session:

- Increase the amount of water you drink for the rest of the day. It will flush your system.
- A warm bath will also help as well as prolong the relaxation effects.
- Try to have as much "downtime" as you can.
- Walk a little bit (or a lot, depending on the kind of bodyway session you have) to allow your muscles and structure to feel the changes they've just gone through. Also, if you feel light-headed or disoriented, you want to be sure you're steady enough before you go out.

Whereas some people want to sleep afterward or spend the rest of the day resting quietly alone, others feel energized, even restless because of a new surge of energy, and want to move. Do what your body wants—stretch, dance, go for a hike. Remain sensitive to what it is feeling and wants, but don't overdo it and get hurt.

Don't feel discouraged if, after a good session, you find your shoulders creeping up around your ears again. It's not a signal that the bodyway didn't work after all. That you're even noticing is a good sign. It gives you the opportunity to relax your shoulders, shift your posture or stand up, stretch, and move about because you realize you've been sitting too long and have started to strain. Or it may be that your shoulders are up around your ears for some good reason that you don't understand yet.

Remember to make an entry in your body wisdom journal.

# Experience: Body Wisdom Journal

Before and after sessions are good times to make entries in your journal. To stimulate your thoughts, you may want to review ☞ the questions in the Experience on p. xxii–xxiii of the Introduction. Here's a simple sample of what an entry might look like. You can write a few key words that will cue your memory or go into elaborate details, according to your personal style.

**February 2, 1996**

**Before my appointment with ___.** *I don't feel comfortable. My lower back hurts. I'm still angry after that fight with ___ yesterday. I didn't sleep well last night. It's been a rough week anyway. I'm tired of getting so pissed every time I feel criticized for something. This morning I dreamed about a fire in the basement of an old building. I couldn't get to the phone in time to call the fire department. I had to run out and let it burn behind me. I overslept, felt groggy all day. Kept drinking coffee at work. I'm jangled now.*

**During the session.** *At first I couldn't settle down. My lower back was still bothering me. Halfway through, I started yawning and finally took some big, long breaths. When ___ went deep into my lower back, everything felt like a tight knot. Then the area got hot. The knots loosened some. Suddenly an image and a feeling flew out. I saw my father bent over with pain in his lower back when I was a little girl. I remember feeling his suffering and wishing I could do something about it. How much of what is going on now has to do with what happened to him then?*

**After the session.** *When I got up to walk around the table, I really felt my feet touching the floor. My whole body felt lower, but not shorter, kind of weighted from the center. The jangling was gone. I need to cut down on coffee. I don't feel angry. I want to talk to ___ in a different way.*

---

suggestion, the 'resistance' holds the seeds of what would be more appropriate to the client's own process."[8]

It is violent for someone to label you as "resistant" or "in denial" rather than accept where you are. It's a lack of trust in your moving at a pace that's appropriate to your evolution. If you *are* resistant to that work or to that practitioner, maybe it's for a good though inexplicable reason. Don't let others, even friends, coerce or influence you just because of their own preferences.

In the mid-1970s I had a friend who, as a devoted student of Aikido, kept recommending it to me. At the time, I was partial to Yoga. Though I knew it would disappoint him, I declined his invitations. Then in 1993, on my own, I went to an Aikido dojo (training hall) to observe. As I watched the students practice the rolling, I felt the energy of it in my body and knew that someday I would study Aikido.

You may also run into resistance when you're working with a practitioner who insists on leading you rather than following your lead. One practitioner kept asking me to verbalize what I was experiencing inside as she worked with me. "What is the mental or emotional component?" she asked. "What color or shape does it have? If it had a voice, what would it say?" All these cues were distracting me from being able to notice whatever might appear spontaneously, the way dreams do. I went along with her to see what would happen. However, when she asked me to have a dialogue with a family member (who wasn't there), I said I'd rather not do it aloud. I sensed my response was not what was expected, that I was being a difficult client, but I didn't care—I have a right to my privacy.

And so do you. Don't be afraid to speak your mind if something doesn't feel right to you. Just say, "This is not working for me." If you're someone who has been afraid of conflict, this is a great opportunity to change a behavior pattern. If your wishes were ignored and your body violated early in life, speaking up is also a chance to take back your power. The experience of feeling that in your body is something you can call upon in other situations as well.

After this particular session, I realized I was bothered that the practitioner applied her specific language and worldview to me as she did to any other client. Her words and her way of looking at things didn't match my own; she didn't meet me on my ground. Though she didn't say so, I imagined her labeling me "blocked," "in denial," or "resistant" because I didn't respond the way I was "supposed to," that is, according to her paradigm.

I'm not saying that guiding a client is the wrong approach—not at all. Many practitioners employ this skillfully, but it is only one way. It has its time and place, depending on the client's need or preference. This is especially true if you are not well versed in paying attention to your own inner process—noting thoughts, feelings, images, and sounds that lead to insights. Having someone keep you focused is helpful. However, practitioners should be sensitive enough to work accordingly—to follow your lead, not impose their agendas. The art of therapy is becoming attuned to your actual experience and to the uniqueness of your individual life expression, not fixating on principles, theories, and methodology.

I say that because on a different occasion, while lying on someone else's table, I found myself filled with longing in response to the music playing. When I expressed that aloud, the therapist simply asked what that feeling was. After I told her, she probed no further, sensing that I could stay with it on my own. In fact, at a certain point during the session, an unexpected insight appeared. Had she talked me through the session, I probably would have missed it. The insight was so valuable that it led to a shift in thinking about a major relationship in my life. In the silence and privacy of my own body and mind, I received, unbidden, exactly what I needed; noth-

No one is an expert on another person's life.

—Eugene Gendlin

We grow more quickly and effectively if we first acknowledge and celebrate our strengths rather than "working on the problem."

—Jean Houston

Most people are looking for a quick solution for their difficulties—from the outside. They don't even realize they have an inside. Everything is from the outside in, rather than from the inside out. They want to be spoon-fed. Some people never learn to feed themselves.

—Hannah Fraenkel

ing like that had happened in the session in which the practitioner insisted on directing me.

Trust your body's wisdom in guiding you away from where you don't belong or don't want to be yet. This is part of developing discernment. If something doesn't ring true for you, honor that. Don't assume that practitioners always know better than you or that all their observations are valid. Sometimes they have a negative effect.

Here are two examples. An Alexander teacher told me of a time when she went for a massage. The therapist was working so hard on her shoulders that she found it too painful and complained. "Well, just let it go," he yelled at her, as though such an aggressive response could force her to relax. She knew he was wrong to blame her and decided not to work with him again. In a different situation, while receiving a Shiatsu session, my friend Bill overheard another practitioner tell his client, "You're so stiff in the neck. Relax. Let go." She firmly replied, "Yes, you're right. That's why I'm here, for you to work on my stiff neck, not talk about it."

One small caveat about resistance. It could be useful to look at what it might be masking. For instance, if you find yourself jumping from practitioner to practitioner without giving anyone or any approach a chance, ask yourself whether you're looking for instant results and unattainable perfection. Try writer Natalie Goldberg's advice: "Stay with something because that's how you deepen your life; otherwise, you are always on the surface."

## ENDING THE BODYWAY RELATIONSHIP

How long you maintain a relationship with a body therapist depends on several factors. You may find that one session is all you need or want and you never call that person again, especially if you live in another city, state, or country (if you had the experience on vacation). Or perhaps you don't care for the particular approach or practitioner and choose to go elsewhere. You also could be involved with a body practitioner or movement therapist for as long as you are benefiting from the experience. Some performers and athletes have their own personal massage therapists and receive a session daily. Other individuals consider weekly or monthly sessions essential to their well-being. Still others incorporate one or more classes in Yoga, T'ai Chi Chuan, or Aikido in their weekly regimen.

How often you see a practitioner, how long you continue, and when you terminate services are up to you, your finances, and the nature of the work you select. One practitioner might advise you that the benefits to be derived are cumulative and thus greater than in a single session, just as the occasional run or tennis game doesn't have the same effect as regular practice. Another might explain that the particular method is a long-term learning process, not just a one-time relaxation or Band-Aid approach. Take the information an experienced practitioner offers, but remember that the decision is always yours. Don't let anyone convince you to go beyond what is comfortable, satisfying, beneficial, or affordable for you. And don't let anyone become possessive of you.

I realize that all these precautions might sound like the warnings of an overprotective mother trying to keep you from any harm in life. Living involves trial and error. You have experiences that are pleasant and fulfilling as well as ones that are unpleasant and unsatisfying. By encouraging you to check for deep pools or shallow spots and rocks before jumping in, I'm not saying, "Don't swim." What I am saying is, go into bodyways with some awareness. But by all means jump in, go swimming, and have a great time.

> It is a language of the body that is being learned.
>
> —Richard K. Heckler

# CHAPTER 5

# Deciding on a Bodyway

One country . . . one ideology, one system is not sufficient. It is helpful to have a variety of different approaches. . . . We can then make a joint effort to solve the problems of the whole of humankind.

—Dalai Lama

Shiatsu people say it's your ki that needs attending to. Neuromuscular therapists contend it's your trigger points. Rolfers, Hellerworkers, and Myofascial Release therapists claim it's your fascia. Therapeutic Touch practitioners maintain it's your energy field. Still others declare it's your craniosacral rhythm.

Are they contradicting each other? Which one should you believe? And which one is right for you?

Actually, nobody's wrong. When practitioners look at your body, they each see or feel a different picture: a network of fascia, conduits of energy, bands of muscle, channels of lymph. When this picture is skewed, they try to adjust it through a variety of methods: compressing, stretching, unwinding, rubbing, mobilizing joints or fluids, modulating energy, and so on. Some approaches may give you immediate relief of pain and help heal an injury faster. Others will facilitate awareness of how you move. Still others will enable you to recognize how the body provides information for emotional healing as well.

## NOT ONE BUT MANY

No one bodyway is the answer or formula for taking care of your body. For every therapeutic principle propounded in a particular bodyway, there is another that is its opposite. One has you lie down, while another has you stand up. One wants you to release feelings, while another says to contain them. One emphasizes the pelvis as the key element in alignment, while another concentrates on the head/neck relationship. One focuses on breathing out, while another highlights breathing in. "Keep your eyes open." "Close them." "Hold it." "Let go."

I am not completely devoted to any one bodyway. I have been enthusiastic about different ones at different times, and I have found value in all of them. However, some practitioners (like missionaries or salespeople) would lead you to believe that their particular system is *the* answer to your ills. Don't believe them! It could be true, but something else might work too. As historian, philosopher, and novelist Theodore Roszak has pointed out: "It's been characteristic of every school of therapy to generalize its peculiar insight to the point of making it exclusive and universal. It's a matter of getting carried away with one's big, new idea." [1]

Each bodyway developed within the context of a culture and the personality of its founder, who had his or her own blind spots. Thus, each system has both strengths and shortcomings in its distinct and illuminating view of how we function and what it means to be human. But that perspective reflects the preferences of the person who created it. Many body pioneers evolved their systems as a result of confronting their own restrictions. Their particular condition and prior experiences led them to explore the workings of their own bodies with much greater awareness until they found how best to operate. ☞ See, for example, the stories of Moshe Feldenkrais, page 233, F. M. Alexander, page 218, Ilana Rubenfeld, page 359, Elisabeth Dicke, page 165, and Yamuna Zake, page 186.

All of the bodyways have the potential to be useful, if appropriate. In India several different medical systems coexist, including allopathy, Unani, and Ayurveda. In an emergency, Western allopathic medicine is the treatment of choice. If you're hemorrhaging from a deep cut, herbs will not stanch the blood quickly enough for you to survive. But for chronic conditions and long-term benefits, Ayurveda and Unani may be preferable. If you have a headache, you don't sign up for surgery (unless there's a brain tumor). Indians know that a plurality of healing modalities covers all the bases. Exclusively relying on or overidentifying with one alone closes you off to what the others have to offer.

Another way of looking at the many bodyways is in terms of the arts. For example, pottery, painting, drawing, and sculpture all use different materials—clay, paper, canvas, marble, charcoal, paints—but the underlying creative process itself remains the same in every art. This is also true in bodyways. While they are all different ways of working with the body, healing as a process remains the same: What was static or blocked gets moving again; where there was separation or fragmentation, there is now unity or wholeness. "True systems all heal," says anthropologist and writer Richard Grossinger, "even if they begin at different points and work through different levels." [2]

But one may serve you best in what you're seeking help for at a particular time. Since no one approach can do everything for you, and because there are so many available today, selecting which one to work with may

Considering all of the marvelous tools of one kind or another that humans have invented during recent decades (and before, for that matter) one is struck by the fact that none of them is so complex, potentially perfect, or wondrous as the human body.

—Isaac Asimov

## What Do You Prefer?

**Knowing your preferences can help you in choosing a bodyway.**
- **Are you more at ease in one-on-one exchanges or in groups?**
- **Do you like attention focused exclusively on you in private sessions, or do you learn better in a class situation?**
- **Are you uncomfortable being alone in a room with someone?**
- **Do you prefer to be a passive receiver and let someone else take over, or do you want to know what's going on and be involved in the outcome?**
- **Would you rather work with a method that is self-directed or with one that is teacher-directed? Do you need a structure imposed from without to keep you focused?**
- **Do you want an orderly series of appointments, or would you rather wait and see what happens?**

seem confusing and daunting. Practitioners themselves often disagree on how to deal with certain conditions and which bodyway would be most effective in reaching a certain goal. But there are several ways you can go about deciding which bodyway to try. How you choose depends on a combination of factors, including your personality and physical preferences.

### PERSONALITY

When you want to travel, how do you pick where to go? Do you need nothing more than a captivating photograph to send you to the phone to make reservations? Or do you carefully weigh one country, state, national park, island, or mountain range over another by reading everything you can get your hands on? Do you also attend a slide or film show, buy a video of the place, and ask others about their travels there? Do you take off spontaneously, or do you study language, customs, geography, and history before you ever get on a plane? Neither way is right or wrong, only a reflection of different personalities.

Those same personal needs styles affect how you choose a bodyway. You can close your eyes and let your finger stop on a page somewhere in this book and then go try whatever it pointed to—Body-Mind Centering®, Chi Kung, Myofascial Release, or Kinetic Awareness. You may see an ad in your local newspaper announcing that a Myotherapist has come to town and decide to experience Trigger Point Therapy. When a friend spontaneously invites you to join her in an Aikido class, you might think, "Why not?" and go along.

You can also read through all the sections of Part III and notice that one bodyway in particular calls your attention; something about it appeals to you. If you feel the need to investigate it thoroughly before making an appointment, you can learn more about the approach by reading additional materials listed in the "Resources" section. You might find videos to view or a live demonstration to attend. You can also ask friends for details. But remember that their experiences are theirs and yours will be yours.

It doesn't matter how you go about it, as long as you know your style and are comfortable with it. Plunge in or research first—do what works for you. Choose what you're attracted to, not what you think is more elite or fashionable, or what your family, friends, or ethnic group would approve of. Over time, you will develop the ability to distinguish what you want, even if curiosity alone is what motivates you to try something different.

What's important is that you allow yourself to embark on a journey of self-discovery. Bodyways represent a vast resource for broadening your psychophysical range. Although some bodyways may seem puzzling and feel awkward or uncomfortable at first, they provide an opportunity to stretch yourself and develop a more balanced life. For example, if you consider yourself a hedonist and you always choose a bodyway because of its sensual, pleasurable appeal, try another kind that rewards you in a different way. If you're someone who operates in a highly structured manner, sample a bodyway that shakes up your sense of order. If you tend to have your head in the clouds and can't seem to pull things together, look for a bodyway that can help you get grounded and centered. If you engage in strength training, try a movement art that adds flexibility and fluidity to your fitness regimen.

# Experience: Automatic Patterns

While sitting in a chair, cross your arms at your chest. Did you cross right over left or left over right? Whichever you did is your automatic pattern. Now cross in the other direction. Which is more comfortable? Which feels awkward or strange? Try the same thing by crossing at your ankles and knees. Do you always cross from the same direction?

Clasp your hands. Does your right thumb rest on your left or vice versa? Is that crossing the same as with your legs?

Now stand up. While standing, notice to which side you shift your weight. Do you tend to twist your torso always to the left or to the right?

Are you doing all your crossing in life from the same direction? Bodyways can help you achieve balance by letting you see what that's about and by giving you a taste of other possibilities.

## PHYSICAL PREFERENCES

Why is your brother drawn to Aikido, your partner to Contact Improvisation, your best friend to Yoga, but you exult over T'ai Chi Chuan? Is it merely a quirk, or is there a physiological basis to your attraction to different bodyways? According to former dancer and choreographer Betsy Wetzig, we each have a home base in neuromuscular patterns that predispose us to one approach or another. ☞ See "Wetzig Coordination Patterns," page 271. You're born with some physical preferences and later develop others. They determine what you're comfortable with and thus why you choose some activities over others. They're also instrumental in deciding for one bodyway over another.

Yet even if you know what you prefer, the condition you're dealing with may call for something different, perhaps the kind of bodyway you're least comfortable with. For many years I was partial to action and deep pressure in a session, but gradually I learned that in some instances light, sustained holding of energy points is what I need, and now I often prefer it. Sometimes less is more. I've come to recognize that it's not just a case of different strokes for different folks, but different strokes for different occasions for the same person.

# Experience: What Is Your Physical Style?

If you're not already familiar with your physical preferences or style in touch and movement, the following questions will acquaint you more with how you use your body, where you move in the space surrounding you, and what your general movement qualities are.

1. Do you seek movement or stillness? Are you athletic, desiring vigorous workouts? Would you rather lie around and not exercise? When you move, are you fast, moderate, or slow? Do you tend to move in a linear way or a random one? Are your movements more extended or more contracted? Do you like to precisely control and shape your movements? Do you tend to move forcefully or lightly? How flexible are you? How strong are you?

2. Do you not feel touch unless it's heavy and penetrating? Do you tend to be ticklish unless someone applies deeper pressure? Do you prefer a light touch? Does even the lightest touch cause you pain? Do you get uneasy when touch is sustained, or is steady pressure reassuring? Touch can also move in different directions—straight or on a diagonal, in a circle, or in a spiral. It can be smooth, like a sliding motion, or rough, with a lot of friction; it can be twisting, grabbing, or pinching. As you experience these kinds of touch, notice your responses to them, and you will learn what your preferences are.

## WHAT ARE YOU LOOKING FOR?

When approaching bodyways for the first time or the tenth time, there are four issues to consider: curing and healing, treatment and education, goal and process orientations, and short- and long-term benefits. Being honest with yourself about where you stand may make the difference between satisfaction and disappointment in your experiences. Each of these goals exists on a spectrum, and neither end of the spectrum is inherently better or worse. Sometimes you need to work with one before you can work with the other.

### Curing and Healing

Are you looking for a quick fix of symptoms, or are you interested in perceiving them as agents of change? Symptoms can serve as clues from the unconscious that lead you to what the body needs and what lifestyle changes they call on you to make. But symptoms also can be so painful that you don't have the presence of mind to explore them.

Gardening is a useful metaphor for understanding the difference between seeking symptomatic relief, on the one hand, and trying to get at underlying causes of hurt and caring for the hurt area, on the other. When your vegetables grow small, disease-ridden, and lacking flavor, you have two choices. On the spot, you can add chemical fertilizers to boost growth and spray pesticides to kill the bugs that are invading the plants. Or you can provide a healthier, stronger environment to begin with, which takes time. By loosening and aerating the soil before planting, you provide room for the roots to grow deeper and find moisture. By adding manure and letting it break down in the soil, you make the dirt richer and more productive. By companion planting, you allow the plants themselves to assist each other to grow well and repel insects. By leaving an area fallow instead of cultivating it continuously, you let it rest and restore itself.

The choice is between attacking and nourishing. You can see your body as an enemy that has to be conquered, or you can consider it a friend that needs to be cared for and supported so that health and well-being will flourish. As sages the world over have affirmed for centuries, love is the greatest healer there is.

That's why it is important to approach bodyways with a gentle attitude of nurturing that which is already good and wise within you, rather than with an aggressive stance—"I'm going to get in there and fix what's wrong." Healing is not about angrily or resentfully judging—"I've got a bad knee." That's like getting annoyed with a plant because it grows crooked around a rock in the soil where the seed sprouted. Instead of blaming the plant—after all, it's adapting the best it can, given the circumstance—remove the rock if you can.

The whole concept of "fixing" and "broken" suggests an insensitivity to the process nature of the world.

—Rachel Naomi Remen

The conclusion is always the same: Love is the most powerful and still the most unknown energy of the world.

—Pierre Teilhard de Chardin

## Treatment and Education

Real, solid growth and
education are slow.
Look at a tree. We
don't put a seed in the
ground and then stick
our fingers in the earth
and yank up an oak.
Everything has its time
and is nourished and fed
with the rhythms of the
sun and moon, the
seasons.

—Natalie Goldberg

Do you want to be the passive recipient of someone's ministrations or an active learner? Are you interested in a practitioner as an educator who can help you learn more effective ways of being in your body for all your activities? Sometimes you need someone to help you enough so that you can then participate more consciously.

Although I favor process-oriented education for long-term benefits, there are times when all I want to do is relax completely and let someone else take over, or when I want to get rid of my restriction so I can function normally. For example, one day I found that each time I tried to sneeze, yawn, or take a deep breath, a sharp pain stopped me short. It was as though something were gripping the ribs in my back and keeping my chest from expanding. I sensed that a muscle spasm was behind all of this. While I could have investigated what it was trying to tell me or how I was moving to bring it on, I also knew that I needed help right away because the less fully I could breathe, the less oxygen all of my body systems, including my brain, were receiving.

For immediate attention to my difficulty, I went to see a Neuromuscular Therapist, who worked with the trigger points that were maintaining the spasm and restriction. After only one treatment I was back to breathing regularly instead of gasping for air. If that condition had recurred, I would have worked with a somatic educator to learn what pattern I was repeating to activate the trigger point. I also could have chosen a convergence therapy to see if there was an unresolved emotion behind the muscle spasm.

## Goal and Process

A good traveler has no
fixed plans
and is not intent upon
arriving.

—Tao Te Ching

Are you interested only in getting there—whatever the end result you want—or are you eager to experience the trip? Do you see life as a "there" to arrive at or as a never-ending learning process? When you are engaged in process, reaching goals becomes secondary or altogether unimportant. Yet having a goal is also what motivates you to seek a bodyway to begin with.

Whatever your physical difficulty, whether new or chronic, it's important not to approach it as a nuisance to be rid of. That frequently intensifies the pain or bothersomeness. The first step in becoming engaged in a process rather than speeding forward to reach a goal is to be *willing* to acknowledge and accept the pain or difficulty.

F. M. Alexander, the Australian actor who originated the Alexander Technique, called the desire to go after a goal without paying attention to how it is reached *end-gaining*. We seek the result without considering the means of moving toward it. It's the difference between will and willingness. To will is to order and direct something to happen, to rigidly confine yourself to only one result, whereas to be willing is to be open and flexible to possibilities, to be inclined to see what unfolds. While it helps enormously to approach body disciplines with willingness rather than end-gaining, bodyways can also be instrumental in making that shift. It can help you change from hankering after only what comes at the end to savoring each moment en route.

The next time you find yourself suddenly tight, anxious, and rushed, stop to check in with yourself. You're probably fixated on goal rather than engaged in process. Have you lost touch with your body? Are you in another time zone instead of in the present? Do you want to be finished with lunch, or are you relishing each mouthful? Do you wish to arrive as soon as you set out on a trip, or do you enjoy the scenery along the way?

## Short-Term and Long-Term

Do you want results immediately even though they might not last, or can you be patient in order to bring about lasting changes? A Chinese proverb says, "Patience is power; with time and patience the mulberry leaf becomes silk." Quick results may enable you to build initial confidence in bodyways. Long-term results can result in profound transformation.

When you try a bodyway and don't get instantaneous satisfaction, that isn't necessarily an indication that it isn't right for you. Give it a chance. Bodyways generally don't work the way a drug does. Many take longer because there's an ongoing process involved. You can get your neck "fixed," or you can relearn how to be in your body and move with greater ease to keep from developing a "bottleneck" between your head and the rest of your body. The more you reeducate yourself—the more you learn to see, feel, and hear with your whole body—the less likely you'll be to incur injuries. Curing appears easier and faster, but in the long run, healing is what will keep the symptoms from popping up again and again. Healing is not a one-shot deal and it involves more than the particular part that may be painful or limited. Writer Ronald Kotzsch's story of what happened to a woman named Susan illustrates how true this is.

In 1978 Susan fell hard down the newly waxed stairs of her country home. When medical doctors were unable to help, she took her recurring face, neck, lower back, and sacrum pain to body therapists. Chiropractic treatments provided only temporary relief, so she started a series of twelve sessions and home exercises in the Feldenkrais Method. The gentle approach not only relieved the pain in her lower back, but it also showed her there are many ways to move, and that how we move affects how we feel.

Ten years after her accident, Susan suddenly had an extreme attack of vertigo. Again, conventional medical treatment offered no hope. Unfortu-

If the drive to change is fueled by self-loathing, then all too often the result of so-called improvement will be a deeper sense of failure. But if, first, you can make peace with your own flawed being, then good things will already have started to happen.

—Thomas H. Rawls

Success is a journey, not a destination.

—Ben Sweetland

Time is an enormous factor in healing. . . . Many elements shape how a person unravels health and physical problems.

—Rosie Spiegel

The body becomes the wisdom to understand what we need to do in terms of our healing journey.

—Clyde Ford

nately, neither chiropractic nor acupuncture provided a lasting remedy, either. Finally, Craniosacral Therapy made the vertigo disappear.

All those painful years taught Susan that how we use ourselves—sitting, standing, walking, talking—has an effect on the whole body. Even though everything was going well, she decided to learn how to use her body better so that she could feel and function better overall. She undertook training in the Alexander Technique and found that it enabled her to understand her body in ways she never would have known. It also has affected and improved everything she does. At the age of fifty, she is more agile than she was at thirty.[3]

Susan is a good example of someone who deeply learned from her journey of healing. For her, change came about from a combination of quick, short-term efforts that brought immediate but short-lived relief and an ongoing course of reeducating her body and mind. Her active participation was as important as external intervention, if not more so, and ultimately proved more interesting and satisfying than merely attaining a cure. However, it is also possible that while chiropractic and acupuncture treatments did not cure Susan of her symptoms, they might have set in motion, at a deep place, the spark of healing that took years to show good effects.

Susan's story illustrates several other points. No one technique is the surefire answer for all people under all conditions. Some people get lasting relief from chiropractic or acupuncture, while others do not. Some people get the results they need from only one body therapy, while others mix several approaches because they build on or complement each other. Susan's combination worked well for her, but Acupressure, Hellerwork, and Kinetic Awareness might just as easily have been the winning blend. There are infinite varieties, and you will work out your own sequence. Success has less to do with what's "right" and more to do with what's right for you and at what time and with which practitioner.

## SCOPE OF PRACTICE

In addition to the issues discussed above, there are other considerations to keep in mind when deciding on bodyways. Presently, there are three ways of looking at the scope of practice of all of them: *relaxation, remediation,* and *holism.*[4] Each perspective represents a different lens through which the practitioner views and works with your body. They are not exclusive; rather, they are interrelated, just as body, mind, emotions, and spirit are.

### Relaxation

Relaxation has less to do with treatment of specific conditions and more to do with personal service. Compared to the other two levels of practice, this one requires the least amount of training and technical expertise. It is founded on the fact that biologically we all need safe, nurturing touch and safe connection. The goal of a session is to provide you with a relaxing, stress-reducing, pleasurable, and sensual (but not sexual) experience through sensitive touch.

However, even though a bodyway does not aim to relieve particular dysfunctions, such as insomnia, constipation, hypertension, depression, and indigestion, research indicates that by diminishing stress on your entire system you help alleviate these and other conditions. When you're relaxed, you're also more likely to stay healthy and avoid disease. Tiffany Field, Ph.D., director of the Touch Research Institute at the University of Miami Medical School, oversees various studies on the impact of massage on adults and children suffering from dermatitis, post-traumatic stress disorder, burns, abuse, asthma, and other physical traumas. At the core of all of them, says Field, is stress of one kind or another. By decreasing anxiety and activity of the sympathetic nervous system, you also reduce pain and the conditions stress is associated with.[5]

## Remediation

Alleviation of pain and correction of dysfunction are the purposes of a variety of body therapies. The practitioner does a clinical assessment or evaluation in order to investigate the nature of your pain and be able to apply the appropriate treatment. Although some of the methods are similar to those used for relaxation, they require more precise knowledge of anatomy and physiology and hand techniques because the work is specific rather than general. While remedial or corrective body therapies do not necessarily aim for either total relaxation or whole-body change, both might accompany the relief of pain and a particular condition.

## Holism

The holistic approach seeks neither relaxation nor remediation as its goal, but both tend to be positive side effects. "Curing" is not the intention. Instead, the objective is a higher level of organization, structure, function, and well-being. Holistic practitioners achieve this through balancing a particular body system—energy, neuromuscular, or myofascial, for instance. A practitioner might work on the connective tissue system of your body to improve your structure and posture, which in turn results in better overall functioning and even psychological transformation and disease prevention. In a holistic way of seeing things, every part of your body and every aspect of your being is connected and affects every other part. Nothing is wholly separate and independent: If you alter any one dimension of a system, you

When you touch a body, you touch the whole person, the intellect, the spirit, and the emotions.

—Jane Harrington

influence all the others. What changes your structure changes your function, and also changes your mind and heart.

One way to look at it is through the Asian concept called "the Diamond Net of Indra." Picture yourself as a vast net, with a multifaceted diamond at every nexus. Each facet of each diamond reflects every other diamond. If you shake one part of the net, the entire net reverberates. The holistic level is where the practitioner's attention, even more than intention, is vital and where your involvement or leadership in your own personal healing or evolution is essential.

### A Triple-Lens Look

You can use this three-lens explanation not only to help you decide what kind of bodyways you want or need but also to understand how the particular one you try helps you or doesn't go far enough. One approach is not superior to another unless it better suits your purpose. If what you want to do is lie down and relax after a hard week and enjoy the sensual pleasure of oil being rubbed on your body, you don't need to sign up for a series of Hellerwork sessions. Likewise, if you're interested in structural changes, a massage that does not penetrate to the fascia will not do the trick. And if you've just run a marathon or biked a century, you want a session that helps flush waste products from your muscles and speeds your recovery time. Don't use a hammer when you need a screwdriver.

Take back pain, if that's what you're dealing with. One day your lower back feels really sore and you want to be sure it doesn't put you in bed and keep you from working. You may decide that all you need to do is

## Experience: Everything Is Connected

Stand up and walk around the room or through the house. Be as relaxed and loose as you can. How easy is it to move? Notice how you feel. Then stop. Now tighten part of your body. For example, tighten your right fist. Holding that tension, try walking again. What happens? Can you swing your arms freely, or does your whole right side get stiff? Does your throat tighten, too? Does your step change? And how do you feel overall? Is it possible to smile genuinely when your fist is a big knot?

Try this with any other part of the body—squeeze your buttocks, clench your jaw, suck in your belly—and see what happens. How we are in one part of the body can't help but affect the rest of the body. And how we feel physically can't help but affect how we feel emotionally.

relax, for you've been under a lot of stress and your back happens to be your Achilles' heel. You know that if you do Yoga daily and get massaged regularly, you tend to be less tense and more flexible, both of which keep the discomfort at bay. Or you may be in pain that requires specific treatment, perhaps to release trigger points. You want attention and relief right now. But if you want to examine why it keeps recurring, then look for a holistic approach, from either a functional or structural perspective, that works with the ways body structure, movement, and behavior all influence one another. Instead of focusing solely on your lower back as the source of trouble and pain, you would take into account your entire bodily organization. You might also try a convergence therapy that allows you access to and understanding of emotions that may lie beneath your physical symptoms.

Understanding the differences among relaxation, remediation, and holism will prepare you to determine not only which bodyway you want to work with but also whether the practitioner you've chosen is working on that level. Let's say you decide on a holistic approach such as Rolfing, but soon enough you realize that the practitioner operates from a remedial perspective. Don't blame the system for not being holistic. Instead, recognize that simply because it was conceived and organized as holistic doesn't mean that each person who trains in it will then practice it that way. You may also find that the practitioner of a remedial system works in a holistic way.

Remember, it's not the technique alone that will give you what you want, but the right combination of method, your relationship with the practitioner, the practitioner's approach, and your level of openness, readiness, and involvement. Also, keep in mind that we don't really know exactly what's working in every situation. Don't discount the placebo response. Personal service, attention, and caring touch all have a powerful effect and may be as important as the technique itself. In the case of many bodyways, we have no definitive research data to prove that the mechanism involved works, only anecdotal evidence. The great results may have as much to do with human warmth as anything else.

> The power of love to change bodies is legendary, built into folklore, common sense, and everyday experience. Love moves the flesh, it pushes matter around. . . . Throughout history, "tender, loving care" has uniformly been recognized as a valuable element in healing.
>
> —Larry Dossey

## MODELS AND CATEGORIES: DIFFERENCES AND SIMILARITIES

As a consumer, whether shopping for food or shopping for bodyways, you need to be able to identify kinds, not brands. When you walk down a supermarket aisle looking for frozen green beans, it may not matter whether you get S&W or Green Giant. But it will matter if you pick up rutabagas or okra instead. Brands are constantly changing, but green beans are still green beans. Once you understand the fundamental differences between

Suddenly I realized the degree of denigration and neglect of the body and emotions in myself and our whole society. I began to see that the body was not just an instrument for aggression and seduction, but a source of information and knowledge that you just can't bullshit. . . .

—George Leonard

one vegetable and another, you don't have to let new labels confuse you.

To get a sense of the how and why of a bodyway, it is helpful to look at the model it's based on: Western (structure and function) or Eastern (energy). The Western way of understanding the structure and function of the body is based on anatomy and physiology. It's all about differentiation and integration: the degree to which you're composed of discrete parts and the extent to which those parts work together and enhance one another.

What are the different parts? Various kinds of tissues become your muscles, bones, fascia, blood and lymph vessels, nerves, organs, glands, and the fluids that run through all of them. They make up every system in your body: muscular, skeletal, nervous, circulatory, endocrine, digestive, respiratory, excretory, craniosacral, and reproductive. Bodyways based on the Western model address specific physical systems. For example, structural practitioners work with connective tissue called fascia to organize your structure in alignment with the force of gravity. Functional practitioners educate your neuromuscular or sensory-motor system to expand the range of your movement and thus affect how you function. Other therapists may focus on your lymphatic network to enhance circulation and relieve edema.

The Eastern or energetic model sees the body as an energy system. Although in almost all of the bodyways based on this model practitioners work with your actual physical structure, they concentrate on your body's fields, lines, flows, and channels of energy. They are concerned with how evenly and unimpededly energy circulates through you.

To untrained eyes and hands, this energy is invisible, intangible, and immeasurable, especially when compared to the visible, palpable, and measurable tissues and fluids that Western approaches are concerned with. But to skilled practitioners of energetic bodyways, energy is real. Energy and structure/function are complimentary ways of understanding what's going on in our body. Consider for example this story about a Tibetan doctor.

Yeshi Dhonden, the Dalai Lama's personal physician, was taken on rounds at the Yale Medical Center in New Haven, Connecticut. He employed the Chinese method of pulse diagnosis—reading the energy, or *chi*. ☞ See "The Chinese Tradition," page 274. The Western doctors used all manner of technology to investigate the same patient's anatomy and physiology. Yet both came up with the same conclusion. According to Dhonden, winds had been coursing through the woman's body; currents in the blood were breaking against barriers and eddying. All were signs of an imperfect heart whose deep gate had been blown open before she was born. The hospital staff confirmed this as congenital heart disease—an intraventricular septal defect with resultant heart failure.[6] Different language, same condition.

Although there are major differences in the concept of the body held by each kind of approach and in the techniques used for attaining their goals, the division between East and West is not a strict one. Energetic work influences our structure and physiology, and structural/functional work influences our energy. In fact, today few practitioners work strictly one way or another, for the overall dynamic of the field is now rich with overlap and convergence. North America is a big salad bowl of people from every part of the world who have been tossed together. Each group brings not only its customs, language, and spiritual tradition, but also its healing practices and the worldview that supports them. All of that is reflected in the eclectic nature of bodyways.

Western bodyways vary in which physical aspect they address to achieve specific and overall improvement, but all of them deal with the same basic anatomy and physiology mapped out by Western medicine. Eastern bodyways vary, according to their cultural origins, in their anatomical maps of the energy body and in the way they stimulate or smooth out energy for particular conditions as well as total well-being.

To help you get a handle on the many different bodyways, I have grouped them according to the fundamental model that informs them. The Western section includes massage and other hands-on techniques, structural approaches, functional approaches, and movement arts in which you, not the practitioner, initiate movement. The Eastern section includes

## Hands-On and Movement Arts Categories

### Western Model—Structure and Function:

**Traditional massage and contemporary therapies**
**Structural approaches**
**Functional approaches**
**Western movement arts**

### Eastern Model—Energy:

**Chinese tradition**
**Japanese tradition**
**Indian tradition**
**Other energetic systems**
**Eastern movement arts**

### Convergence Systems—Physical/Emotional Integration

The messages that make up our emotional and mental life must be routed through the tissues of the body.

—Robert Marrone

the hands-on and movement arts of the Chinese, Japanese, and Indian traditions as well as the outgrowth of Western-created energetic bodyways. The section on convergence approaches synthesizes elements from several Eastern and Western systems, in order to deal with and integrate emotions that emerge when working with the body. While emotions can arise in any body session, not all bodyways have the intention of dealing with them, nor are the practitioners prepared to do so.

Convergence is the direction in which the entire bodyways field seems to be moving. The trend today is to be more comprehensive by including movement and emotions. Practitioners recognize that when you don't learn how to move differently and don't resolve emotional issues underlying your physical conditions, true change or healing is elusive.

Although these categories are useful for understanding distinctions, keep in mind that your body itself does not make such arbitrary separations. It does not distinguish between "I'm getting Western Aston-Patterning® now" and "This is an Eastern Shiatsu session." Neither does it recognize the differences between systems within the same category, such as Rolfing and Hellerwork, which are both structural approaches. What your body knows on the most basic level is that it is receiving sensory impressions—pain, tingling, pressure, stretching, heat, and so on. Beyond that, what we know about the systems is conceptual.

The systems themselves fall into divisions, both by category and within a category, through the language their creators and practitioners use to describe their intentions and techniques and where they place emphasis. For instance, even though all functional approaches have the same goal and use similar tools, such as focused awareness, *what they emphasize* in describing what they do and how they do it is different.

Structural and functional approaches also are neighbors. Physically, they both deal with our posture and its relationship to gravity and with even or balanced distribution of tension. But they come from opposite perspectives—structure affects function vs. function influences structure. They address different body systems—myofascial vs. sensory-motor. And they use different levels of manipulation—deep vs. light (or none at all).

It is true that each system produces a different body. A body trained in Yoga is not the same as one practiced in T'ai Chi Chuan. As Dub Leigh, who studied with some of the best-known somatic pioneers, has said:

> The well-processed bodies turned out by Rolfing, Feldenkrais, and Zen Bodytherapy are quite different. Ida's processed bodies have a lift, a lightness that reminds me of a bullfighter. Moshe's processed bodies have more mobility and appear fluid in almost all configurations. Zen processed bodies are grounded. They

seem almost unmovable by any outside force, yet they have a smooth gliding motion and never seem to lose their grounded-ness with the universe.[7]

Despite these differences, all still strive for a client's functional econ-omy and freedom on every level of being, and thus a certain basic similarity still results. I'll let Leigh speak again:

> All of the above well-processed bodies house psyches that are much more emotionally mature and optimistic than the non-processed. They live mostly in enthusiasm, cheerfulness, interest and contentment. When appropriate, they can move down to anger, fear and grief. Only rarely, under unusual conditions, will they drop down to despair, resentment, self-abasement or apathy. When they do, they bounce back fast. They do not "muck around" in any of the negative emotions.[8]

## MIXING AND MATCHING

It doesn't matter which bodyway you try first, and there's no final one to wend your way toward. You don't necessarily begin with Yoga and mas-sage and end up with Aikido and the Alexander Technique. There's no hi-erarchy here. Rather, in a kind of cross-fertilization, each bodyway informs all the others you engage in. One may affect you at a certain level of your being, while another might have a healing effect on a different aspect, and both could influence yet other levels. In most cases, the various approaches are not mutually exclusive but can be used in combination, simultaneously or sequentially. However, some are more compatible than others. If you're already involved in one bodyway and wonder what else you might experi-ment with, reading through the different sections can give you a sense of which mix and match well and which might unnecessarily confuse your body as well as waste your time and money.

I prefer to cross categories rather than scramble my body with, let's say, more than one structural or energetic approach at a time. For example, if I'm receiving sessions in Aston-Patterning, I don't mix them with Heller-work, Rolfing, or Myofascial Release at the same time. I would fully expe-rience one before moving on to another. The reason for being careful about what you mix is simple. Imagine the Rolfer or Hellerworker as a sculptor working with clay. Once he moved the clay of your body around, you wouldn't want another artist to distort the shape he's already created. If you're receiving energetic work, think of it as having an electrician come to your house to adjust the wiring because it was shorting out in certain

> The body is what we came into the world with and what we leave behind. And in between there is only a growing awareness and under-standing that starts with the body and goes on from there.
>
> —Olivia Vlahos

# Experience: Mapping Your Body

To help you identify your needs or goals, as well as to be able to communicate them to a practitioner, it's useful to have a sense of what's going on in your body . Fill in the body outlines as you ask yourself the following questions, but don't limit yourself to them. If you come up with something else, by all means use it.

Before you read the questions, slow down by taking a few deep breaths with your eyes closed so that you can focus inwardly. When you feel ready, open your eyes and read a question. If it helps you to feel more, close your eyes again. Do whatever you need—walk, sit, lie down—to sense what's happening in your body.

• Do I feel balance in my body? Are the top and bottom halves, front and back, right and left sides equally developed, strong, and flexible? Note any area that feels massive, weak, flexible, or rigid.

• Where do I feel limited or restricted in my movements? Where am I anxious and tight or tense and fearful? Write in what matches your feelings.

• Where do I feel free and relaxed? Where am I easy and comfortable in my body?

• Where do I feel pain? What does it feel like? Does it burn like a hot poker? Is it sharp as a knife? Is the ache as heavy as a truck? Does it pierce like needles? Does it have a particular color? If you have difficulty describing it, just write "pain" in that area.

• Where do I not feel anything? Note places of numbness.

• Is a part of my body trying to tell me something? What is the message?[9]

rooms. You wouldn't want another electrician to then undo that work and run the circuits a different way.

Certain combinations are advantageous. For example, movement practices are a useful accompaniment to structural approaches because they can help reinforce and maintain the changes gained through the hands-on work. Movement instills new proprioceptive information about your new ease and freedom and makes relief more long-lasting. It also can facilitate letting go in an area of your body that a practitioner might find impossible to release or that would require invasive, intolerable pressure. Some systems offer movement and structure in tandem: for example, Feldenkrais Functional Integration with Awareness Through Movement, Rolfing with Rolfing Movement Integration, and the Trager with Mentastics. Energetic systems that balance you overall might be helpful in preparing you for deeper fascial work. General massage is usually compatible with most anything if you need an easy, soothing way to relax. One woman, while going through her Rolfing series, scheduled a massage every other week for her pleasure and relaxation; she also kept up her Yoga practice.

You may experience a bit of mixing and matching in the practitioner you're already working with. Body therapists often learn a variety of approaches to complement their main work. For example, my Rolfer also studied craniosacral work and checked my craniosacral rhythm at the beginning and end of each session. Another Rolfer combines Structural Integration with Hanna Somatic Education because he finds them synergistic. Both cultivate balanced and free movement, but one does so through the web of fascia, while the other works through sensory awareness and mastery of movement. Yet another Rolfer blends Rolfing with Yoga.[10]

## MEANDERING LIKE A RIVER

In reading through the categories, you may be tempted to match your body symptoms to the bodyway you think will successfully relieve them. That's not unreasonable. You want to gain a measure of security and control over what feels chaotic—pain, dysfunction, limitation. You fear you'll have to live with this. You hope someone will make it go away. When you choose by ordered categories, you are looking for predictability.

But bodyways often work in mysterious ways. You may choose one with a particular goal in mind but come out with a benefit you never anticipated. You also may not know rationally or logically what you're looking for, but something unconscious could be guiding your choice. You don't have to know why. It's important to stay open to other possibilities, for you may need something entirely different than what you think you want.

I decided to try Rolfing again fifteen years after I'd experienced my first sessions. During that period, my body had suffered a number of running injuries, a fall down a flight of stairs, and other stresses, not to mention getting older. I decided on Rolfing because I knew I was structurally off balance—my right shoulder, arm, and hip were lower than on my left side—and I wanted to be more symmetrical. While I never got completely aligned—I still hang lower on my right side—something more important happened about midway through my series. For years I had been estranged on and off from my family, especially my sister. Somehow the work on my chest opened my heart, too. When I went to see my family, I had a reconciliation with them and have been on warmer terms ever since.

That's why I'd like you to consider another, more creative way to approach bodyways: Playfully explore and experiment in the unknown. Don't worry about finding the "right" one. Let yourself be led by the unexpected or "accidental" and see what happens.

If you could rise high above your own life or have a retrospective view, you would see that changes and healings do not lie at the end of a straight line. You may think that the simplest, quickest way to find relief from your symptoms is to find the "right" technique. But I urge you not to become fixated in a search for the single system that will give you immediate, satisfactory, permanent results; it doesn't exist. Sometimes you do happen on the appropriate practitioner and bodyway at the right time. More commonly, you move like a river, meandering through the landscape, branching and rejoining as you course toward deeper waters.

## DEVELOPING AN INTERNAL SENSOR

Experimenting with different kinds of bodyways can afford you the opportunity to develop an internal sensor, to reclaim the voice of your "inner physician," "inner guide," "inner healer," or "inner teacher." In the same way that you learn the language of musical instruments, you can also begin to learn the language of your body. You become sensitive to what your body needs or wants without a mental idea of what that should be. The more you become attuned to the music of your body, the more you recognize what type of movement your body is calling for at a particular time. Let me describe how this works for me.

One summer day, when I drove down the narrow dirt road through the woods where I lived while writing this book, the sun momentarily blinded me as I came out of the shade, and I didn't see someone coming. I slammed on my brakes, but slid down the gravel into his vehicle anyway. The front of my car got pushed in, but luckily neither of us was visibly hurt. Still, I knew that the shock had registered in my body and psyche. After reporting the accident, I reflected on what I needed—definitely some-

I want to awaken that still, small, wise intuitive voice in all of us, that voice of our own body that we have been forced to ignore through our culture's illness, misinformation, and dysfunction.

—Christiane Northrup

# Experience: Asking Your Body What It Wants

Once you're acquainted with the bodyways described in Part III, you can check with your body to see which approach it is interested in or thinks could be especially effective. As needs and goals change, you can ask again and again.

Lying down or sitting up, close your eyes. Breathe normally, without forcing anything, until you feel your mind is settled and your respiration slows. Then silently, internally, ask your whole body or the particular area where you feel pain, discomfort, or restriction what it wants. You can ask a general question, such as "What would help you the most?" If nothing comes up—as a word, image, or feeling—you can be more specific and ask for a yes or no. For example, "Would an overall relaxation session soothe you best?" or "Do you want an energy balancing?" or "Will deep therapy be most satisfying?" or "Is it time for structural realignment?" or "Are you ready to learn how to move differently?" and so on.

If you're feeling pretty good and would like to enhance what already functions fairly well, you can ask a different kind of question. For example, "Which approach would enable me to fulfill my potential as a runner?" "What will help me feel lighter and more graceful as I dance?" "What can I do to keep from stiffening as I get older so I can stay active?"
☞ See also "A Guided Journey to Body Wisdom," page 51.

---

thing soothing so that the trauma would not take up permanent residence in my body. I was fortunate in that my friend Linda was visiting and available to do a craniosacral unwinding. It released the impact from my body and I never had any repercussions, except financial, from the accident. Other gentle bodyways might have accomplished the same thing.

At another time, I had difficulty falling asleep and was not waking up rested. I had a post- rather than pre-menstrual migraine and felt a dull pressure around my right eye. The base of my skull was sore on the right side. My eyes tired easily and my neck and shoulders kept tightening. Since I had gone hiking and swimming during those days, I knew a lack of exercise was not to blame for my poor sleep. I wasn't aware of any particular worries, either, for all was going well in my life. So what was it? I realized that I felt off-kilter in my neck and shoulder area but not in a muscular way. This was a call not for massage but for a balancing of my craniosacral rhythm. Immediately after a session, there was a shift. My sleep returned to its normal, easy pattern and the migraine no longer lingered.

As a contrast, let me share a different experience, one that didn't beg for craniosacral work. I had a lot of discomfort in my right hip whenever I

You are in search of inner peace but you hate your body and senses. You long for inner joy but develop hostility towards the body which is a means to that joy, as though it were your most formidable enemy.

—Swami Muktananda

rode in the car or rolled over in bed, but not while walking. It began after I switched from a regular exercycle to a recumbent one and also sat twisted while talking to an aerobics instructor at the fitness center. My hip was already a sensitive area, full of memories of physical trauma, including a fall down a flight of stairs. I knew this time I needed to address the muscles engaged in creating the discomfort. To induce them to let go, I chose Neuromuscular Therapy. The massage therapist applied pressure to trigger points and also artfully integrated several other methods. The overall effect was relaxation and relief.

This is not to say that energy work couldn't lead to a release of spasm as well, immediately or soon after. Three days after a Jin Shin Do session, suddenly my tight left shoulder let go and I heard a pop in my neck. Finally I could turn my head all the way to the left again.

Keep in mind that my sensor works only for me, not for my friends or clients, which is why you have to evolve your own. While doing so, you will also find that you come back to bodyways you tried years before. When my friend Maria originally did Yoga, it was no more than physical exercise, whereas now it leads her to greater body awareness. Because her body knowledge has expanded during her years of meandering, she is experiencing Yoga differently so many years later. As the ancient Greek philosopher Heraclitus said, you can't step twice into the same river.

Any doorway you walk through first will lead you to many others. As you experiment, you will gradually empower yourself to make your own decisions. Over the years, the more you do this, the more adept you become, and the more your body becomes your friend and ally in living with greater ease and comfort, with greater well-being. This allows you to prevent exhaustion, pain, and disease, or at least to ameliorate it. Also, by staying with the sensed experience—staying inside your body rather than in your head—of whichever bodyway you try, your intention moves inward rather than outward. You're concerned more with how good you feel than with how good you look or how much you achieve.

This is a lifelong process, and at times it can be frustrating because it involves zigs and zags rather than moving in a direct line. Learning the language of your body develops from an enduring commitment to know yourself, to undo the physical and emotional patterns that limit your sensitivity and authentic expression.

Seeing within changes one's outer vision.

—Joseph Chilton Pearce

# CHAPTER 6

# Psychological Dimensions
# of Bodyways

It would be easy to consider bodyways as something strictly physical. Indeed, many started out that way, and some have remained so. But the influence of psychology looms large in this field. Psyche and body are part of the same continuum—what affects one affects the other. Rare is the body practitioner or somatic educator today who doesn't have some understanding that where there's a physical difficulty, there's also an emotional counterpart, or vice versa. Learning more about the psychology of bodyways can help you better understand that during a session more than your physical structure is being touched.

## THE THERAPEUTIC TRADITION

*The unconscious, repression, armor, libido,* and other terms are commonly used today to discuss mind and body interaction. They originated early in the twentieth century with two Austrian doctors, Sigmund Freud (1856–1939) and his disciple-turned-renegade, Wilhelm Reich (1897–1957). These men changed the course of both our thinking and our ways of working with the body to influence the mind. But the tradition was already there to draw on.

In other cultures around the world, the "talking cure" (psychoanalysis), as we know it, has never been the treatment of choice in healing so-called mental problems. First, in these other worldviews there is no

> Whatever the explanation of how emotional and bodily changes are linked, it is as profoundly true that we are as much affected in our thinking by our bodily attitudes as our bodily attitudes are affected in the reflection of our mental and bodily states.
>
> —Mabel E. Todd

Many of our psychic maladies are in fact caused by the overactive mind, and exclusively analytic therapies may deepen the quagmire.

—Shaun McNiff

separate mind that gets sick; body, mind or psyche, and spirit are one. Second, though words may be spoken, as in chants or incantations, no one intellectually probes the past in an impersonal relationship between doctor and patient. Indigenous groups use massage, herbs, movement, song, and music, but no analysis. They include physical means, whether the disturbance is physical or mental, for they make no distinction between the two. Their healing rituals do not address only one aspect of a person's life. No one would say, "It's all in your head."

In contemporary Western society, to deal with emotional or mental difficulties we generally take our head to a psychotherapist's offices and leave our body at the door. This wasn't always the case. The ancient Greeks healed mind and body through a combination of baths, diet, herbs, massage, exercise, and other natural remedies. This was as true for a person suffering from melancholy as for someone afflicted with fever, headaches, or epilepsy.

In the late nineteenth century, some European and American physicians dismissed language as the way to reach their "mental" patients and tried physical measures. For example, massage was a standard part of the regimen in treating neurasthenia, an emotional disorder prevalent among women and characterized by such symptoms as a tendency to fatigue easily, lack of motivation, and feelings of inadequacy. At Salpêtrière Hospital in France, Jean-Martin Charcot (1825–1893) used massage and hypnosis for hysteria. At a sanatorium in Baden-Baden, Germany, the Hungarian Georg Groddeck (1866–1934) bathed, massaged, made bone adjustments, and prescribed exercises for his patients in order to communicate with what he called the *It* (later to be known as the *id,* the unconscious part of the psyche). A pioneer of psychosomatic medicine, he wrote to Freud that he saw no separation between bodily illnesses and psychic illnesses. The body became the royal road to the psyche.

## The Unconscious

Emotion always has its roots in the unconscious and manifests itself in the body.

—Irene Claremont de Castillejo

It was Freud who first proposed the existence of the unconscious, that hidden part of human nature which breaks into awareness through dreams, slips of the tongue, and disconnected acts. The unconscious is like a vast, uncharted territory where instinctual needs for survival and desires for satisfaction roam free, uncontrolled by reason and logic. Although we appear properly civilized on the surface, following society's rules and regulations, in the unconscious we act and respond spontaneously. However, outward good manners do not cancel out true longings. We internalize whatever events shape us—emotions, shocks, and frustrations register physiologically in the body—and reenact them throughout life. Anthropologist Richard Grossinger describes this:

So no matter what a person's attitude or expressed moral position, it is formed only of raw instinct. The ideological avoidance of sexual acting out, for instance, does not end the matter. The desire stays within the organism unconsciously and is expressed in some other activity which compensates exactly even though it may not have specific sexual content. Civilization, with its etiquettes and repressions, offers no sanctuary against primary desires and original pain. A later life of ease and pleasure does not alleviate the terrors and agonies of childhood; unexperienced pain limits pleasure without the person even being aware of it.[1]

*And the body is the expression of the personality; it expresses the way the person experiences himself and lives in the world.*

—Hannah Fraenkel

## Repression

Freud said, "In the unconscious nothing can be brought to an end, nothing is past or forgotten."[2] Whatever we suppress—push down or sweep under the rug—early in life to survive and meet with social approval becomes *repressed* when we have no way to resolve the conflict at the time.

*We wear our attitudes in our bodies.*

—Patti Davis

How many of us had to hold down fear of an angry and critical parent, smother rage at an abuser, endure dependence on a parent, bite back jealousy and rivalry toward a sibling, perform to satisfy parents' unfulfilled desires, or set aside our own needs to act as caretaker for a parent made incapable by illness, depression, or alcoholism? We had to exclude such feelings from our conscious awareness, memory, or recall. Otherwise, we'd be forever pained, or we'd feel threatened by the possibility that these feelings would overwhelm the "normal self" we developed in order to manage in the world. Those feelings became skeletons behind a locked door to which we threw away the key. We learned to defend against them by distorting how we see ourselves and others and by limiting our movements and self-expression—in short, by altering our life experiences.

But, as you probably know, and as Freud pointed out, ultimately repression is not successful. The unresolved emotions appear in disguise, slipping out in dreams and art, leaking into jokes, manifesting themselves as physical symptoms, and haunting relationship patterns. Chronic depression or anger may bring you to a psychotherapist; chronic body difficulties may bring you to a bodyways practitioner.

Being touched on a practitioner's table or maintaining a Yoga asana may unexpectedly open the closet door. Suddenly a memory surfaces from ten, twenty, thirty years ago, and along with it come emotions. Finally having access to the hidden information and feelings enables you then to work consciously to assimilate it. Once you're aware of it, you no longer have to use up so much energy to hold it down. You can see it for what it is rather than as an unknown bogeyman that holds sway over you. You can respond differently than you had to long ago, and you can become free to live your life without that shadow following you around.

## BODY EGO

Psychological insight and understanding are rarely sufficient to create change.

—Stanley Keleman

Although psychoanalysis turned into a "talking cure," its founding father, Freud, stated from the outset that the development of the ego—our sense of self—is above all the development of a body ego or body self. Child psychologists would later refer to this early stage as the sensory-motor period, when bodily sensations inform us of our very being and the world around us before we ever know language.

Not experiencing certain sensations in the body limits ego development, the way lack of rain stunts the growth of vegetables. For example, if, as an infant, you did not experience enough body sensations of support against gravity—being held, rocked, picked up, and laid down—your ego, in a parallel way, would not have grown in self-support. Later in life, you might be "weak in the knees" or have frail legs, ankles, or feet. Merely analyzing the difficulty for intellectual insights would not be powerful enough to bring about change. Experiencing the necessary bodily sensations and any attendant, previously withheld emotions—having them register as real—is what would make the difference. Sensations bring awareness to the present. You know something about yourself you didn't know before. You see how an old pattern has operated and can envision a different possibility. You then have a choice to act on it and integrate this new pattern.

### Libido

In addition to the unconscious and the body ego, Freud gave us *libido*. Although we're quick to define it as "sexual drive," it's much more than that. It is our basic drive, our life force that gets shaped into sexual drive. It's our emotional or psychic energy derived from primal biological urges. As babies we display libido in our desire to suckle, to suck our thumbs, and to know things with our mouths. Genital sexuality is no more than a later phase in this developmental process.

### Seduction Theory

Whatever else place means, it means first and foremost where the flesh is and where human dwelling occurs.

—Robert Kugelmann

Freud was keenly aware of the body. He recognized it as the source and location of our experiences—where we live. In doing so, he laid the groundwork for focusing on the body in psychotherapy, but he never actually went beyond that. Given the taboo-riddled climate of the Victorian and post-Victorian eras in which he lived, it's not surprising that some of his earliest ideas never took root. For example, in 1895 and 1896, in listening to his women patients, Freud discovered that early sexual traumas, not heredity, lay at the core of their neuroses. He was the first psychiatrist to believe their memories of abuse instead of dismissing them as fantasy or hysterical lying.

But when Freud revealed this revolutionary theory of mental illness in his first major public address at the Society for Psychiatry and Neurology in Vienna in April 1896, he met with silence. His colleagues strongly discouraged him from publishing "The Aetiology of Hysteria," telling him his reputation would be damaged. For defying their advice, he subsequently suffered condemnation, ostracism, and isolation. In 1905 Freud publicly retracted his so-called seduction theory and said that his women patients had been fantasizing instead. This allowed him to participate again in medical society, but until recent years caused medical practitioners to suppress reports of sexual abuse, especially by women, and to question their validity.[3]

Nevertheless, Freud sowed a seed that, in turn, inspired others to develop new approaches for including the body in psychotherapy. One of Freud's most well known pupils, Sandor Ferenczi of Hungary (1873–1933), was an early champion of body awareness, concentrating on muscle tone and posture. The major proponent of body awareness, Wilhelm Reich, was influenced by Ferenczi.

## Wilhelm Reich: Character Armor and Orgone

Reich broke with traditional psychoanalysis and made the body his primary focus. He pioneered the connection between neurosis (or psychological rigidity) and muscular tension (or physical rigidity), known as *character armor*. This armor builds up in the body like layers of calluses. If you walk around barefoot, eventually you develop skin thick enough so that you don't feel rocks, thorns, and other sharp materials when you step on them. In the same way, your body develops tension strategies or holding patterns to protect against feeling certain emotions, traumas, stresses, and memories.

From early on, we experience the conflict between our instinctual urges (including sexual ones, such as masturbation) on the one hand and the demands of family, society, and religion on the other. To inhibit or deny the urge, we tighten the muscles that would carry out the impulse. If, as a child, every time you reach out, you're told no or pushed away—especially when child-rearing practices teach that touch and affection will spoil children, make them weak, dependent, and undisciplined—you learn to stop your muscles from carrying out your need to be held. You also suppress the sadness or rage you feel, stifling your breath and stiffening your muscles to stem an outburst of sobs or screams. Eventually you no longer know when you're sad or angry. If you habitually contract to hold back actions and feelings, you wind up with neurotic behavior and chronic spasms that block the flow of energy through your body and may lead to physical disorders. As you cut off the source of pain, you also cut off the source of pleasure.

Reich considered that flow to consist of measurable bioelectrical energy (his student Alexander Lowen would later call it *bioenergy*). He

There is no neurosis without a secret corporeal disorder or transformation that organizes it.

—François Dagognet

There is something crazy about a person who is out of touch with the reality of his or her being—the body and its feelings.

—Alexander Lowen

All feelings, both positive and unpleasant, come out of the same faucet. To turn down the faucet on pain is to slow the flow of pleasant feeling as well.

—Gay and Kathlyn Hendricks

dropped Freud's "libido" for "orgone." His basic premise was that dissolving the armor of muscle spasms would allow the orgone to move freely. By going beneath the protective layers you come to the alive, pulsing, feeling core of the person. In particular, Reich fixated on full-body orgasm—energy streamings from head to toe—as its expression. As far as he was concerned, unless this orgastic experience happened, the patient was still neurotic.

Today, except for orthodox Reichians—M.D.s called *orgonomists*—body-oriented psychotherapists do not limit themselves to Reich's theories of orgone and orgasm. They work beyond the strong reflex movements of birth and orgasm to affirm the primary pleasure of being alive. They embrace the life-force energy known in Chinese traditions as *qi* (pronounced "chee") and in Japanese traditions as *ki* (pronounced "kee"), and strive to promote its unimpeded flow throughout the body. In India, psychological dysfunction is related to energetic disturbance in the seven energy vortices—*chakras,* or wheels—of the subtle body. ☞ See sections on chi and chakras, pages 274 and 297.

Another way to understand character armor is as your personal history embodied—all of your physical and emotional pains written on your body, their marks left in the form of cumulative restrictions of breathing and mobility. Each one of us has such an imprint, some more dramatic than others.

Writer Susan Griffin relates a particularly moving example, the story of a Japanese woman she met on a trip to Hiroshima. When the bomb exploded on August 6, 1945, Yoko, only two at the time, was thrown through the air and out a window. Although she does not remember the blast, her body does: She still has two small scars on her face where the glass was embedded. Her mother, very badly burned, died two weeks later of radiation sickness; her father's body disappeared. For the children who survived, it became a life of privation—no electricity, no heat, barely any food or clothing, and illness. One sister, sick from radiation exposure, had to go to the hospital. A brother abandoned them. Yoko eventually moved among five different relatives, feeling a burden to them all. She had no room or bed of her own, only a corner, carried her few belongings in a scarf, worked till late at night, and heard them argue over who would take her next.[4]

"Such a childhood settles into flesh and bone," reflects Griffin. "It can be seen. It is not invisible but present in the line of shoulders, the measure of breath, a hand moving to lips, words spoken or unspoken, so that even a story not told is told over and over again in mimed gestures of shyness and fear and conscribes a place in the body which holds this old suffering."[5]

Reich would have seen Yoko's character and armoring in an arrangement of seven major body segments, somewhat similar to the seven chakras, rather than individual muscles or nerve pathways. Each segment

The events from your past are now inscribed upon the tablet of your flesh, and today your body shows your life story so clearly.

—Joseph Heller

Primary muscle patterns being the biological heritage of man, man's whole body records his emotional thinking.

—Mabel E. Todd

is a ring of tension that encircles the body and includes the internal organs. From top to bottom, which is how he proceeded, Reich would have observed and worked with what was around her eyes (ocular segment), mouth, chin, jaw, and throat (oral segment), neck (cervical segment), chest, arms, and hands (thoracic segment), diaphragm and surrounding organs (diaphragmatic segment), abdominal muscles, sacrum, and lower back (abdominal segment), and pelvis, genitalia, rectum, legs, and feet (pelvic segment). Constriction in any one segment, as in any one chakra, disrupts the longitudinal flow of energy through the body. The release of one segment paves the way for release in another.

*The body tells the clearest what we want to hide the most.*

*—Marion Rosen*

Reich was revolutionary in moving away from excavating a patient's past through dreams and free association. Instead, he looked at the person's character and history presented right in front of him. Instead of painstakingly reconstructing traumatic moments, he saw the trauma as it still existed in every breath taken and every gesture made.

He developed a variety of nonverbal techniques for dissolving muscular armoring and evoking catharsis (strong emotional expression and release).[6] Because his treatment directly involved the body's vegetative or autonomic nervous system, he called it "vegetotherapy." First he had the patient strip down to underclothes. Visually he could diagnose what words never revealed. "As soon as the patient ceases to talk, the bodily expression of emotion becomes clearly manifest," he said.[7] To get things moving, he had patients breathe deeply. He deeply pressed, pinched, rocked, or stroked their muscles and organs. Reich would encourage people to actively express

## Chua Ka

According to Oscar Ichazo, founder of the Arica School for the development of human consciousness, the idea of the body storing emotions existed long ago. Legend has it that in ancient Mongolia warriors used a system of body manipulation before going into battle to release traumas and painful experiences held in their bodies as muscle tension. In Chua Ka, the body is divided into twenty-seven regions, or "zones of karma." Each one can serve as a depot for a different fear. For example, the lower back retains the fear of losing. Once the warriors massaged out these old injuries and fears, they were ready to act.

Chua Ka means "to sculpt out." You do this by applying firm pressure to the muscles, using a ka stick (a flat massage tool), and rolling the skin. These three techniques loosen the skin and muscles and release connective tissue all the way to the bone. Relaxation sets in; stress and trauma go out.

To be fully incarnated means to experience again all those nasty feelings that people move into their heads to avoid.

—Anita Greene

themselves vocally, facially, or with their whole body, screaming, pushing, pounding, kicking, and banging. He also worked with gagging, coughing, and yawning reflexes, and made patients maintain stressful positions.

All of these techniques helped arouse and release repressed sexual and emotional energies. Often they stimulated patients to reexperience long-forgotten episodes and the emotions that accompanied them—anguish over a parent's death during childhood, humiliation and anger over treatment by a former employer, and so on. Reich emphasized that the patient did not talk about the past but actually relived it, for first came the emotion and then the memory appeared.

The purpose of releasing the repressed tensions and feelings was for the person to feel greater physical vitality and aliveness, with energy coursing up and down the body, and respiration becoming full and deep. But for such changes to continue, Reich was clear that a patient had to adopt a new lifestyle. It was not enough to do analysis or physical exercises; the person had to eliminate the causes of armoring—the defensive attitudes and actions behind it.

## Body Reading

Like the Rosetta stone, for those who know how to read it, the body is a living record of life given, life taken, life hoped for, life healed.

—Clarissa Pinkola Estés

Reich's vision and division of the body into these armor segments spawned the practice of body reading—interpreting someone's personality or character by what the body reveals in muscle tone, skin tone, movements, proportions, tensions, and posture. For example, in their book *The Body Reveals,* Ron Kurtz and Hector Prestera, a medical doctor, describe individuals who have overexpanded chests as fearful of taking in energy from the outside, including relationships. Such people stay within the bounds of rules and schedules, a rigid system of attitudes about how to act, and a rational, logical, intellectual framework that does not include emotional and intuitive aspects. In *Emotional Anatomy,* somatic psychologist Stanley Keleman associates the opposite posture of a collapsed structure—sunken chest, sagging abdomen, and protruding pelvis—with a helpless, obedient, despairing, apathetic character.[8]

Don't be surprised if a therapist looks at your body, reads it, and gives you a mini-biography. But keep in mind that these body interpretations reflect each system's theory and typology. Someone else might interpret a different emotional history in your physical structure, just as each artist renders a scene through different eyes.

Before you speak . . . your body speaks for you.

—Isabelle Anderson

Above all, don't let anyone control you by labeling you as one type or another or telling you what you're feeling or holding in any part of your body. Whether or not therapists are accurate is not the issue. What's crucial is whether they are helping to educate you—that is, draw out of you what you know—or enable you to experience for yourself what they're observing

# Experience: Emotions in Your Body

If someone suggests that one part of your body houses a particular emotion, don't accept it as gospel, but do stop to consider whether it might be valid. Become aware of what you are feeling there. Focus on the quality of that area. Is it comfortable, warm, tight, cold, queasy, heavy, painful, soft, or numb? Does an image or color come up? When you pay attention to that area, do you suddenly think of a person or an incident? Do you have a memory of something? What is the feeling connected to it—anger, love, grief, remorse, conflict? Try to know for yourself what your body might hold there.

in you. Unless you come to know what's in your body through your own insight and experience, how can you develop the power of body wisdom?

## Growth of Body-Centered Therapy

By the time Reich left Scandinavia for the United States in 1939, he had already influenced many professionals in the psychology field in Europe. For example, Fritz Perls, who studied with him before they both had to escape Germany in 1933, many years later was instrumental in bringing Gestalt therapy to America. It centered around the basic idea that losing touch with our bodies and feelings leads to suffering, and healing comes from recovering self-awareness. Reich's effect continued even after his death in a federal prison in 1957, having been censured for his radical ideas and experiments.[9] Some of Reich's students strictly followed his tradition. Others developed their own therapy styles, inspired not only by his groundbreaking work but also by other models, including Western movement and dance as well as Asian martial arts and meditation practices. In turn, they generated even more therapies that have sustained the body-oriented tradition, but in divergent ways.[10]

Like any originator of a system, Reich had his blind spots. Others partially modified his methods or worked differently altogether. Somatic educators also affected therapy styles. For example, Gerda Alexander, the creator of Gerda Alexander Eutony, was very much against an aggressive way of working to break down a person's resistance and force maturation. She felt it weakened individuals still more, instead of helping them to stand on their own feet. Some therapists, most notably in the Lomi and Hakomi methods, moved away from vigorous catharsis to a gentler way of allowing emotional expression; they also integrated mindfulness practice from Buddhism.

Still others came from a Jungian tradition. Like Reich, Swiss psychiatrist Carl Gustav Jung (1875–1961) separated from Freud and developed a whole other school of analysis. Jung played an enormous role in the development of psychotherapy, introducing a host of concepts, such as archetypes, collective unconscious, shadow, anima and animus, into the field and even into common parlance. Several therapists influenced by Jung added a somatic component to their work. For example, Arnold Mindell evolved Dreambody, Process-Oriented Psychology.[11]

In general, the newer therapies have softened. They don't rip away a person's defenses but rather acknowledge them as survival strategies and help build healthier ones that are more appropriate to the present. They also recognize the flip side of hypercontracted muscles—hypotonic or underdeveloped muscles—as a different response to stressful situations.

Somatic psychotherapies have grown in popularity, with many to choose from in America and Europe. They continue to be profoundly influential in bodyways. However, whereas bodyways begin with the body, the body-based psychotherapies begin with the psyche. Still, instead of being leagues apart, certain psychotherapies and body therapies are increas-

## Some Body-Based Psychotherapies and Their Originators

| | |
|---|---|
| GESTALT THERAPY | Fritz Perls |
| BIOENERGETICS | Alexander Lowen |
| RADIX | Charles Kelley |
| CORE ENERGETICS | John Pierrakos |
| GENTLE BIO-ENERGETICS | Eva Reich |
| LOMI SCHOOL | Robert Hall |
| BODYNAMICS | Lisbeth Marcher |
| PRIMAL THERAPY | Arthur Janov |
| FOCUSING | Eugene Gendlin |
| HAKOMI | Ron Kurtz |
| DANCE THERAPY | Marian Chace |
| SENSORY INTEGRATION | Jean Ayres |
| SOMATIC PSYCHOLOGY | Stanley Keleman |
| ORGANISMIC PSYCHOTHERAPY | Malcolm Brown |
| PESSO SYSTEM/PSYCHOMOTOR | Albert and Diane Pesso |
| BODY-CENTERED THERAPY | Gay and Kathlyn Hendricks |
| DREAMBODY, PROCESS-ORIENTED PSYCHOLOGY | Arnold Mindell |
| HOLOTROPIC BREATHWORK | Stanislav Grof |
| INTEGRATIVE BODY PSYCHOTHERAPY | Jack Lee Rosenberg and Marjorie Rand |

ingly drawing closer, not unlike how different branches in education and medicine have merged into multidisciplinary departments, such as psychoneuroimmunology. Practitioners at both ends of the continuum are borrowing from one another. Those in bodyways learn psychotherapeutic skills to deal with their clients' emotional difficulties while handling their bodies. Those in psychotherapy learn body techniques to reach hidden emotions.

Whatever bodyway you engage in, your psychic structure will be touched or moved at the same time that your body is getting massaged or going through a Yoga routine. Most body and movement therapies assume that the body has a long memory, that it holds history.

## REMEMBERING THROUGH THE BODY

Any trauma—accident, injury, surgery, sexual, physical or emotional abuse, war, difficult birth—may surface spontaneously as a memory years, even decades, later during a bodyways session. This phenomenon of memories seeming to reside in the body rather than purely in the brain is variously called *body memory, tissue memory, cell* or *cellular memory,* or *somatic memory.*

These terms do not appear in any standard English-language dictionary (yet) and have no agreed-upon definition. The juxtaposition of such words as *body* and *memory* even seems a contradiction. Who among us wasn't taught that memory is a mental function? But in our journey beyond the Cartesian mind-body dualism that has informed our thinking since the seventeenth century, we can no longer believe that memory, emotion, and feeling are only in the brain. Intrepid mind-body researchers are providing the evidence to change opinion.

Foremost among them is Candace Pert, Ph.D., former chief of brain biochemistry at the Clinical Neuroscience Branch, National Institute of Mental Health. Pert found that neuropeptides—chemical substances such as beta endorphin—and their receptors appear not only in the brain, but throughout the body. She calls them "the keys to the biochemistry of emotion."[12] They form a communication link between the brain, the immune system, and our emotions. A lot of this chemical interaction takes place at nodal points where sensory information (touch) comes in, such as the dorsal horn of the spinal cord, and where neuropeptide receptors are located.

Pert's work expands the concept of the primitive limbic system—the seat of emotions in the brain—to the whole body. Memory researchers, such as Marvin Mishkin, Ph.D., chief of the Laboratory of Neuropsychology, National Institute of Mental Health, have been able to follow the flow of information from sensory receptors on the skin through the spinal cord

Your body is just the place your memory calls home.

—Deepak Chopra

and brain stem into different areas of the brain. There information activates the limbic system to lay down memories—in this case, images of tactile experiences. In other words, memory doesn't occur by itself in the brain, nor is it confined to a particular site in the brain. It depends on communication with everything that is happening in the body. Billions of neurons (nerve cells) and trillions of synapses (connecting points) are our body's telephone lines.

"Memory resides nowhere, and in every cell," says Saul Schanberg, Ph.D., professor of pharmacology and biological psychiatry at Duke University Medical Center. "It's about two thousand times more complicated than we ever imagined."[13]

Various bodyways professionals explain body memory according to their own understandings. For example, Ilana Rubenfeld, originator of the Rubenfeld Synergy® Method, says, "The skin and muscles and nervous system record all the memories of how we were handled from the womb all through life. Body memory is a holding pattern, the muscles remembering a particular event or series of incidents in a pattern of tension [in response to abuse, injury, illness, shock, fear, anger]."[14] Such holding patterns can be embedded even before we're capable of verbalizing and understanding what is happening. That's because we know the world first through our bodies—through our senses, especially touch.

Clyde Ford, D.C., founder and director of the Institute for Somatosynthesis Training and Research, describes how our bodies remember through our sense perceptions:

> Somatic tissue functions as a secondary storage facility for the brain. An automobile accident shows us how this takes place. The sound of screeching tires, the sight of an upcoming tree, the touch of an out of control steering wheel are the sensory cues which cause us to hold our bodies tight and to experience fear in the few moments before impact. After impact, the continuing spasms and lingering fear are, in effect, stored images of these original cues. Here muscle spasm is a form of somatic memory arising from three different sources—seeing, hearing and touching.[15]

Other somatic practitioners shy away from using such terms as *body memory* because the whole idea of memory is presently under revision among scientists. Peter Levine, Ph.D., originator of Somatic Experiencing®, says, "Despite millions of dollars and the dedication of top people in the world to solve the problem of where is memory, they're no further than psychologist Karl Lashley was in his 1930 experiments with rats, when he said, 'I can't find it.' Memory per se doesn't exist."[16]

However, Levine adds, there are operations that all derive through the body sense—that is, something happens and the body responds. For ex-

Our bodies remember it all: our births, the delights and terrors of a lifetime, the journeys of our ancestors, the very evolution of life on earth.

—Kat Duff

ample, if there's an explosion, you'd probably react with contraction—shoulders go up and legs go limp—and then the body returns to where it was before. But if you're traumatized by the event, your responses won't complete. "It's like a snapshot—things look stuck in position," says Levine. "The 'body memory' is the frozen or incomplete response."[17]

John E. Upledger, an osteopath who teaches Craniosacral Therapy, finds that the tissues retain memory of the position your body was in when an injury or accident took place. He explains that the "energy of injury" can go farther into the body than the external location of injury. For example, a blow on the foot or ankle might go through the leg all the way to the pelvis. When it reaches its maximum penetration, it stops and forms a localized "ball" of foreign or external energy that doesn't belong there. If your body is unable to disintegrate it for normal healing to occur, the energy is compacted into a smaller and smaller ball in order to minimize the area where tissue function is disrupted. Eventually it becomes compressed into what he calls an "energy cyst." To release the energy from that cyst, your body needs to be in the precise position it was in when the external energy first entered. At that site, a practitioner will feel heat peak as a "therapeutic pulse" crescendoes. As that pulse decreases, a cooling occurs, followed by a lessening of pain and perceptible relaxation or softening of body tissues. You then might report an emotion such as fear or anger and a vivid memory of an accident or injury related to that area of your body.[18]

Touch alone, however, does not necessarily trigger the memory. The right conditions must be present. Being comfortable with a bodyways practitioner is crucial. You need to trust the person enough to be able to let down your defenses. Lying down helps, too. It can put you into a deeply relaxed state where you feel more vulnerable and your unconscious is more accessible. It also eliminates gravity's effect on the body, which allows the therapist to distinguish between muscular tension required to stand up and tension that is part of chronic armoring patterns. And you must be psychologically ready—that is, you must feel safe enough—to deal with the memory. "In order for the system to allow such memories to surface," says Paul Linden, Ph.D., the creator of Being In Movement®, "it has to know that the person has been strengthened enough to be able to face and survive the memories."[19]

Knowing that it's possible for you to be retraumatized, sensitive therapists do not push you, but respect, guide, and trust your body to make the decision on how much to wake up. Blocking out the memory may have been the means of surviving the original trauma. Unblocking it and releasing its tension calls for consensus between what Upledger calls the "censor" and the "efficiency expert" operating inside you. The censor wants memories to stay buried so as to protect you from hurtful information. But keeping the lid on exacts a price—pain, disability, unhappiness, chronic anger, irritability, lack of self-esteem, and so on. The efficiency expert prefers to

The skin is no more separated from the brain than the surface of a lake is separate from its depths; the two are different locations in a continuous medium. . . . The brain is a single functional unit, from cortex to fingertips to toes. To touch the surface is to stir the depths.

—Deane Juhan

The body tells the story. It is, in fact, a living autobiography.

—Elaine Mayland

In our bodies, in this moment, there live the seed impulses of the change and spiritual growth we seek, and to awaken them we must bring our awareness into the body, into the here and now.

—Pat Ogden

have memories brought to the surface and resolved, knowing it would lead to all kinds of healings—of depression, anxiety, bad relationships, addictions, eating disorders, career struggles, and physical ailments.

Many practitioners warn against eliciting memories through strongly cathartic methods. They create a dependency on continuing catharsis, says Levine, because in a sense the catharsis becomes a high. You get relief by releasing energy, even exploding with endorphins and catecholamines (adrenalinelike substances). But a couple of hours, days, or weeks later, you can be back in the trauma vortex, needing to release again, and thus setting an addictive pattern. Levine believes these methods also encourage the emergence of so-called false memories.[20]

The whole question of whether memories are true or false hinges on recent theories about how the brain works. Contrary to a long-standing popular myth, we do not accurately remember people, places, things, and events, according to Israel Rosenfield, M.D., author of *The Invention of Memory: A New View of the Brain* (Basic Books, 1988). They are not imprinted permanently on our brain, the way a video camera records events and leaves no room for imagination or prevarication.

The research of Nobel prize–winning neuroscientist Gerald Edelman suggests that memory is a creative or reconstructive act rather than a perfect reproduction of what was. Instead of calling up carefully filed and stored traces, as in a computer, the brain uses procedures that restructure the past in terms of present needs and desires. It chooses images, sounds, other sensations, and interpretations registered in the past, then combines them to produce what we call a "memory." This memory may be a veridical depiction of something that happened. But just as easily it can be a personal creation, using data from various incidents.[21]

What makes it feel so real, scientists say, is the arousal of the limbic portion of the brain, which mediates emotions. Particularly in trauma, the associated emotions and sensations are intense, and because of that the experience is fragmented, says Levine. Consequently, only fragments of a remembered traumatic event are likely to be entirely accurate. Other parts may be derived from elsewhere.[22]

Levine explains that when the nervous system is aroused, it goes through the basket of stored images to try to explain the arousal. Some correlate well with what actually happened; others are a mixture of many different things. For example, if you're aroused while reading a magazine or watching a movie or talking with a therapist, all of that goes into the basket as well. As a result, the next time your nervous system is aroused, your experience may involve all of these things—the real event, the movie, something the therapist said.

"It comes up more like in a dream," says Levine. "We don't consider dreams literal, but when we're awake and have arousal associated with different images, it feels like memory. The more activation, the more it feels like a true memory. But all memory is a waking dream."[23]

The ultimate goal of working with body memories is neither remembering facts nor reexperiencing emotions. Healing requires changing our relationship to our memories. Transformation comes from investing the traumatic event with a new meaning—Rubenfeld calls it "rescripting." It necessitates replacing unsuccessful episodes with successful ones and imprinting new neuromuscular patterns. And in the process, we establish or reestablish somatic, emotional, and psychological resources.

## THE PRACTICE OF AWARENESS

Some of the body-centered psychotherapies have incorporated awareness practice as a way to bring clients closer to their living experience rather than staying removed from it in their intellect. Borrowing this focus from somatic and movement education as well as meditation, they help clients to center their attention in their own bodies. It is equally useful in bodyways. You can apply it to enhance any session or, for that matter, anything else that you do, whether lying down, standing, sitting, or moving.

Awareness practice will enable you to increase your attention and aliveness in the here and now. It will also develop and strengthen your self-confidence. The philosophy of such practices is that "you are the world expert on your life, your body, and your mind, or at least you are in the best position to become that expert if you observe carefully," says Jon Kabat-Zinn, associate professor of medicine of the Division of Preventive and Behavioral Medicine at the University of Massachusetts Medical School.[24]

Spiritual traditions have been teaching awareness practices for millennia. There is nothing esoteric or sectarian about them, and they have no relationship to any religious dogma. They are neither Eastern nor Western but universal—the direct and immediate awareness of your sensory experience, exactly as it is, from moment to moment.

Awareness does not have to be formalized as a meditation practice, but if you have no experience in it, Mindfulness Meditation is a good place to start. Although the Buddha originally taught it in India twenty-five hundred years ago, today you can find it not only in Western retreat centers but also in health programs. Both anecdotal reports and research evidence indicate the therapeutic psychological and physiological effects of meditation, including reduction in blood pressure, cholesterol, and the severity of asthma, migraine, and chronic pain.[25] At the University of Massachusetts Medical Center's Stress Reduction Clinic, which he founded and directs, Kabat-Zinn teaches Mindfulness Meditation to patients to help them cope with chronic pain, illness, and stress.

The mind's first step to self-awareness must be through the body.

—George Sheehan

Awareness, insight, and indeed health as well, ripen on their own if we are willing to pay attention in the moment and remember we have only moments to live.

—Jon Kabat-Zinn

# Experience: The Practice of Mindfulness

You can begin with the instructions that follow or try others ☞ listed under "Resources," pages 130–131. To become more skillful, it is important to have the guidance of a competent teacher. You can find such individuals through retreat centers listed in "Resources." Remember, your body is to you what an instrument is to a musician. Until you become well practiced and masterly, whether of the flute or of mindfulness, it is helpful when someone more experienced has a hand in your training.

Start by sitting with your eyes closed, preferably in a quiet place where you won't be interrupted or distracted. Choose a time when you can feel most present, alert, and at ease, a time when your schedule is not pulling you into the future and excessive tiredness is not pulling you into sleep. Later, you can try the practice anywhere with eyes open: waiting for a red light to change or traffic to move, standing on line at a supermarket, washing dishes, or walking in the woods. At first, set aside fifteen minutes; then, as you can, add five to ten minutes to each sitting, working up to one hour.

Breathe naturally, without forcing. This practice is not a breathing exercise, but rather the cultivation of awareness by observing the bodily sensations that arise within the movement of the breath. Neither is this a meditation that uses an image or mantra to develop concentration (as in Transcendental Meditation, or T.M.).

Sit comfortably on a chair or cushion on the floor. Keep your back straight, in an alert, yet restful position. This is a posture of dignity, rather than rigidity. Let your hands comfortably repose together in your lap or separately on your knees. Allow your eyes to close gently. Allow your breath to come and go naturally—to breathe itself—for several minutes. Then take a few moments to check for possible tension in various areas of your body—eyes, forehead, jaw, neck, shoulders, chest, hands, pelvis, knees, feet. Bring a gentle awareness to each place, letting it relax and soften.

Begin to notice where in your body you can feel the movement of the breath most distinctly while still allowing the breath to remain natural. This may be in the abdomen,

The simplest way to define mindfulness is to say it is nonjudgmental attention to everyday things in your life. Foremost is the breath—the changing bodily sensations around your abdomen, chest, or nostrils during an in-breath and an out-breath. You may observe lightness, pressure, expansion, warmth, heaviness, or coolness.

Mindfulness is also awareness of your five senses—hearing, touching, seeing, tasting, and smelling. It is awareness of bending your body as you go to sit down, leaning forward as you get out of a chair, lifting your feet as you walk, placing a dish in the sink, or raising a toothbrush to your mouth. And it is awareness of the passing parade of thoughts—planning a dinner, worrying about finances, remembering an argument, or rehearsing what you'll say to your employer. In mindfulness, you note all these things with-chest, or at the tip of the nostrils. It is important to choose only one of these areas and maintain it as the "primary anchor" of mindfulness because it serves as the basis for calmness to arise.

Now bring awareness to the beginning of an "in" breath, sustaining mindfulness there as much as you can until the end of the "in" breath. Do the same with the "out" breath. You may find it helpful to make a silent mental note of "in" or "rising" as you experience the in-breath, and "out" or "falling" as you experience the out-breath. This technique of mental noting strengthens your practice by clearly connecting awareness with the physical sensations of the breath. It also helps in focusing your attention more precisely.

After a few breaths, your mind will probably wander to one of the six sense doors (the five physical senses and the mind). As soon as you are aware of this, acknowledge where you are present in that very moment with a silent mental note about whatever is actually happening—wandering, thinking, hearing, pain, itching, coolness, sadness, happiness, smelling, fantasizing, etc. This wandering of the mind is normal. It's important to be compassionate and patient with yourself. Just remain relaxed, yet alert, and be willing to begin again and again. Gently bring mindfulness back to the primary anchor of the breath, experiencing each breath as fully as possible and continuing to note "in/out" or "rising/falling."

Try to maintain balance in your practice. By neither striving too much nor leaning toward laziness, you may encounter joy in this exploration. Over time, this training stabilizes your attention and builds energy. You can gradually cultivate inner calm and centeredness within the changing rhythms of the breath and, by extension, within the changing rhythms of life. From this inner calm, you can clearly comprehend skillful thought, speech, and action in the world, which can lead to incalculable peace and understanding.

—Courtesy of Kamala Masters, Vipassana teacher.

out condemning, criticizing, blaming, pushing away, interpreting, belittling, berating, elaborating, comparing, translating, liking, or disliking them. You don't label these as good or bad, right or wrong, better or worse. You directly experience whatever processes are going on in your body and mind. You shift from living in the realm of concepts, ideology, conditioning, and running commentaries to cultivating a life of fully experiencing the physical truths of the body.

In doing so, you have the opportunity to stop looking at yourself as a problem to correct and see the goodness, strength, and intelligence you can nourish. Mindfulness Meditation is not a self-improvement project. We don't use it "to throw ourselves away and become something better," says American Buddhist nun Pema Chödron. "It's about befriending who we are already."[26]

My task is really not
to change myself but to
become familiar with
who I am.

—Maureen Cook

Yet the precise awareness of exactly what you are doing moment to moment without judgment provides the spaciousness in which transformation can occur. In the present moment, the only moment you ever have, you learn to hear your original voices, the voices that are not conditioned by all the shoulds and fads. In stillness and in movement, you learn to be at home in your body in a natural, spontaneous way. You feel the physicalness of being alive—your feet pressing on the ground, a cool breeze caressing your skin, warmth suffusing your chest, tightness grabbing your gut, your arms slicing through water. Sensitized to your body, you become attuned to subtle things, to deeper layers, and thus to the body's wisdom. You catch imbalances earlier. You don't wait until you're past the point of no return and in a state of disease. You hear the message and act accordingly.

It's like being a redwood house along the coast of northern California. Even when left unpainted and exposed to the salt air, rain, and sun, the redwood does not get destroyed, but turns a characteristic, beautiful gray. However, if that house was painted, it would have to be scraped and repainted over and over in order to maintain a certain look because the elements would eat through the colors. Through mindfulness, you can get down to your unpainted self, and you can weather whatever conditions come to bear on you. You too can remain naturally beautiful.

When engaging in any of the bodyways, awareness of your body is an essential tool in your healing journey. You begin to notice that your attention, not your effort, is what brings success. Relaxed attention, or the right amount of awareness, is like holding an egg: If you grasp it too tightly, it will crack; if you hold it too loosely, it will drop and break. Whether you do T'ai Chi, Yoga, Aikido, or Continuum, through such awareness you know how much effort is appropriate. Appropriate effort is what practitioners of the Alexander Technique, Feldenkrais Method, Hanna Somatic Education, Kinetic Awareness, and other functional approaches teach. As the Taoists say, you will learn how to let "not doing" be your doing.

To be aware is the unity
of knowing and doing.

—Seymour Kleinman

## RESOURCES:

Mindfulness Meditation is also known as Insight Meditation or Vipassana.

**Books:** Joseph Goldstein, *The Experience of Insight: A Simple and Direct Guide to Buddhist Meditation* (Shambhala, 1993); Joseph Goldstein and Jack Kornfield, *Seeking the Heart of Wisdom: The Path of Insight Meditation* (Shambhala, 1987); Jon Kabat-Zinn, *Full Catastrophe Living: Using the Wisdom of Your Body and Mind to Face Stress, Pain, and Illness* (Delta, 1990); Thich Nhat Hanh, *The Miracle of Mindfulness: A Manual on Meditation* (Beacon, 1992).

**Audiovisual:** Dharma Seed Tape Library, Box 66, Wendell Depot, MA 01380, (800) 969-SEED for catalogue; "Guided Body Scan Meditation" and "Guided Sitting Meditation," audiocassettes by Jon Kabat-Zinn, from Stress Reduction Tapes, P.O. Box 547, Lexington, MA 02173, or Institute of Noetic Sciences, (800) 383-1586; "The Inner Art of Meditation," Jack Kornfield, 6 audiocassettes, and "The Present Moment: A Retreat on the Practice of Mindfulness," Thich Nhat Hanh, 6 audiocassettes, both through Sounds True, (800) 333-9185; *The Mindful Way,* videotape by Bhante Gunaratana, 50 mins., VHS, Bhavana Society, (304) 856-3241, fax (304) 856-2111.

**Retreats and classes:** There are many retreat centers and classes in North America. For listings here and abroad, see *Inquiring Mind,* a semiannual journal of the Vipassana community, P.O. Box 9999, North Berkeley Station, Berkeley, CA 94709, (by donation, $10 or more); and *Vipassana Newsletter,* P.O. Box 51, Shelburne Falls, MA 01379.

In the Northeast, contact Insight Meditation Society, 1230 Pleasant St., Barre, MA 01005-9707, (508) 355-4378, and Vipassana Meditation Center, P.O. Box 51, Shelburne Falls, MA 01370-0051, (413) 625-2160, fax (413) 625-2170. In the Southeast, Southern Dharma Retreat Center, Route 1, Box 34H, Hot Springs, NC 28743, (704) 622-7112. In the Northwest, Northwest Dharma Association, 311 W. McGraw, Seattle, WA 98119, (206) 286-9060. In northern California, Spirit Rock, P.O. Box 909, Woodacre, CA 94973, (415) 488-0164, fax (415) 488-0170, and California Vipassana Center, P.O. Box 1167, North Fork, CA 93643, (209) 877-4386. In southern California, Vipassana Support Institute, 4070 Albright Ave., Los Angeles, CA 90066, (310) 915-1943.

# PART III

# A Guide to Bodyways

C H A P T E R     7

# How to Use This Guide

This guide to bodyways is born of more than twenty years' involvement. At first I read about bodyways and tried to practice them on my own. Then I attended classes and workshops. In some cases, I also entered training programs so that I could be a practitioner and teacher, privately as well as at retreat and fitness centers and educational institutions. Many of the people I have studied with and/or been "handled" by have become well known and respected in their particular systems. For a historical and cultural understanding of the role bodyways has played, I did extensive research into the history of Western and Eastern medicine and indigenous healing arts around the world. I also observed and spoke with native practitioners in many different cultures, and experienced the work myself. As a contributing editor to *East/West* (now *Natural Health*) and *Massage Therapy Journal,* I had the opportunity to interview individuals recognized for their innovative contributions to the field. I have been writing about them or other therapists, methods, cross-cultural traditions, and trends since 1980.

My impressions of bodyways are based in part on the people whom I have worked with and interviewed over the years and while preparing this book. Descriptions of the different systems' theories, techniques, and benefits are derived from how their founders and practitioners have expressed them. If some of the ideas sound esoteric, keep in mind that they often are metaphors for more intangible realities of the body. If, for whatever reasons, a particular way of understanding the body doesn't appeal to you, don't dismiss the practice simply because of that. Whether the body has seven segments or seventeen, energy channels or blood vessels, doesn't matter. No single theory is the absolute truth about the way we function. These interpretations are not my own; I have tried to report them accurately, and my descriptions were reviewed by leading practitioners of each method.

To know oneself as a body is more important, at this moment in history, than to read the words of all the wise men who have ever lived.

—Marco Vassi

*Our body heals best when we're living in the present.*

—Christiane Northrup

While the introductory overview for each category of bodyways is my own synthesis, how I've categorized the different bodyways is also based on the systems' self-referential explanations. These categories are not a clear-cut straitjacket that rigidly confines bodyways. Rather, they constitute an imperfect form that is open to debate and change. In many cases, a particular practice easily could belong in one or another category. For instance, Body-Mind Centering, the Mensendieck System, the Pilates Method, and others in the chapter "Functional Approaches" could appear instead in "Western Movement Arts"; Zero Balancing could be in "Convergence Systems" or "Other Energetic Systems"; Being In Movement could fall into "Functional Approaches," "Western Movement Arts," or "Convergence Systems."

## WHAT'S INCLUDED, WHAT'S NOT, WHY NOT

You probably will recognize the names of some bodyways instantly, while others may be new to you. The better-known systems are usually the core from which others have emerged and expanded, combined, synthesized, cross-fertilized, or diverged in some way. Think of this core system as a tree that grows branches. But keep in mind that even the trunk sprang forth not on its own but from roots in the ground. Every new bodyway that arises is based on what came before it. For example, Rolfing is the tree from which all structural approaches have grown, but osteopathy was a major influence on Ida Rolf.

I've included little-known practices so that you can learn about those I consider rising stars in the field. Also, a few are more available in Europe or Asia but not nearly as prevalent in North America. In several instances, despite repeated efforts, I had difficulty gathering information about various practices altogether, and thus they don't appear here. And with so many new systems emerging each year, I probably missed some. But in no way have I intended to slight any practice. I welcome being informed of other bodyways. Nevertheless, it's impossible to describe, or even mention, every single therapy or discipline that has arisen lately or is popular in another part of the world. Doing so would have made this book as unwieldy as an encyclopedia. The test of time will show us which endure because they truly have something effective to offer.

As I explain in "Deciding on a Bodyway," the Western group of practices consists of massage and other Western-style methods, structural approaches, functional approaches, and movement arts. The Eastern group encompasses Chinese, Japanese, Indian, Thai, and Kurdish energetic practices, along with Western-generated versions and Eastern movement arts. A third group, convergence systems for physical-emotional integration, borrows and combines from both.

Originally I wanted to include body-based psychotherapies as well, for in working with the psyche, they include the body's behavior. However, after much research and discussion, I realized that they deserve a book of their own. For the same reason, I have left out as well mystical traditions that incorporate the body, such as Kabbalah and Sufism. However, the chapter "Psychological Dimensions of Bodyways" examines how the development of psychology informs bodyways and lists body-centered psychotherapies. It also discusses the practice of awareness, or Mindfulness Meditation, for it is integral to functional approaches and useful for all bodyways.

Nor have I incorporated certain systems that once were innovative and relatively unknown but which have become, in some cases, mainstream modalities. These include osteopathy, chiropractic, biofeedback, and physical therapy. Osteopathy was created by Andrew Still, a mid-nineteenth-century doctor who was disillusioned with the medical practices of his era. It is based on the theory that disease is due chiefly to a loss of structural integrity, which can be restored by manipulation. In addition to a regular medical education, which allows them to prescribe medications and treat infectious disease, osteopaths spend hundreds of hours studying the muscular and skeletal systems. Like Still, Daniel David Palmer believed that the body, when in balance, would heal itself. Palmer was a magnetic healer before he invented chiropractic in 1895. He developed specific levered manipulations of the spine to relieve impingement on the nervous system caused by subluxations (displacements) of the vertebrae. Chiropractic is now a primary health-care profession. In 1905, after researching the practice of *napravit* in Czechoslovakia, American chiropractor Oakley G. Smith founded yet another manipulative therapy, naprapathy, which focuses on the connective tissue rather than bones.

Biofeedback training uses machines to track and reflect such bodily functions as heart rate, muscle tension, brain waves, hand and finger temperature, and skin conductivity to help you gain greater conscious control over your autonomic (involuntary) nervous system. Physical therapy grew out of massage therapy for rehabilitation of injured World War I soldiers. Today physical therapists combine both hands-on and mechanical means to treat a variety of conditions in clinical settings.

Three more systems that do not fit here are naturopathy, homeopathy, and aromatherapy. Naturopathy emphasizes a wide range of natural healing agents and avoids drugs and surgery; body manipulation is only one aspect of treatment. Homeopathy, founded by eighteenth-century German physician Samuel Hahnemann, has no hands-on component. It treats disease symptoms by administering minute doses of substances that in large amounts would otherwise cause them—the Law of Similars, or like treats like. Aromatherapy uses aromatic essential oils extracted from wild or cul-

So the discipline is to bring yourself back to the experiences and expression of your body, fully and constantly.

—Barbara Dilley

As the breathing deepens, the whole body comes alive, ready for action.

—Mabel E. Todd

tivated plants. Some bodyways practitioners employ such oils in massage and for inhalation in the room where they work for certain physiological effects, such as sedation or stimulation.

The art of breathing is essential in personal development and optimal health and integral to bodyways. It is also easily a book unto itself. (☞ see "Breathwork Resources.") Different breathwork practices encourage different kinds of breathing for different ends: to energize and enhance alertness, relax and reduce tension, deal with emotions, release blocked energy, free creativity, and balance the nervous system. Body practitioners generally include attention to the breath in their work.

## BREATHWORK RESOURCES:

Our breathing reflects every emotional or physical effort and every disturbance.

—Moshe Feldenkrais

For information on Holotropic Breathwork (deep and rapid breathing co-ordinated with dramatic sounds and rhythms to induce psychedelic states) contact Stanislav Grof, M.D., Holotropics, 38 Miller Ave., Suite 158, Mill Valley, CA 94941, (415) 721-9891. For the work of Ilse Middendorf, considered Europe's premier authority on breathing and its relationship to physical movement and health, contact The Middendorf Breath Institute, 198 Mississippi, San Francisco, CA 94107, (415) 255-2174. For information about *pranayama,* or yogic breathing, ☞ see "Yoga Resources," page 350.

**Books and audiocassettes:** Jonathon Daemion, *The Healing Power of Breath: An Introduction to Wholistic Breath Therapy* (Prism/Avery, 1989); Jane Huang, *The Primordial Breath, vol. II, An Ancient Chinese Way of Prolonging Life Through Breath Control* (Original, 1990); Gay Hendricks, *Conscious Breathing: Breathwork for Health, Stress Release, and Personal Mastery* (Bantam, 1995); and "The Art of Breathing and Centering," 60 mins. audiotape, Audio Renaissance, (800) 266-2834; Ilse Middendorf, *The Perceptible Breath* (Junsermann Verlag, 1990), book and two audiocassettes, Feldenkrais Resources, (800) 765-1907 or (510) 540-7600; Carola Speads, *Ways to Better Breathing* (Felix Morrow, 1986); Carl Stough and Reece Stough, *Dr. Breathing: The Story of Breathing Coordination* (The Stough Institute, 1981).

## BODYWAY ENTRIES

In each chapter, a discussion of the foundation underlying each group of bodyways precedes the individual entries. These discussions give you an overview for understanding the philosophy that makes these bodyways similar and seeing what distinguishes them from another category of practices. The entries themselves indicate how bodyways within a group are also different from one another.

Entries explain the theory behind a major system, the goal or intention of the work, the techniques used to attain it, practitioner training, and the benefits reported. I have noted where there's a body of research to support these claims. Some entries include Experiences, to give you a taste of the practice. There are also occasional anecdotes and mini-biographies of the individuals who created particular methods. At the end of each entry you will find Resources: related books, periodicals, audiovisual materials, institutes, schools, and associations. The listing is not comprehensive; rather it is a beginning to help you get started in your exploration. Because the field is evolving so rapidly, the information in the entries, especially as regards training and resources, is subject to change.

Because of space constraints, I do not describe each and every bodyway in detail. The extent of coverage varies for several reasons. In some cases, the bodyway is the foremost or original version among a group of similar practices, or it is long-established and widespread, with practitioners or teachers available across the country. In other cases, a therapy or system may not be as well known, but it has the potential for growth and represents the cutting edge in the field. In yet other instances, a particular method is simple and straightforward enough not to need a lengthier explanation. The number of words devoted to any one bodyway does not constitute an endorsement of how effective or preferable it is. Only you can be the judge of that as it applies to your own likes and needs.

# CHAPTER 8

# Western Structure and Function:

## Traditional Massage and Contemporary Therapies

The body is in itself organized to recover, so if you help the circulation to normalize, and recover the sensitivity by stimulating the skin, then the body begins to recover in its own way. The brain needs stimulation from the body.

—Gerda Alexander

Western bodyways practiced today are based on an understanding of human structure and function as it has evolved in Western medicine. It is founded on both empirical and scientific information. Generally, experimental research follows and confirms the clinical experiences and observations of many different health practitioners. Scientific knowledge has emerged (and continues to emerge) through a long process of reducing the whole to its constituent units, then determining the purpose of each one and how they all interrelate. In medical schools even today, aspiring physicians learn about the body by dissecting a cadaver, the way mechanics study how an engine operates by dismantling it down to the smallest screw.

## COMPARING MEDICAL MODELS

In contrast, physicians of traditional Eastern systems have learned almost exclusively by observing living human beings. This difference is reflected also in the diagnosis, explanation, and treatment of illness. Western science explains the body and how it works in impersonal, physiochemical terms. Using an engineering approach, it regards our health difficulties as mechanical trouble, which requires technical manipulation of faulty parts. Whereas the Eastern energetic view sees a disorder as reflecting imbalance in the whole body, rather than as signaling only individual symptoms, Western medicine treats the condition by addressing a particular body part—for instance, the eyes, stomach, or heart. Eastern medical traditions strive to reestablish the flow of a person's overall life energy so that the body's ability to heal itself can overcome the illness.

Neither the Western approach nor the Eastern approach is wholly right or wrong. The body is neither entirely a conglomeration of discrete elements nor only a flow of energy. Each represents a different side of the same coin. In the language of physics, we are both particle (a piece of matter) and wave (moving energy). Eastern bodyways begin with the premise that a person has an energetic structure and function. The starting point for Western bodyways is the body's material structure and function. Nevertheless, a major principle for both approaches is circulation. If any system—energy, respiratory, digestive, or muscular—gets blocked, stagnates, or stops working altogether, it will adversely affect movement in the others.

Even though Western bodyways are based on the sciences of anatomy and physiology, that does not mean their practitioners necessarily see you as a human machine, an aggregate of components that together make up various systems. To a great extent, the concepts of interconnectedness, energy, and mind-body interaction now pervade Western practices. Body therapists know that no part or system works in isolation. Since everything in the body is interdependent, handling one aspect—muscles, for example—has to influence favorably other areas as well, such as increasing circulation of blood and lymph, soothing nerves, or realigning bones. A shift in the energetic structure can translate into a shift in the physical structure and vice versa.

All of the body's systems literally touch and affect one another. You can feel this by using one hand to grab the opposite arm. What do your fingers feel? Are you touching only skin? If you feel thickness, you're also contacting muscle. If you press deeper, you feel the hardness of bone. The fact that you sense the pressure of your grip means that nerve endings are receiving and transmitting. If you notice the color of your skin change, you've touched your blood vessels. And you were also pressing on lymph vessels.

## The Soft Tissues

The aim of Western bodyways is to improve functioning of these different systems. Most of them do so by accessing the soft tissues of the body—muscles and fascia. In contrast, chiropractic and osteopathy adjust the hard tissues, or bones.

The muscles body therapists manipulate are the type called skeletal or striated. They're the ones that make up your body's shape. Unlike smooth muscle tissue, which is present in the walls of visceral organs and blood vessels and which contracts involuntarily, skeletal muscles are under your conscious control. Because they attach to bones at joints, when they contract, bones move. Their rapid, short-term, strong contractions depend on nerve impulses. Without messages from the nervous system, these muscles atrophy and die. Skeletal muscles are the primary focus of most massage.

Although we tend to think of muscles as composing the greatest percentage of body structure, connective tissue, or fascia, is the most widely distributed of all the body's tissues. It appears everywhere. As a binding tissue, it joins one type of tissue to another: organs to organs, muscles to bones (as tendons), and bones to other bones (as ligaments).

Superficial or subcutaneous fascia, which lies directly below the skin, stores fat and is richly embedded with nerve endings. Bindegewebsmassage is concerned chiefly with this layer. Deep fascia is a three-dimensional continuous web of tough connective tissue from head to foot. A thin, fibrous sheath or envelope, it surrounds and supports skeletal muscle, nerves, blood vessels, organs, even cells themselves. ☞ See illustration on page 189. Most structural bodyways, such as Rolfing, manipulate deep fascia. The deepest fascia encases the central nervous system and the brain, forming the dura mater (the tough, fibrous membrane that envelops the brain and spinal cord) of the craniosacral system. Connective tissue also plays a role in the production of new blood corpuscles, the removal of worn-out ones from the bloodstream, and immunity against disease.

## It's All in the Emphasis

Each of the Western methods puts its attention on a distinct body system with the intention of relieving certain dysfunctions and achieving well-being. For instance, Manual Lymph Drainage restores movement in the lymphatic system, while Trigger Point Therapy addresses the neuromuscular system. To give you a better sense of how Western bodyways can help you, I've gathered them into separate chapters, rather than listed them in an A-to-Z manner. Each grouping reflects a different orientation.

In this chapter we'll examine everything from general massage to highly specialized massage therapies that tend to be pathology-oriented, diagnosis-related, and treatment-specific. Some of them originated with medical doctors. In the chapters that follow, we'll look at the various approaches that emphasize your body's structure and those that concentrate on how you function or move. We'll also examine Western movement arts. This division should enable you to decide on which way of working might best suit your needs.

## RESOURCES:

**Books:** For a better understanding and experience of your anatomy and physiology: N. Elson and Wynn Kapit, *The Anatomy Coloring Book* (HarperCollins, 1977); Wynn Kapit and Robert Macey, *The Physiology Coloring Book* (HarperCollins, 1987); Mabel E. Todd, *The Thinking Body* (Dance Horizons, 1959); Andrea Olsen and Caryn McHose, *BodyStories: A Guide to Experiential Anatomy* (Station Hill, 1991); Irene Dowd, *Taking Root to Fly: Ten Articles on Functional Anatomy* (Contact, 1990); Deane Juhan, *Job's Body: A Handbook for Bodywork* (Station Hill, 1987).

# Massage

Does your back lock up in spasm, your head ache, your feet hurt, your jaw clench? Do your legs cramp, your joints stiffen, your shoulders tighten? Are you lacking healthy touch in your life? Do you hate your body and treat yourself poorly? Are you grieving over the loss of a loved one? Are you tied up in knots? Do you need to lose or gain weight? While not a panacea, massage can help to some degree directly or indirectly in all of these conditions.

*Massage* is only a seven-letter word, but this manipulation of soft tissues has performed wonders for thousands of years throughout the world. It is the great-great-great-great-grandmother of all the other bodyways because it is a primal, instinctive act to make yourself or someone else feel better through touch.

Massage has been the practice not only of massage professionals but also of medical staff, midwives, sports trainers, shamans, and teachers of dance and martial arts. Native Americans from Argentina to Alaska have used it during pregnancy, in healing ceremonies, and in the treatment of psychological disorders. Ancient Greek, Roman, and Arabic physicians prescribed it for everything from insomnia and gynecological problems to paralysis and hysteria. Their medical treatises note in detail how and when massage should be administered, including as part of a sports regimen.[1] Even today, writers continue to quote the advice of Hippocrates (ca. 460–ca. 377 B.C.E.), the father of Western medicine, from *On Articulations:* "The physician must be experienced in many things, and among others, in friction. Friction can bind a joint that is too loose and loosen a joint that is too rigid."

However, despite its effectiveness, in the West massage fell out of popularity at different times for a variety of reasons. The Catholic Church regarded the body as a repository of sin. It condemned any practices that might be construed as pleasurable or erotic and might thus lead to further transgression. Many of the "witches" that burned at the stake during the Middle Ages were undoubtedly midwives and other healers who included massage in their work. Still, despite the long, strong arm of the Church, by the 1600s several physicians, especially the French surgeon Ambroise Paré, revived interest in the therapeutic benefits of massage.

Starting in the 1800s, a renaissance of massage finally took hold in the Western world, with only brief intervals of disfavor. As a result of the work of Per Henrik Ling of Sweden and Johan Georg Mezger of Holland, many medical doctors in North America and Europe referred their patients for massage treatments. Some even did massage themselves and wrote about it extensively in books and medical journals. After the Civil War, two Swedes opened the first massage therapy clinics in the United States. The one in Washington, D.C., included among its clientele members of Congress and Presidents Benjamin Harrison and Ulysses S. Grant.

In the early decades of the twentieth century, a nurse's training included massage. It was also the foundation from which physical therapy developed during World War I. But when the pressure of time and the high cost of medical attention increased, health professionals opted for technological advances over labor-intensive hands-on work. For a while, massage nearly became a forgotten healing art in America. With the flowering of the alternative health-care field, we have been experiencing another rebirth of massage, including among nurses and in hospital settings.

Today we have a multitude of massage therapies—everything from the traditional Swedish system to contemporary variations that are deeper or lighter, more specific or more generalized. Among them are sports massage, Vodder Manual Lymph Drainage, Trigger Point Therapy, Esalen, Bindegewebsmassage, Pfrimmer Deep Muscle Therapy®, and Craniosacral Therapy. Some stick strictly to Western anatomy and physiology; others reach beyond a purely medical or remedial approach to encompass emotional and spiritual aspects as well.

The term *massage therapist* may indicate that the practitioner does a basic Swedish massage or, more likely, combines several kinds. Every time I learned a new system, I mixed and matched techniques according to what my clients preferred or needed and what I enjoyed doing.

How massage therapists work reflects the kind of training they've had. Programs vary greatly from school to school in terms of methods taught, classroom and internship time, and depth and breadth of knowledge. Someone who provides a relaxation massage does not need as much education as someone who works with athletes to help condition them and recover from injuries. A basic course in massage would include the fundamental Swedish routine and may incorporate other practices. In some places certification can come after 150 hours; in others, instruction can range up to 2,200 hours. Massage graduates add additional skills through workshops, for example, in Neuromuscular and Craniosacral Therapies.

> The human body . . . A chemical laboratory, a power house. Every movement, voluntary or involuntary, full of secrets and marvels!
>
> —Theodor Herzl

## SWEDISH STYLE

Swedish or "traditional" massage is a combination of Ling's and Mezger's movements and strokes. It was the standard that nurses and physical therapists learned and applied in medical treatment. It was also popular in health spas and sports and country clubs. The stereotype we used to see in movies was of a hefty Scandinavian woman pummeling a person on the table or a sports trainer taking care of his prizefighter.

Nowadays massage therapists come in all different sizes and shapes and from all walks of life. To affect your body's structure and function, they rely on an assortment of strokes, manipulations, or movements, the way a painter begins with a palette of primary colors and blends them to achieve the desired effect. For example, massage therapists apply the classic Swedish strokes at varying depths and rhythms according to the results they seek, including stimulation, relaxation, and rehabilitation. They also take into account such factors as age, health status, strength, and certain conditions—premature birth, pregnancy, rigorous athletic regimen. Depending on how they work with you, you may need to be only partially undressed.

Based on experience and laboratory studies, massage therapists report that Swedish massage provides help for many ailments, too numerous to mention all. It achieves this because pressure applied to the skin and the contents beneath it sets up a chain of reactions through the whole body. The skin is our largest organ and is as important as the brain, heart, and lungs in keeping us alive. ☞ See box on skin, page 53. Stimulating the tissues through rhythmic pressure, stretching, and percussion has an effect on skin texture and appearance, blood vessels, lymph vessels, sensory receptors, sweat glands, muscles, fascia, bone, and, through reflex action, even visceral organs and respiratory structures.[2]

For example, if you suffer from indigestion or constipation, working

# Classic Swedish Strokes

Effleurage, or stroking, can feel like water gliding and rippling over your body. Practitioners work with their palms, thumbs, fingertips, or forearms. Repeated rhythmically with light or superficial pressure, this even, long, flowing stroke has a lulling or hypnotic effect that leads to relaxation. When firm or deep in a centripetal direction—toward the heart—it stimulates circulation in the area stroked. As fresh blood flows to the tissues, it nourishes them with more oxygen and other nutrients. Movement of lymph also increases. Stroking additionally prepares the tissues for deeper work by warming them up. The soothing or sedating effect on muscles and nerves induces sleep and decreases pain.

Pétrissage, or kneading, is the rhythmic picking up of muscles away from the bone, then squeezing, pressing, and rolling them. Practitioners use both hands or two thumbs alternately to grasp the tissue to provide a continuous motion either in one place or while traveling gradually along a leg, an arm, a shoulder, etc. A more vigorous stroke, it improves blood circulation on a deeper level than effleurage. It helps reduce edema and decongest muscles by flushing out fluids and metabolic waste products and replacing them with a fresh supply of blood. It stimulates nerve endings, invigorating dancers and athletes before performance, and it cleanses tissues afterward to prevent stiffness and soreness.

Friction, or rubbing, consists of circular, linear, or transverse strokes done with the thumb, fingertips, palm, or heel of the hand. When superficial, it moves only over the surface of the skin. Deep transverse or cross-fiber friction, as in the Cyriax technique, penetrates beneath the skin and superficial fascia to broaden the underlying muscle by spreading the muscle fibers. It can also free muscles from adhesions and scar tissue formed after an injury. (Damaged muscle fibers often stick together or become glued onto ligaments, other tissues, or bones.) Friction helps loosen joints and tendons as well.

Tapotement is a series of percussive movements delivered as short, rapid strokes only to the fleshy parts of your body. Hacking uses the outside edge of the hand. Tapping uses the fingertips, lightly or firmly. Cupping or clapping uses cupped palms, with the fingers held close together. Beating or pummeling uses either loose or tight fists. In plucking, practitioners pick up small patches of flesh or loosely pinch them between the thumb and fingertips. Each technique has a stimulating or toning effect when applied for a few seconds. However, when prolonged, it leads to overstimulation, even exhaustion, of nerves and muscles.

Vibration with the hand or fingertips creates a rapid trembling, shaking sensation. It stimulates nerves and releases tight muscles; in the abdomen, it activates the digestive organs.

Compression is a rhythmic pumping movement on the muscle to induce it to relax and to sustain an increase in circulation for the reduction of accumulated metabolic wastes.

Range of motion is the passive exercising of limbs to mobilize joints whereby the practitioner rotates, flexes, and extends your body parts.

on the abdominal area can relieve tension and help move the bowels. It is not unusual to get immediate results. On several occasions after I had massaged along their colons, clients had to get up in the middle of a session to go to the bathroom. Percussive movements on the back can help loosen and clear phlegm and mucus from the lungs. Massage near a broken bone—but never directly on it—helps speed recovery by removing waste materials and nourishing the injured area with fresh oxygen and nutrients through increased blood circulation. It also helps keep unused muscles from atrophying and overused muscles from becoming tight and inflexible. For the swelling that develops either from a sprain or because of the reduced mobility that often occurs after surgery, massage can help drain the excess fluid. If you have trouble falling asleep, massage can help sedate your nervous system so you can rest. If you need to be alert, massage applied vigorously can stimulate you.

A University of Maryland study conducted by neurosurgeon Walker Robinson suggests that most over-the-counter pain relievers don't stop what's actually causing tension headaches, only make it easier to ignore the pain, whereas massage therapy is more effective at pain reduction. In another study, Michael I. Weintraub, clinical professor of neurology at New York Medical College, reports that massage dramatically relieved back pain in 86 percent of patients, whereas heat and ultrasound did not go deep enough to get to the source of pain. Several studies also indicate that massage therapy results in substantial cost savings in health care.[3]

> To neglect one's body for any other advantage in life is the greatest of follies.
>
> —Arthur Schopenhauer

# Lubricants

Except in certain techniques, massage therapists lubricate your skin to reduce friction, pinching, and pulling of body hair. They apply any of several kinds of lubricants, each with its own benefits and drawbacks.

Because oil is a slippery liquid that takes longer to be absorbed, it allows for smooth stroking. Vegetable oils—almond, apricot kernel, peanut, sunflower, safflower, olive, sesame, coconut—are the healthiest for the skin, though they can leave stains, and some may have a strong smell. Mineral oil (also known as baby oil) is clear, odorless, and does not stain. However, since it is a refined derivative of petroleum, it is not recommended for body use.

If oil feels too greasy, ask for lotion or cream. Lotion is soothing, but most brands contain some alcohol, which evaporates quickly and leaves a cooling sensation. That means the massage therapist has to keep reapplying the lotion in order to glide on your skin. A good compromise is mixing oil and lotion together. If you're allergic to both products, try powder or choose a bodyway that does not require any lubrication.

A body is forsaken when it becomes a source of pain and humiliation instead of pleasure and pride.

—Alexander Lowen

The most popular all-around benefit of general massage, of whatever style, is reduction of tension and stress. In a study of patients suffering from chronic inflammatory bowel disease (ulcerative colitis and Crohn's disease or ileitis), which stress exacerbates, massage therapy diminished the frequency of pain and disability episodes.[4] Other research demonstrates that massage lessens anxiety in child and adolescent psychiatric patients and also relieves depression. And even though it can't cure catastrophic illnesses, massage can provide the solace of feeling cared for. In a Touch Research Institute study with HIV-positive men, not only did their anxiety and stress levels go down, but also their level of natural killer (NK) cells rose—an indicator of an increase in immune response.[5]

What occurs as a result of massage is a shift in the autonomic nervous system. Activity of the sympathetic nervous system goes down—that is, the portion that mobilizes your body in arousal or emergency situations (fight-or-flight situations) by increasing heart and respiratory rates, shifting blood flow from the skin and visceral organs to the skeletal muscles, elevating blood sugar and adrenaline levels, and causing you to sweat and your pupils to dilate. On the other hand, activity of the parasympathetic nervous system goes up. This is the portion of the nervous system that is involved in processes of nurturing and rebuilding by slowing your heart and respiratory rates, shunting blood back from the skeletal muscles to the digestive organs, and stimulating secretions of the gastrointestinal tract, liver, and pancreas, which leads to peristalsis and emptying of the bowel and bladder. By reducing stress, massage can positively influence all of the body's systems.

## Enhancing Your Massage Experience

During a session of massage (or other bodyway), use what you've learned about yourself from earlier Experiences to help awaken neglected, despised, or frozen areas of your body, release tension, and receive nurturing. When the practitioner contacts such an area, bring your attention to it. As he or she soothes it with touch, try to give the same caring with your mind's hand. Allow the therapist's hands to give you a kind of connect-the-dots experience, in which touch unites all your different parts into a whole body.

## CONTEMPORARY ESALEN STYLE

Beginning in the 1960s, the Esalen Institute, considered the founding center of the human potential movement, experimented in evolving a more contemporary Western style of massage. At spring-fed hot baths on a cliff overlooking the Pacific Ocean at Big Sur, California, practitioners eschewed the strictly Swedish method, which they considered somewhat impersonal, clinical, mechanical, and vigorous. Instead, they created a more personalized, sensual, holistic approach that came to be

## Caution: Contraindications

Deep pressure, rubbing, and manipulation may aggravate specific ailments unless massage is recommended as tangential or complementary treatment. Such ailments include:

Broken bone, fracture, dislocation, or severe sprain
Acute infection
Inflammation of tissues and joints (when they are red, hot, swollen, and painful)
Injury or abrasion of the skin and skin diseases
Hemorrhaging
Large hernias
Cancerous tumors
Torn ligaments, tendons, or muscles
Cardiovascular conditions—advanced arteriosclerosis, aneurysms, severe varicose
    veins, thrombosis, acute phlebitis, embolism
Advanced diabetes
Osteoporosis
Frostbite
Kidney disease
Hypertension

A highly trained, knowledgeable massage therapist will know what to avoid completely, when to modify pressure, and how to work around, rather than directly on, the condition in order to provide therapeutic benefits. Whenever in doubt, talk to a doctor who is familiar with both bodyways and your particular disorder so you can make your own informed decision. You don't have to deprive yourself of touch if it is light or if you use practices that contact the energy field around your body but not your skin directly. They may be useful, soothing, and comforting, and they cause no harm. ☞ See Chapter 13: "Other Energetic Systems."

associated with general stress reduction and mind-body-spirit unity. As a personal service rather than a medical treatment, it fulfilled a different kind of need—to experience the sheer pleasure of nurturing touch. For fragmented bodies living in a fragmented world, it imparted a sense of wholeness.

An Esalen relaxation massage (or Swedish-Esalen style) uses the basic Swedish strokes but emphasizes the long, flowing, gliding movements for their sensual, sedating effect. Since this kind of massage does not address specific conditions, except the need to relax, don't expect a health assessment before your session. Depending on what facilities are available, you might be able to take a sauna or soak in a hot tub first to help soften your muscles. Unless you're more comfortable in underwear or a bathing suit, you'll lie naked on a padded massage table. The practitioner will drape you with a sheet or towels and uncover each area to be massaged. (Aromatic oils or lotions made with special herbs will enhance the relaxation process. If you have allergies, check first to avoid a reaction.)

The massage may begin with your feet or your head, the front of the body or the back, and proceeds until every part of you (except breasts and genitals) is stroked and kneaded. Practitioners follow their own sequences and rhythms. By the end of the session, you should feel pleasantly soothed. Although a relaxation massage is not the kind you need to heal a sports injury or alleviate a structural dysfunction, a state of deep rest and calm has an overall therapeutic effect. As anxiety and stress hormones diminish, your body can function more efficiently and pain can decrease. The good feelings from massage also may be due to a release of endorphins, the body's own opiates.

A simple relaxation massage is also what you can learn to share with loved ones. It's a great way to show your caring and concern for friends and family members and to exchange intimacy with your partner.

RESOURCES:

**For information and practitioners:** American Massage Therapy Association (AMTA), 820 Davis St., Suite 100, Evanston, IL 60201-4444, (708) 864-0123, fax (708) 864-1178 [request "A Guide to Massage Therapy in America," a free 24-page pamphlet]; Associated Bodywork and Massage Professionals (ABMP), 28677 Buffalo Park Rd., Evergreen, CO 80439, (303) 674-8478; International Massage Association and National Association of Massage Therapy, 3000 Connecticut Ave., NW, Suite 102, Washington, DC 20008, (202) 387-6555, fax (800) 776-NAMT, (202) 332-0531; Associated Massage Therapists, QWL Services, 124 W. 93rd St., New York, NY 10025, (212) 222-4240, fax (212) 222-4208; Massage Therapy

Resource Network, (312) Massage; National Association of Nurse Massage Therapists (NANMT), 1720 Willow Creek Circle, #517, Eugene, OR 97402, (800) 336-2668.

**Research:** If you're interested in what research is revealing about massage, you can stay abreast of the findings by subscribing to *Touchpoints,* the quarterly publication of Touch Research Institute (TRI), the world's first scientific facility devoted to the study of touch, at the University of Miami School of Medicine. TRI conducts dozens of studies on the effects of massage on people of various ages—from cocaine-exposed and HIV-positive infants to adults dealing with fibromyalgia, hypertension, or repetitive motion syndrome. It also abstracts research carried out at other institutions. Send $10 to *Touchpoints,* Touch Research Institute, Dept. of Pediatrics (D-820), University of Miami School of Medicine, P.O. Box 016820, Miami, FL 33101.

**Periodicals:** *Massage Magazine,* P.O. Box 1500, Davis, CA 95617, (916) 757-6033 or (800) 872-1282; *Massage Therapy Journal,* AMTA quarterly, see "For information and practitioners," above; *Massage and Bodywork Quarterly,* ABMP quarterly, see "For information and practitioners," above.

**Books:** Armand Maanum and Herb Montgomery, *The Complete Book of Swedish Massage* (Harper & Row, 1988); George Downing and Anne Kent Rush, *The Massage Book* (Random House/Bookworks, 1972) (this is the original all-time bestseller [more than 1 million copies sold] on the massage style developed in California); Lucinda Lidell et al., *The Book of Massage: The Complete Step-by-Step Guide to Eastern and Western Techniques* (Fireside/Simon & Schuster, 1984) .

**Videos:** "Massage for Health," hosted by Shari Belafonte, with instructions by Mirka Knaster and James Heartland, 65 mins., includes a 38-page booklet by Knaster (Healing Arts Home Video), (800) 254-8464; "Massage for Every Body," 90 mins., Swedish Institute (Increase Video/Wishing Well Distrib.); "Massage for Beginners: A Cayce/Reilly Massage Video Workshop," Vicki Battaglia, 60 mins. (A.R.E. Bookstore, [800] 723-1112).

> His body became indescribably touching to him and of no further use than to be purely and cautiously present in.
>
> —Rainer Maria Rilke

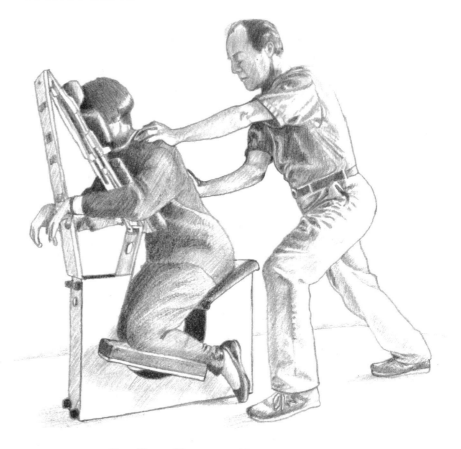

## ON-SITE/SEATED/CHAIR MASSAGE

If you want to experience the beneficial effects of massage but you're un-comfortable with taking off your clothes or having oil on your skin, there's another option. Fully dressed, you can sit facedown in a specially de-signed, padded chair that allows massage therapists access to your muscles and joints. They can fold up and carry this chair anywhere—store, health club, airport, office, home, school. Using a combination of techniques—percussion, pressure points, range of motion, and others—they can help you release stress or rehabilitate such discomforts as neck pain and TMJ disorder.

Some massage therapists work exclusively with a portable massage chair, having learned the technique as part of their overall training in a massage school, in an introductory workshop, or through a separate certifi-cation course. Others use the chair for out-calls and use a table in their of-fice practice. Presently in New York and Las Vegas (and planned for other cities), at the Great American Backrub Store you can walk in off the street, sit down, and enjoy a session.

RESOURCES:

**For instruction, practitioners, and videos:** Seated Massage Experience, Raymond Blaylock, (800) 868-2448; Skilled Touch Institute, David Palmer, 584 Castro St., #555, San Francisco, CA 94114, (800) 999-5026 or (415) 472-2011.

## PREGNANCY MASSAGE

Pregnancy is a time to be pampered. Just being pregnant demands a lot of physical effort. All of a woman's body systems are working twice as hard to sustain another being. When you're pregnant, the extra and unevenly distributed weight keeps shifting your center of gravity, creates aches and pains in different parts of your body (especially the lower back, neck and shoulders, and legs and feet), and makes it more cumbersome to move and harder to rest for long.[6] The major changes that pregnancy generates in your body and psyche call for special attention. Prenatal massage can help reduce these difficulties as well as comfort and affirm you during this significant life transition.

Even when there are no specific aches, massage acts as an overall tonic. It increases body awareness and gives you a chance to learn how to relax in preparation for labor. In sedating your nervous system, massage facilitates the release of endorphins, leading to a state of deep relaxation, which also affects your baby in utero. Focusing on your body in a positive way can engender self-acceptance at a time when it would be too easy to think of yourself as "fat and ugly."

Massage also can have a rejuvenating effect if you work during your pregnancy. By increasing both blood and lymph circulation, it brings more nutrition to all parts of your body, including the placenta, and aids in the removal of waste products. This can translate into greater energy, less fatigue, and reduced swelling. If moving about is limited or impossible because of a medical condition, massage is an alternative for stimulating circulation, stretching muscles, and keeping joints flexible.

There was a time when pregnancy alone was considered a contraindication for massage, but doctors now agree that massage can be beneficial, unless it is administered aggressively. For example, slow, gentle circling of the abdomen and at the lower back and sacrum is soothing, but there should never be any vigorous rubbing. Nor is deep pressure acceptable in any other part of the body if it causes pain. Beginning in the second trimester, lying supine may not only be uncomfortable, it also can be dangerous. In this position, the baby's weight could

*We have the body we have because it is precisely the vehicle in which we can best do what we came to do.*

*—Christiane Northrup*

# Experience: Soothing the Lower Back During Pregnancy

For lower back discomfort, try the soothing touch of circular stroking. Having your partner or a friend do this for you will give you a sense of what a whole-body massage during pregnancy can offer. It's also a nice way of sharing a special bond with your partner.

If you are the one to receive the massage, lie on one side, with rolled-up towels or pillows placed wherever their support would make you more comfortable—under your belly and breasts, between your knees, at your head and neck.

If you are the one to give the massage, kneel by the woman's buttocks, facing her shoulders. Warm a little oil or lotion between your hands, then with flat palms apply the lubricant by moving clockwise on the sacrum and lower back. One palm stays continuously on the skin while the other crosses over. Applying firmer pressure can make this move useful also during labor contractions.

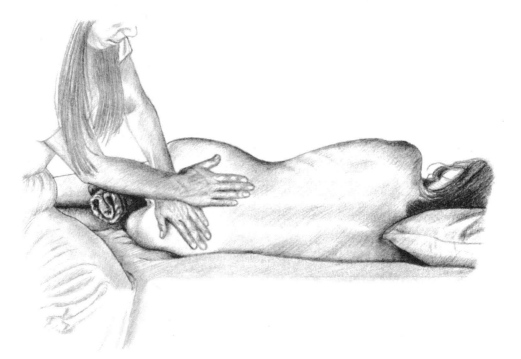

Palming the Sacrum Clockwise

compress major blood vessels (such as ascending vena cava) against the spinal cord and result in a marked decline in blood pressure.[7] In the later stages of pregnancy, when the hormone relaxin loosens the joints in preparation for childbirth, only careful handling—no yanking or jerking of the joints—is safe. It is advisable to avoid massage if you experience morning sickness, nausea, vomiting, diarrhea, vaginal bleeding or discharge, abdominal pain, high blood pressure, or deep venous thrombosis.

Around the world, postpartum massage is as much a time-honored tradition as prenatal massage. It helps relieve the fatigue and tension incurred by the strenuous effort made during labor and delivery. It also aids in "figure control" and toning the uterus. Massage can strengthen muscles and prevent weakness due to inactivity, particularly if you're confined during pregnancy and in need of convalescence afterward. As you face the challenge of mothering, you can appreciate the physical and emotional reassurance and nurturance you can get from postpartum massage.

There is no massage school set up exclusively for teaching pregnancy massage. Some practitioners receive pointers as part of their overall massage training; others attend additional workshops with instructors experienced in this specialty.

*Turning the attention to the body is the beginning of the process of compassionate self-care.*

—Stephen R. Schwartz

### RESOURCES:

**For instruction and practitioners:** National Association of Pregnancy Massage Therapists, 4200 Marathon Blvd., #330, Austin, TX 78756, (512) 323-5925; Bodywork for the Childbearing Years with Carole Osborne-Sheets and Kate Jordan, Somatic Learning Associates, 8950 Villa La Jolla Dr., #2162, La Jolla, CA 92037, (619) 436-0418 or (619) 748-8827; Elaine Stillerman, Swedish Institute, Inc., 226 W. 26th St., 5th fl., New York, NY 10001, (212) 924-5900, fax (212) 924-7600; Claire Miller-Pohlen, Nurturing the Mother Workshops, 36316 Foxfire Dr., Chapel Hill, NC 27516, (919) 929-4253.

**Books:** Gordon Inkeles, *Massage and Peaceful Pregnancy: A Daily Book for Mothers and Fathers* (Perigee/Putnam, 1983); Elaine Stillerman, *Mother-Massage: A Handbook for Relieving the Discomforts of Pregnancy* (Delta/Delacorte, 1992); Kate Jordan and Carole Osborne-Sheets, *Maternity Massage* (Somatic Learning Associates, 1995); Bette Waters, *Massage During Pregnancy* (Research Triangle Publishing, 1995).

## Infant and Child Massage

*After all, touch is the language of the body.*

—Clyde Ford

We live in times that are rife with fear about the most negative form of touching—child abuse. Too many children are mistreated physically, sexually, and emotionally. The loving touch of massage is a way to help ensure that the next generation grows up with a foundation of trust and caring, which are vital in developing a positive sense of self.

Baby massage is a continuation of pregnancy massage outside the womb and a primary way to establish parent-child bonding, especially between fathers and breast-fed infants and between parents and adopted children. It also helps caretakers get to know a baby better and develop confidence in handling her or him. Because touch is a baby's first major form of communication, children can quickly sense the message that others convey when touching them.

Infant massage has been growing in popularity in the West during the last twenty years, since the publication of French doctor Frédéric Leboyer's photographic essay of a mother massaging her baby in Calcutta, India.[8] It is a widespread practice in Asia, the Pacific Islands, and other parts of the world, where massage is generally part of the baby's bath routine. The mother, other female relative, or the midwife is the hands-on practitioner. From their own experiences, these women know that massage helps infants grow healthy and strong, as well as eat and sleep better; it soothes irritability, eases digestive difficulties, and relieves colic and other discomforts. Historically, some cultures—for example, the Maoris and Hawaiians—also used massage to correct deformed body parts, such as clubfoot, and to mold different features to attain certain standards of beauty and prepare the child for future activities, such as dancing.

Today, studies indicate that massaging premature babies enables them to catch up in their neurological, physical, mental, and motor development.[9] It also prevents preemies from developing pneumonia and helps release birth traumas and tensions associated with cesarean section and forceps.[10] Infants born to cocaine-addicted and depressed mothers exhibit fewer postnatal complications and stress reactions when they receive massage.[11]

After infancy, massage has been shown to improve blood-sugar levels in diabetic children. The relaxing effects of massage can help special-needs children gain better balance, posture, rhythm, and coordination as well as become less hyperactive and improve in behavior and schoolwork. ☞ See "Improvement of Skills," page 17. Similar benefits occur also in children without mental retardation or physical disabilities. Fifteen years ago I gave a session in Trager to my friend Jo Lynn's two-year-old daughter. I soon got unexpected glowing reports. The director

# Infant Massage Experience

To have a fun and intimate time with your baby, place him or her on a pad in front of you as you sit cross-legged or kneel. If you sit leaning against the wall, skip the pad and let the baby lie on your legs, head pointing toward your feet. Make sure the room and your hands are warm. Slowly and gently spread a little vegetable oil (you don't want lotion or mineral oil to get in the baby's mouth) all over your baby's body, except the face.

Use flat palms or only fingerpads, since there is little surface area to cover and your movements will be small. With both hands, first glide up the chest, then down around the ribs; repeat three times. Then begin at the right hip with your right hand and move diagonally to the left shoulder and down the side; with the left hand move up and across to the right shoulder and down the side. Synchronize these movements so that they create a wave motion; repeat three times. Before proceeding to an abdominal stroke, repeat the first move—glide up the chest and come down around the ribs. To massage the belly, alternate your hands as you gradually circle clockwise, pressing slightly, as though to empty the stomach. If the baby's legs are bent toward the abdomen, that will keep the area soft while you massage. Stroking the torso can help digestion and elimination and also move gas bubbles through the system.

If your baby arches his or her back or otherwise fusses, try again later. Infants may tolerate only the briefest of massages and may want to suckle right away. Once they get a little older and start to move around, make massage a game instead of trying to keep them still.

---

of the child-care center said Sara had been her calmest and most well-behaved self ever, getting along better than usual with the other children. And going to bed that night had not been an ordeal because she requested, "Mommy, Daddy, do what Mirka did." She even directed them how.

If you're interested in learning how to massage your own baby, there are classes and books. A session with a professional first could insure that you get started with the right moves and become alert to your baby's individual preferences for a firm or light touch. You could work with a massage therapist who has experience with babies and children, with a certified infant-massage instructor who has undergone massage training specifically for infants but is not necessarily also a licensed massage therapist, or with a childbirth educator.

Remember, in whatever ways massage (or any bodyway) is fruitful for adults, it will be worthwhile for children. We are all born with the same anatomy and physiology and subject to accidents and injuries, aches and pains, structural imbalances, emotional disturbances, and the rest. If you turn to bodyways to help yourself, you can also let them help your children.

## RESOURCES:

**For instructors and practitioners:** International Association of Infant Massage (IAIM), 5660 Clinton St., Suite #2, Elma, NY 14059, (800) 248-5432 or (716) 684-3299; Diana Moore, International Loving Touch Foundation, Inc., P.O. Box 16374, Portland, OR 97216-0374, (503) 253-8482, fax (503) 666-8974; Canadian Institute of Baby Massage, P.O. Box 354, Station S, Toronto, Ontario M5M 4M9 Canada, fax (416) 488-3716.

**Books:** For a basic introduction, Teresa Kirkpatrick Ramsey, *Baby's First Massage* (1992), a booklet available through AMTA, (708) 864-0123. Also Frédéric Leboyer, *Loving Hands: The Traditional Indian Art of Baby Massage* (Alfred A. Knopf, 1976); Amelia Auckett, *Baby Massage: Parent-Child Bonding Through Touch* (Newmarket, 1988); Tina Heinl, *Baby Massage Book: Shared Growth Through the Hands* (Coventure/Sigo, 1991); Vimala Schneider McClure, *Infant Massage: A Handbook for Loving Parents* (Bantam, 1982); Healthy Alternatives Inc., *Tender Touch: A Guide to Infant Massage* (Healthy Alternatives, 1986); Wataru Ohashi, *Touch for Love* (Ballantine, 1986)—Shiatsu (Japanese) massage for babies; Marybetts Sinclair, *Massage for Healthier Children* (Wingbow, 1992); Claude Lavoie, *Le massage des enfants: Guide pratique* (Montreal: Louise Courteau, 1989).

**Videos and audiotapes:** "Baby Massage," 30 mins., Cumberland Gap Productions, 635 W. Main St., Louisville, KY 40202, (502) 587-7348. IAIM (see "For instructors and practitioners," page 157) has various videotapes on massage for infants, children, and young adults, and for those who have been traumatized or have special needs. The International Loving Touch

Foundation, on page 157, also has several videos. "Pediatric Massage: For the Child With Special Needs" (book and 117-min. videotape in English and Spanish for massage professionals), Kathy Fleming Drehobl and Mary Gengler Fuhr, Therapy Skill Builders, 3830 E. Bellevue, P.O. Box 42050-TN3, Tucson, AZ 85733, (602) 323-7500.

---

## SPORTS MASSAGE

Exercise and massage have been a winning combination ever since the ancient Greeks and Romans practiced them together. Athletes received massage first to prepare them for action and later to relieve the fatigue and soreness from a vigorous workout, and also to help heal injuries. Europe and the former Soviet Union continued the tradition and helped spread its popularity abroad. Today there are few world-class athletes, dancers, and gymnasts who don't use massage as a regular part of their fitness and conditioning routines. And they do it for the same reasons as in earlier times: They want to increase their endurance and speed their recovery time so they can perform better and sooner. For example, after runner Mary Decker Slaney discovered massage in 1981, she set eight world records and won several national and world championship titles.

However, you don't have to be an Olympic contender for sports massage to make a noticeable difference in your own life. Added to a routine of stretching and warming up, it may promote greater flexibility. It loosens muscle fibers, breaks up fibrosis to lengthen shortened muscles and prevents adhesions from forming, relieves swelling, and reduces muscle tension.[12] If you like to compete but get pre-meet jitters, massage will calm your nerves. It will also lead to greater self-awareness. As you learn to recognize your body's signals, you'll be able to avoid overuse injuries, which result when you demand too much of your body too soon. If you injure yourself, massage can help diminish the pain as well as reestablish a full range of motion after tendonitis, ligament sprains, epicondylitis, and other lesions. Some athletes swear massage gives them a brand-new body to work with, for it can restore fatigued muscles more rapidly and thoroughly than rest alone.

Any technique applied to athletes to help them train and perform free of pain and injuries can qualify as sports therapy. Massage therapists blend classic Swedish strokes with such methods as compression, pressure-point therapy, cross-fiber friction, joint mobilization, hydrotherapy, and cryotherapy (ice massage) to meet the special needs of high-level performers and fitness enthusiasts. Especially popular are procedures that use active joint movements, such as proprioceptive neuromuscular facilitation (PNF), active muscular relaxation technique, body mobiliza-

*Awareness, in and of itself, is curative.*
—Robert Marrone

# A Sports Massage Experience

There are many techniques a sports massage therapist uses. Here's one Robert K. King, a past president of the American Massage Therapy Association and author of *Performance Massage,* teaches. Try the "heel squeeze" on a friend or have someone practice on you. It works well on large muscles, such as the gluteals (buttocks), the gastrocnemius (calf), and the hamstrings (back of the thighs).

Intertwine the fingers of both hands and place the heels on each side of the muscle. Keep your hands in line with your forearms to avoid stressing your wrists. Grasp the thick middle part of the muscle between the heels of your hands and squeeze. This gives a two-sided compression to the tissues. You can use the heel squeeze to work the entire length of the leg, front and back.

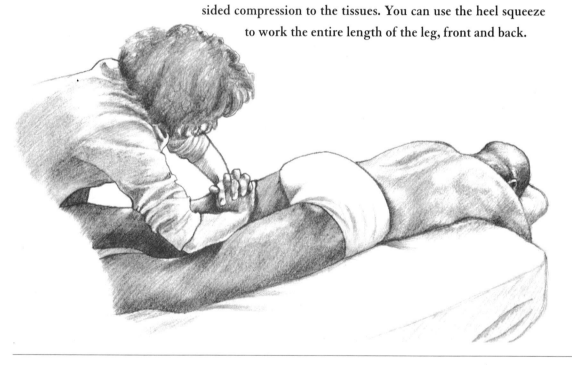

tion technique, and muscle energy technique. An example of combining these many ways of relieving pain and promoting better biomechanical function is the ONSEN Technique, developed by Rich Phaigh, who worked with such Olympic runners as Mary Decker Slaney and Alberto Salazar.

Athletic massage is more specific, more precise, more stimulating, and deeper than an Esalen-style relaxation or general Swedish massage. Depending on the particular sport or performance, different sets of muscles and joints are emphasized. The massage therapists perform will vary depending on whether the session is before or after an athletic event or between competitions. Prior to activity, therapists generally combine light jiggling, compression, and stretching to complement a warm-up. After an event, they work more slowly and include light pétrissage, shaking, and stretching to help relax muscle cramps, unwind, and remove waste products from muscles.

Sports massage therapists need training beyond that required for a general Swedish session. In 1985 the American Massage Therapy Association (AMTA) established a sports massage certification program that includes written and practical exams testing practitioners' knowledge of both theory and the skills necessary for safe and effective application of massage to top athletes in pre- and post-competition stages of sporting events. Advanced technical instruction is available through various massage schools. The AMTA National Sports Massage Team consists of state chapter teams across the country; its members work in cooperation with other on-site medical staff.

## RESOURCES:

**For practitioners and instruction:** AMTA National Sports Massage Team, (708) 864-0123; Sports Massage Training Institute, 2156 Newport Blvd., Costa Mesa, CA 92627, (714) 642-0735; Kurashova Institute (Russian sports massage), P.O. Box 6246, Rock Island, IL 61202, (309) 786-4888, fax (309) 786-8687. Check with sports medicine clinics or athletic rehabilitation institutes as well.

**Books:** Robert K. King, *Performance Massage* (Human Kinetics, 1993); Jack Meagher and Pat Boughton, *Sportsmassage: A Complete Program for Increasing Performance and Endurance in Fifteen Popular Sports* (Station Hill, 1990); Rich Phaigh and Paul Perry, *Athletic Massage* (Fireside/Simon & Schuster, 1986); Myk Hungerford, *Beyond Sports Medicine: Injury Prevention and Care Through Sports Massage* (Sports Massage Training Institute, 1994); Joan Johnson, *The Healing Art of Sports Massage* (Rodale, 1995).

**Videos:** "Athletic Massage: Therapeutic Massage for Sports and Fitness," Rich Phaigh, CVT Productions, (800) 284-4403; "Clinical Sports Massage," Benny Vaughn, CSM Video, (404) 457-5136; "Russian School of Sports Massage: Kurashova Method," 3 videos, 60 mins. each, (916) 757-6033.

## MASSAGE FOR THE ELDER YEARS
### (GERIATRIC MASSAGE)

In traditional cultures, several generations live together, with each one performing an important role in the family, often including the pleasant responsibility of massaging the children from birth on. In turn, as the children grow, they massage those who took care of them. But in our highly mobile Western society, we tend to live far from family, with generations separated from one another. Even when distance is not a barrier, we lead such hectic lives that we often neglect our elders. Yet the human need

# A Hand Massage Experience

In a nursing home I taught a group of residents to share hand massage. Because you don't need to use a massage table or ask the person to undress, it's a simple and easy experience. Massaging the hands can be especially rewarding for someone who suffers from arthritis, but only if you do it when the joints aren't inflamed.

Let the person's hand rest in your lap so that there's no muscle strain. Warm a little oil or lotion in your hands and then apply. Holding the hand, palm down, between your hands, use your thumbs to stroke upward from the knuckles and outward, moving in opposite directions. Then, with alternating thumbs, smooth up in the depressions between the metacarpals (hand bones) till you reach the wrist. Turn the hand over and lace your fingers through his or hers so that you can keep the palm open and give the fingers a stretch. In this position, make small circles in the palm with your thumbs. Release your fingers and now one at a time, take hold of each finger with your thumb and index finger to twist and squeeze gently from the base to the tip. Hold the whole hand between yours before you move on to the other hand.

to be touched with caring doesn't diminish with age. Whether we're seventy years old or seven months old, it's vital to our physical and emotional well-being.

Massage can help assuage the isolation and loneliness many older people feel, revitalize connectedness to others, and reaffirm self-esteem. Massage also provides physical stimulation to help ease certain conditions that often accompany growing older. Circulation slows down, the skin becomes thinner, bones turn brittle, muscles have less tone and joints less flexibility. Rheumatism and arthritis lead to pain. Massage and range-of-motion work can increase circulation, mobilize the joints, and improve the condition of the skin. For the sedentary or bedridden person, it provides some passive movement and may reduce edema. Its relaxing effects may also help lower blood pressure and relieve chronic tension headaches.

As in pregnancy, certain precautions are necessary: no massage when there is a cardiovascular condition or joint inflammation due to arthritis, and no pressure on varicose veins. Most massage therapists have a general practice, but a few specialize in geriatric care, having learned it in massage school or through a continuing-education workshop.

RESOURCES:

**For training programs, books, and videos:** Day-Break Productions, P.O. Box 1629, Guerneville, CA 95446, (707) 869-0632.

## RUSSIAN MASSAGE

In Russia, massage plays a major role in medical care and advanced athletic training, according to Zhenya Kurashova Wine, who studied physiotherapy in her native country. Unlike in North America, Russian massage therapists are regarded as medical professionals. The massage therapy department is often the largest in Russian hospitals and clinics because it is crucial to rehabilitation, not only in musculoskeletal dysfunctions but also in cardiovascular, neurological, gynecological, and internal disorders, and in postsurgical situations. Kurashova Wine also worked with top cyclists, rowers, basketball and hockey players, and other high-level performers in what was then the Soviet Union.

Russian massage includes the same strokes as Swedish massage, along with other techniques, such as segmento-reflective massage. ☞ See "Bindegewebsmassage," page 165. However, according to Kurashova Wine, the Russian version is very precise, clinically oriented, and tailored specifically to a patient's condition or an athlete's individual needs. Research in the Soviet Union backs up its effectiveness.

Helped are those who love the broken and the whole, none of their children nor any of their ancestors, nor any parts of themselves shall be despised.

—Alice Walker

RESOURCES:

**For information, instruction, practitioners, and videos:** Kurashova Institute, P.O. Box 6246, Rock Island, IL 61202, (309) 786-4888, fax (309) 786-8687.

# The Benjamin System of Muscular Therapy

The approaches of Austrian psychiatrist Wilhelm Reich, English orthopedist James Cyriax, and Australian actor F. M. Alexander all influenced Ben E. Benjamin in his development of the Benjamin System of Muscular Therapy in 1967. A combination of treatment and education, its purpose is to break down chronic muscular tension and prevent it from returning. It works with mechanical tension that results from poor physical habits and posture, accidents, injuries, surgery, occupational hazards, improper body alignment, and environmental conditions.

This system encompasses deep massage, self-help tension-release exercises, body-care techniques, and postural realignment. Although the method is also useful for relaxation and stress reduction, the precise, detailed vocabulary of seven hundred specific movements is applicable to a wide variety of conditions, including athletic injuries.

Training is a two-year part-time program with specialties in relaxation massage, therapeutic massage, or sports massage.

RESOURCES:

**For practitioners, instruction, videos, and books:**  Muscular Therapy Institute, 122 Rindge Ave., Cambridge, MA 02140, (800) 543-4740 or (617) 576-1300 in Massachusetts.

**Books:** Ben E. Benjamin, *Are You Tense? The Benjamin System of Muscular Therapy* (Pantheon, 1978); Ben E. Benjamin and Gale Borden, *Listen to Your Pain: Understanding, Identifying and Treating Pain and Injury* (Viking Penguin, 1984).

# Bindegewebsmassage

*Bindegewebsmassage* is German for "connective tissue massage" or "reflexive therapy of the connective tissue." The practitioner strokes the subcutaneous fascia, the connective tissue sheath that is not as deep as the fascia addressed in structural approaches, such as Rolfing, Hellerwork, or Myofascial Release. Located between the skin and the muscle, this fascial layer is richly embedded with nerve endings. As a result, the massage sets up a strong sensory stimulation to the nerves in a cutaneo-visceral reflex, that is, from skin to organ, not unlike how acupuncture works. These nerve connections develop as the different layers of the embryo differentiate. For example, the endoderm, or inner layer, becomes the foundation for most of the internal organs, while the ectoderm, or outer layer, gives rise to the skin, the nervous system, and most of the sense organs.

Depending on the area of your body, therapists or doctors who administer this specialized massage use a variety of strokes (fan, hooking, smoothing, etc.) and vary the number of them and the side worked on. They do not use a lubricant. Nor do they push, but rather pull or drag the tissues under their crooked fingers. The sensations you feel may be a cutting, scratching, or dull pressure. In my Bindegewebsmassage session, I felt as though the doctor were precisely etching sharp lines in my skin with a scalpel, yet I felt no pain.

Strokes in specific patterns activate the nerve endings just below your skin. The information then goes into your spinal cord, where it is processed, and comes out as an "improved" information flow to your organs. Because the massage works with the nerves, Dr. Ronald Lavine, a New York City chiropractor who practices this so-called connective tissue massage, believes it should be more aptly named "peripheral nerve massage."

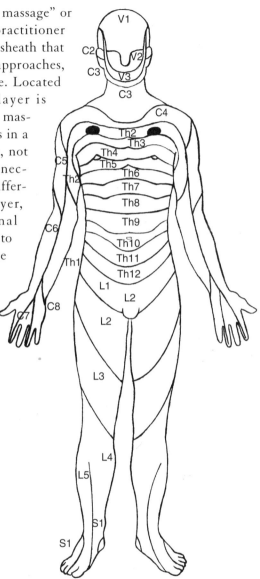

Dermatome Map: The spinal nerve endings in the subcutaneous fascia of each skin zone have a reflex connection to organs in other parts of the body and are involved in different conditions. For example, in headaches segments Th2 through 9 are affected in the front, with the dark areas in Th2 contracted and sensitive to touch; in the back, zones C3–4, Th2–12, and L1–2 would be tense.

You receive the massage in a sitting position unless you're unable to sit up. For treatment of the legs, you lie down. You can even have the massage underwater. Each session always begins at your sacral-pelvic area, called the "basic section," to induce the first reflex effect, which is a boost to your parasympathetic nervous system. Treatment gradually proceeds up to your chest and neck areas. Other zones of dermatomes (areas affected by the spinal nerves in the skin and subcutaneous layer) refer to the liver, heart, stomach, pancreas, ovaries, and so on.

# Elisabeth Dicke

Elisabeth Dicke, a physiotherapist in Germany, discovered Bindegewebsmassage as a result of severe illness. In 1929 her right leg was ice-cold and gray-white and her toes felt as though they were tightly bound by rings. Circulation was so impaired that gangrene appeared imminent. Dicke's doctor was ready to order amputation of her lower leg. This was what a neglected tooth infection had finally come to.

But while lying in bed for five months with extreme pain, not only in her leg but now also in her back, she discovered how to heal herself. Feeling around her sacrum (the base of the spine) and iliac crest (the upper edge of the pelvis, just below the waist in back), Dicke found thickened tissue and increased tension of her skin. She tried to relax it by stroking the area in a pulling motion. Although these parts of her body were supersensitive to the touch, she persisted, and slowly the tension and backache lessened.

Gradually Dicke felt itching and prickling in her right leg, followed by warm flushes. Her "dead" leg was reviving. She continued the stroking and now included her thigh as well. She was able to see her veins again, and she watched them fill with blood. Within three months all her symptoms were completely gone. After a year, during which a colleague continued the treatment for her, she was able to return to work. Finally, all the disorders she had incurred while ill—chronic gastritis, renal colic, chest pains, shortness of breath, swelling of the liver, and heart trouble—cleared up. Somehow massaging in one part of her body had had a positive reflex effect in other areas.

By systematically observing her patients, Dicke confirmed her findings. Eventually she worked out a body map of the skin zones—dermatomes—through which to influence inner organs with an orderly procedure of treatment. She later learned that Henry Head, an English neurologist, had similarly described such a reflex map. Dicke called her newfound technique "massage of the reflex zones in the connective tissue" and clinically tested it with doctors and professors in Germany in the 1930s.

Because of these referral patterns, in European medical circles Bindegewebsmassage is prescribed for a long list of pathological conditions—everything from bronchial asthma and orthopedic dysfunctions to chronic colitis and uterine infections. There are courses of treatment for periarthritis and epicondylitis of the shoulder joint, muscular rheumatism, chronic lumbago, torticollis, ankylosing spondylitis, infantile kyphosis, Sudeck's syndrome, sciatica, paraplegia, Parkinson's disease, migraines, circulatory disorders such as Raynaud's disease, cardiac and respiratory ailments, and diseases of the liver, gallbladder, and kidneys.

Among some therapists, Bindegewebsmassage also serves as a diagnostic tool. If you have pain in one area, they can trace back to the part of your body from which it has been referred and thus determine what your condition might be.

There is an Elisabeth Dicke School in West Germany. Some therapists have been able to learn the system in the United States as well, but I know of no institutionalized training program or regulation of its practice here.

## RESOURCES:

**For practitioners:** Ask local physical therapists and massage therapists for anyone who has been trained in Bindegewebsmassage, or call professional associations.

**Books**: Elisabeth Dicke, H. Schliack, and A. Wolff, *A Manual of Reflexive Therapy of the Connective Tissue, "Bindegewebsmassage"* (Sidney S. Simon, 1978); Maria Ebner, *Connective Tissue Massage* (Williams and Wilkins, 1962).

# Lymphatic Massage

Most massages stimulate movement of lymph as a matter of course, but lymphatic massage provides external pressure specifically to affect this flow. Different versions come from different parts of the world—Ayurvedic from India, Huna from Hawaii, and Vodder Manual Lymph Drainage (MLD), developed by Danish physical therapists Estrid and Emil Vodder in France in the 1930s.

To understand the function of lymphatic massage, it is useful to know the role lymph plays in your body's health. Like its red brother blood, milky white lymph filters foreign matter and removes excess fluid, protein, and waste products from the tissues and transports them to the blood to be circulated and eliminated. If the lymph didn't do its job, you would die from protein poisoning within twenty-four hours.

But unlike the blood, lymph does not have a heart to pump it through the body. It moves along slowly, with assistance from several forces. The contractions of voluntary muscles (which is one reason exercise is so beneficial) and intestinal muscles (in peristalsis) squeeze lymph vessels. The pulsations of nearby arteries massage them, too, and the negative pressure in the chest cavity provides suction. External hands-on stimulation helps increase the passage of lymph, especially when it gets backed up.

Lymph collects at nearly eight hundred nodes throughout the body, with two hundred in the neck alone. When nodes become swollen in the neck, armpit, or groin, the areas feel tender. And when the ankles, feet, legs, arms, and hands become thick with accumulated fluid, you have edema. Lymphedema also may occur following the removal of lymph nodes due to cancer.

Vodder Manual Lymph Drainage is a gentle, precise, and rhythmic method performed especially in clinics in Europe, where it has become the fourth most prescribed massage technique by medical doctors. Therapists and doctors report good results for sprains and bruises, puffiness in the face following cosmetic or dental surgery, and muscular spasms from overuse or chronic tension. It also figures in the treatment of sinusitis, burns, acne, scars, arthritis, emphysema, migraines, tinnitus, trigeminal neuralgia, spinal injuries, and some cerebral disorders. For patients who have undergone such operations as hysterectomy, prostectomy, and mastectomy, clinical evidence indicates that MLD moves fluid when an area can no longer perform this function. If begun before the fifth month of pregnancy, it can serve as a preventive for swelling and stretch marks. Research by European scientists confirms the effects of MLD.[13]

Unlike regular massage, MLD is very light and does not penetrate to the level of your muscles. That's because almost half of your body's lymph lies within the superficial layers below the skin. There is a deeper technique for dealing with spasms in the lymph vessels that drain the muscles. In a session I had, I was surprised that the physical therapist's touch was as gentle as a feather. In the late 1970s, I had learned a different kind of lymphatic massage that called for stronger action, and thereafter I'd assumed that deep pressure was necessary to affect the lymph.

The Lymphatic System

Whether light or deep, MLD uses an on-off pulsing pressure, like a smooth pumping action, which has an immediate lulling, relaxing effect on your autonomic nervous system. It also uses other manipulation techniques—scooping, rotary, and stationary circles. Therapists follow the pathways of the lymph and move in the direction of muscle fibers, the same as that of lymph vessels. MLD can be effective even when the therapist can't work directly on the affected area because of severe burns or other conditions. Massaging the opposite side of the body or near the site can bring the same needed results.

The main source of MLD instruction and treatment is in European schools and clinics. Massage therapists and physical therapists become certified after a four-week training program, part of which is done under medical surveillance. Courses are also available at massage schools in the United States and Canada, where therapists must have at least five hundred hours of massage therapy training or a physical therapy background. The North American Vodder Association of Lymphatic Therapy (NAVALT), formed in 1992, has a mandatory review of practical techniques every two years, and teachers must recertify every year.

## RESOURCES:

**For practitioners and courses:** Contact NAVALT, P.O. Box 861, Chesterfield, OH 44026, (216) 729-3258; your local massage school; or Robert Harris, Dr. Vodder School–North America, P.O. Box 5701, Victoria, British Columbia, Canada, V8R 6S8, (604) 598-9862, fax (604) 598-9841. There is also a National Lymphedema Network (NLN), (800) 541-3259.

**Books:** Since this is highly specialized work, only technical manuals on lymph drainage are presently available, some in German. See H. and G. Wittlinger, *Introduction to Dr. Vodder's Manual Lymph Drainage,* vol. 1, 3rd revised ed. (Haug, 1986); Ingrid Kurz, *Introduction to Dr. Vodder's Manual Lymph Drainage*, vol. 2, therapy 1, and vol. 3, therapy 2 (Haug, 1986 and 1990).

# Pfrimmer Deep Muscle Therapy®

The origins of Pfrimmer Deep Muscle Therapy resemble those of Bindegewebsmassage—incapacity led to ingenuity, which led to healing. Thérèse Pfrimmer, a registered massage therapist and physiotherapist, discovered her technique in 1946, when she was doing all the heavy work of running a large laundry in Ontario, Canada. After she sustained injuries, the doctors told her she would never walk again. She began to deeply knead and manipulate her own muscles. After three months, she was completely cured and walked away from her wheelchair.

Pfrimmer later realized that the answer to many crippling conditions was not in the nerves but in the muscles. She attributed paralysis to two things: When muscles are sealed off from blood circulation, they degenerate and become hard, rubbery, mushy, stringy, or woody; and when the muscles are cut off from lymph, they stick together. Thus the Pfrimmer cross-tissue movements soften hardened fibers in all layers of muscle, clearing adhesions, relieving congestion and inflammation, alleviating pain, improving the range of motion in joints, and releasing entrapment of nerves as well as of lymphatic and blood vessels, thus enhancing circulation in the restricted muscles.

Practitioners state that Pfrimmer Deep Muscle Therapy has proved effective for arthritis, carpal tunnel syndrome, constipation and digestive distress, neck-, back-, and head-aches, heart conditions, joint and muscle pain, occupational and sports injuries, sciatica, tendinitis and bursitis, and whiplash and other traumas from car accidents. They say it also has been helpful in improving dysfunctions caused by amytrophic lateral sclerosis (ALS), Bell's palsy, brain injury, cerebral palsy, fibrositis and fibromyalgia syndrome, lupus, multiple sclerosis, muscular dystrophy, neuralgia, neuritis, Parkinson's disease, polio, scoliosis, strokes, and TMJ disorder.

A variety of health-care professionals practice the Pfrimmer method, including doctors, nurses, chiropractors, physical therapists, and massage therapists. Only two schools are authorized to teach this technique and only to people with a background of at least five hundred hours of anatomy, physiology, hygiene, ethics, and other subjects.

## RESOURCES:

**For practitioners and other information:** Thérèse C. Pfrimmer International Association of Deep Muscle Therapists, Inc., c/o Cindy Gaydos, 269 S. Gulph Rd., King of Prussia, PA 19406, (800) 484-7773, ext. 7368.

**For instruction:** Alexandria School of Scientific Therapies, P.O. Box 287, Alexandria, IN 46001, (317) 724-7745; Pennsylvania School of Muscle Therapy, 651 S. Gulph Rd., King of Prussia, PA 19406, (610) 265-7939.

**Books:** Thérèse C. Pfrimmer, *Muscles . . . Your Invisible Bonds* (Blyth, 1983).

# Lauren Berry Method

The late Lauren Berry was exceptionally straightforward whenever anyone asked what he did. "I'm not a healer and I'm not a doctor," he would say. "I'm just a mechanic." Although he worked as a registered physical therapist, his deep understanding of the mechanics of the body came from childhood experiences with a Finnish doctor who practiced "Swedish gymnastics" and with cadavers in a city morgue, and from his later training as an engineer.

Berry saw the muscles, tendons, and ligaments as the "guy wires" of the body. He found that their distortion was often the major contributor to mechanical problems of the spine and extremities. He also believed that everything in the body is innately programmed to self-correct. But if your natural center of gravity (located in the pelvic girdle on a line between the fifth lumbar-sacral articulation and a point approximately two inches below the navel) is off balance, then everything above and below becomes distorted in order to adapt to a new center of gravity. This interferes with your body's ability to maintain itself.

Therapists who practice the Lauren Berry method use deep massage techniques and soft-tissue manipulation. By releasing spasms, distortions, and adhesions in the connective tissue, skeletal muscles, and smooth muscle of organs, they stimulate the body's natural inclination toward balance and harmony in its structure and function. For example, such correction can quickly restore a knee joint to full, pain-free mechanical function or relieve low back discomfort.

Practitioners of the Lauren Berry Method studied directly with Berry; some now teach the technique to others.

RESOURCES:

To find a practitioner in your area, send a stamped, self-addressed envelope with your request and phone number to Institute of Integral Health, Inc., 1442A Walnut St., Berkeley, CA 94709.

# Bowen Technique

The Bowen Technique is a system developed by the late Tom Bowen in Australia. According to practitioners, when they gently pluck, like a guitar string, certain patterns of tendons, nerves, and muscle fascia, it sets up a vibration that imparts new information to the body and releases a cascade of neuromuscular reflexes. In turn, these reflexes free joints, relax muscles, improve circulation of blood, lymph, and energy, and balance organ systems.

Gene Dobkin, one of several qualified North American instructors, describes the Bowen Technique by what it's not—neither massage nor chiropractic, Trigger Point Therapy, fascia release, lymphatic massage, energy work, or neuromuscular education. There's no pounding, stroking, rubbing, force adjustments, or deep pressure. Instead it is a study in delicacy. It does not probe deeply into the muscles or joints nor does it manipulate bones or the connective tissue beneath muscles. It is never sharp or shocking, and it uses no more than "eyeball pressure" (what you could tolerate on your closed eyelids). No lubricant is necessary, and you can keep your clothes on.

During a Bowen session, practitioners will apply first a three-part sequence of moves along the spine, back, and neck, then follow with the arms and legs. Additional procedures address particular difficulties. The sequence is not unlike the way a piano tuner works, adjusting a few strings to lead to overall harmony. Practitioners will synchronize the moves with your breath and, for greater relaxation, encourage you to sigh as you exhale.

In my own session, after each series of moves, the practitioner left the room so that I could "bake" a few minutes. Each time, I immediately dropped down into a deep state of calm and ease. Afterward, he suggested I drink lots of water and walk (but not engage in a strenuous workout) to remove metabolic by-products and stay flexible. I also was to avoid other systems for a week because they could interfere with or negate the effects of a session, which continue to "cook" for another five to ten days. A second or third session fine-tunes and reinforces the benefits of the first. Only extreme or chronic disorders require extended treatment.

Bowen therapists report success with a long list of ailments, including abdominal, back, sacro-iliac, sternal, chest, coccyx, and diaphragm pain. They work with breast lumps, Bell's palsy, bursitis, carpal tunnel syn-

# A Bowen Experience

To get a sense of how the Bowen move feels, put the thumb of one hand on the center of the biceps muscle (unflexed) of your opposite arm. Moving horizontally, draw the skin back toward your chest. Then push against the muscle for a few seconds. Using gentle pressure, roll over the top of the biceps until you feel the muscle return to its original shape. Don't rub the skin, but rather drag it completely across the muscle.

# Tom Bowen

Tom Bowen, the originator of the Bowen Technique, was born in Australia in 1903. He studied briefly at a medical school but eventually became an industrial chemist. One day in 1952 there was a commotion outside the office where he worked. A workman had fallen off a scaffold and was lying in tremendous pain on the sidewalk. Everyone ran around chaotically while waiting for the ambulance to arrive. When Bowen realized that no one was comforting the badly injured man, he got down next to him, put his hand gently on the man's shoulder, and said things to soothe him. Later, the man reported that the moment Tom touched him, his body filled with a warm glow and all the pain was gone. Although he suffered broken bones and internal injuries, he had no shock from the experience.

As soon as the word spread, people began to approach Bowen for help. They cornered him at work and followed him home at night. Since he could never say no, every night he stayed up until three o'clock in the morning healing them. He quit chemistry, opened a clinic in Geelong, Victoria, and gradually developed a technique that changes the body's structural and functional relationships.

By 1976 this self-taught healer was treating more than thirteen thousand patients a year, with rarely more than two sessions per person. Even after he lost both legs to diabetes, he continued his work from a wheelchair. He died in 1982, and several years later Oswald and Elaine Rentsch, trained and authorized by Bowen, began teaching the technique in Australia and other countries.

—Courtesy of Gene Dobkin, Bowen therapist.

drome, groin pulls, infertility, vomiting, tennis elbow, sciatica, scoliosis, shin splints, asthma, hay fever and sinus conditions, headaches and migraines, frozen shoulder, constipation, Ménière's disease, digestive ailments, hernia, bunions and hammer toes, TMJ syndrome, and disorders of the liver, gallbladder, prostate, ears, and eyes. Therapists also treat infants for colic or birth canal torsion.

Various health professionals—including massage therapists, physical therapists, M.D.'s, nurses, dentists, podiatrists, naturopaths, and acupuncturists—practice the Bowen Technique. Basic training is twenty-eight hours, six months of practice, then fourteen hours more for certification. There is a Bowen Therapy Academy in Australia; certified instructors teach in the United States as well.

RESOURCES:

---

**For information on training and practitioners:** Milton and Deni Larimore-Albrecht, 177 Valley View Dr., Auburn, CA 95603, (916) 823-6336, fax (916) 823-5759; Gene Dobkin's Bowen Seminars, (800) US Bowen.

---

# Trigger Point Therapy

Trigger points are localized areas of hyperirritability in the muscles. They are palpable as lumps or knots, which, when pressed, are extremely sore and refer a sensation to another part of the body. The nervous system is at play here. When there's no stress on the muscle, the nerve endings usually fire at a low, rhythmic rate. But if you do something to provoke the point, such as experience emotional distress or lift furniture that's too heavy, that will trigger neurological activity to speed up and inhibit normal physiological function. This initiates a cycle of spasm, pain, tension, weakness, and limited range of motion in the joints. When the muscle goes into spasm, it shortens, thus also affecting the ligaments and tendons attached to it and the bones they're connected to.

Trigger points can form early, with a birth trauma, or later, as a result of blows, sprains, and strains from accidents and injuries, diseases, overuse patterns in sports and occupations, structural imbalances, and other stresses. They then can lie dormant or latent, even for years, until something stimulates them. Trigger points can create pain not only where they first take up residence in the body but also in distant locations. They do this in specific, predictable patterns in a kind of road map of referred pain. For example, a trigger point in the trapezius muscles (they extend from the neck and shoulders to the middle of the back) can export pain to the base of the skull and the jaw and behind the eyes. Pain can move from one muscle to another, from a muscle to an organ or gland and vice versa, and from one organ or gland to another.

Originally doctors performed Trigger Point Therapy with injections. Janet Travell, M.D., pioneered the practice in the United States after trigger points were identified in Europe in the 1930s. She treated John F. Kennedy's severe back pain when he was a senator and later President. Travell injected points in his back with a saline solution and the anesthetic procaine, then followed with passive stretches and a cooling spray of fluorimethane.

Some M.D.s, generally physiatrists, who specialize in treating physical disorders with heat, water, or manipulation, still employ this "spray and stretch" technique. Others refer patients to physical therapists or to practitioners who do Trigger Point Therapy without drugs or injections—Certified Bonnie Prudden Myotherapists and Neuromuscular Therapists. Such therapists apply pressure with their fingers, knuckles, and elbows, or small T-bars and L-bars. They vary the depth, intensity, and length according to your level of sensitivity and the part of your body they're working on. This procedure defuses the trigger point to break the cycle of spasm and pain.

Therapists explain the mechanism whereby a trigger point lets go in terms of different processes that occur. One of them is a reflex arc. Stress to the point results in excessive sensory input to an area of the spinal cord. In turn, the muscles and visceral organs served by that nerve segment also remain in a state of overactivity and continue to provide abnormal stimulation, setting up a vicious cycle. Pressure may interrupt or override this reflex, decreasing or even eliminating the transmission of pain sensations, the way recording on audiotape can erase what's already on the tape or, at the very least, make the sounds faint. Pressure may also arouse the nervous system to release the body's self-generated analgesics, such as enkephalin and serotonin, which inhibit neurostimulation.

In addition, pressure and friction warm the muscle and increase blood flow, which brings oxygen and nutrients to the tissue and removes pain-inducing metabolic waste products. The warmth diminishes muscular contractions and makes the surrounding fascia more pliable, allowing the muscle to lengthen and decreasing both pressure within the joint and impulses to the spinal cord.

After defusing the trigger point, therapists use gentle stretches and movements to help reeducate your muscles to stay relaxed and free of spasm. Without the added exercises, it's likely that stress will activate the trigger points again and cause muscles to spasm.

Once the trigger points release, the musculoskeletal and nervous systems return to normal functioning. Pain lessens or disappears. As muscles extend again, bones can go back to their natural resting places, too, and give up postural distortions. This also frees nerves that were "entrapped" by spastic tissue.

Trigger Point Therapy offers precise and specific treatment of acute and chronic pain that is muscle-related, including head-, neck-, and backaches, whiplash, TMJ syndrome, Bell's palsy, menstrual cramps, arthritis, bursitis, fibromyalgia, multiple sclerosis, sciatica, numbness, postsurgery distress, carpal tunnel syndrome, and occupational and athletic injuries. The extent of practice and the protocol used vary according to where and how much therapists have trained. There are two major branches of Trigger Point Therapy that have grown from Travell's original work.

*Bonnie Prudden Myotherapy* is a technique that fitness authority Bonnie Prudden developed in 1976, working in conjunction with the medical

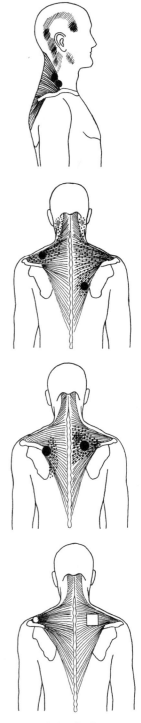

Trigger Points in the Trapezius Muscles

## An Experience in Relieving Trigger Points

One of the ways you can reach trigger points on your own is with a tennis ball. Place the ball in the area just to the right or left of your spine, then lean against a wall. You can also do this lying down, keeping the ball between you and the floor. Slowly roll the ball up and down your back until you reach a sensitive spot. Stay there about twelve seconds, either by pressing your back toward the wall or by allowing the weight of your back to sink into the ball.

If you want to get trigger points on both sides of your spine, place one tennis ball in a long sock, tie off a knot to hold it in place, then insert a second ball and tie off again. The space formed by the knot between the two balls should bridge your spine so that you do not apply direct pressure to the vertebrae themselves.

profession. Certified Bonnie Prudden Myotherapists train for fourteen hundred hours at her Institute for Physical Fitness and Myotherapy before taking board exams. To maintain certification, they must update with an additional forty-five hours every two years. In order to receive treatment, before their first session patients must present a written note of medical clearance from their physician, osteopath, dentist, or chiropractor to ensure that there is no pathological problem that could interfere and that the medical condition is under a doctor's care. Certified practitioners work in hospitals, doctors' and dentists' offices, and in their own pain clinics. Some medical professionals include Myotherapy in their practice. There is also Myotherapy for infants, children, and animals. Another term Prudden uses for her work is *Pain Erasure*.

Neuromuscular Therapists may learn the basics of *Neuromuscular Therapy (NMT)* as part of a massage school program. Those who want more advanced training also attend a series of weekend seminars conducted by certified instructors in the United States and Canada who are massage therapists, nurses, or physical therapists.

### RESOURCES:

**For equipment, instruction, and practitioners:** Bonnie Prudden Institute for Physical Fitness and Myotherapy and Pain Erasure Clinic, 7800 E. Speedway, Tucson, AZ 85710, (602) 529-3979; St. John Neuromuscular Therapy Pain Relief Seminars, 10710 Seminole Blvd., Suite 2, Seminole, FL 34648, (800) 232-4668; Neuromuscular Therapy Center, 900 14th Ave. N., St. Petersburg, FL 33705, (813) 821-7167; National Association of Trigger Point

Myotherapists, 2600 S. Parker Rd., Suite 1-214, Aurora, CA 80014, or 2821 Baxter Rd., #3A, Anchorage, AK 99504.

**Books:** Bonnie Prudden, *Pain Erasure: The Bonnie Prudden Way* (Ballantine, 1985); Bonnie Prudden, *Myotherapy: Bonnie Prudden's Guide to Pain-Free Living* (Ballantine, 1985).

**Videos and audiotapes:** "How to Get Started with Bonnie Prudden Myotherapy," 90-min. video; "Quick Rx for Back Pain," 90-min. video; "Quick Rx for Headaches," 90-min. video; "How to Relieve Pain," 40-min. audiocassette—all available through Bonnie Prudden, 7800 E. Speedway, Tucson, AZ 85710, (602) 529-3979; Neuromuscular Therapy Home Study Video Program (vols. 1, 2, 3, 4), 6 hrs., and client education videos, Paul St. John NMT, 10950 72nd St. N., #101, Largo, FL 34547, (800) 232-4668.

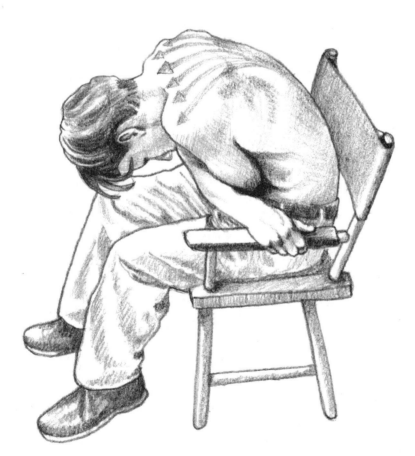

Stretching the Trapezius Muscles

# Trager® Psychophysical Integration

Trager Psychophysical Integration, a creation of Milton Trager, M.D., operates on the principle that you learn to be lighter, easier, and freer by experiencing light, easy, and free sensations in your body. Through their hands, Trager practitioners focus on communicating to your unconscious mind that there is an effortless way of being. To impart that quality, they work in a state of heightened awareness and connectedness, which Trager calls "hook-up" and describes as a meditative process of "becoming one with the energy force that surrounds all living things."[14]

Trager is a combination of hands-on tissue mobilization, relaxation, and movement reeducation called Mentastics. Without using a lubricant, practitioners introduce pleasurable sensory information to the soft tissues by steadily, gently, and rhythmically cradling, jiggling, rocking, vibrating, and stretching your body as you lie undressed on a padded table. There is never any invasion, force, or pain. Practitioners say the message from these sensations enters your central nervous system and triggers tissue changes through sensory-motor feedback loops between the brain and muscles.

The hands-on work sets off waves of motion in your body that lead to an experience of deep relaxation and greater joint and muscle mobility. This encourages freedom from deep-seated physical and mental patterns of rigidity and restriction that inhibit fluid movement, cause pain, and disrupt normal function. Such patterns develop in response to daily stresses or adverse circumstances, including accidents, surgery, and emotional trauma.

Dr. Trager has spent five decades helping people with severe neuromuscular disorders, including polio, multiple sclerosis, muscular dystrophy, Parkinson's disease, and poststroke trauma. He even saved his own wife from life in a wheelchair. According to practitioners, people also come for Trager work to reduce postoperative recovery time (for instance, after mastectomy), back pain, muscular and joint discomforts, and chronic headaches, and to gain greater energy, vitality, and inner peace.

To help maintain and strengthen the benefits of the hands-on experience, practitioners may instruct you in how to do Mentastics. This system of "mindfulness in motion" consists of easy-to-do, slow, dancelike movements—arm and leg swings, shakes, and kicks, and body stretches. He designed them to help his patients recall and re-create the satisfying sensory state induced during the table work.

To become certified in the Trager method, practitioners undergo beginning, intermediate, and advanced training, with supervised practice ses-

# Milton Trager

Unlike some innovators in the bodyways field, Milton Trager did not start off with a life-threatening illness. His method developed gradually and unusually.

Born in Chicago in 1908, Milton moved with his family to Miami when he was sixteen and frail. He took a job as a mail carrier, and every day after work he built up his body by running and doing gymnastics on the beach. This movement and meditation at the ocean became the foundation of what he later called Mentastics—a combination of "mental" and "gymnastics."

By the age of 18 he was training to be a professional boxer. After each workout his manager would give him a massage. One time the trainer looked so tired that the budding fighter offered to work on him instead.

"Hey, kid, how'd you learn to do that?" the trainer asked him.

"What do you mean?" he answered. "You taught me."

"I've never done anything like that to you. I'm telling you, you've got hands."

Young Milton was so elated that he went home and said, "Lie down, Pa, I think I can fix your legs up." His father's sciatica, acute for two years, was completely gone after two sessions and never reappeared. After this first success, Trager roamed his neighborhood looking for aches and pains to work on. He was only nineteen when his first polio victim walked—a sixteen-year-old boy who had been paralyzed for more than four years. Trager quit boxing to protect his hands and worked as a dancer and acrobat. And he Tragered.

In 1946 Trager tried to use his GI Bill benefits to get a medical degree, but seventy medical schools turned him down because of his age. Finally he took off for Mexico to study at the Universidad Autónoma de Guadalajara. When the interns there found out that he worked with infantile paralysis, Trager was called to do a treatment. Doctors, professors, the mother superior, and some of her nuns lined the room. On the table lay a four-year-old girl who had no function from the waist down. Trager started playing with her foot and she soon felt something. After forty minutes, the girl was able to move her foot and twitch her leg. The mother superior and her nuns dropped to their knees and crossed themselves. Within three weeks, the girl was walking. The university organized a clinic for Trager, in which he worked throughout his medical training.

In 1959, Dr. Trager opened a private practice in Waikiki, Hawaii. It wasn't until 1973 that he gave his first public demonstration, at Esalen, where he met group leader Betty Fuller. She convinced him to teach her his work, and she organized the Trager Institute to train others. Four years later, Dr. Trager closed his Hawaii practice to devote all his time to the growing number of students and to demonstrating his work at hospitals, medical schools, and training centers in the United States and Europe.[15]

# A Mentastics® Experience

Mentastics are not exercises but rather mentally directed movements. In exercise, your goal is increased tone, strength, endurance, or speed, all of which take effort. Mentastics are an effortless process of developing feelings of freedom, lightness, or softness. Dr. Trager recommends that when you do Mentastics, allow the movements to come from your mind by asking, "What can be lighter . . . and lighter than that? What can be softer . . . and softer than that?"

You can incorporate these movements easily into your daily life. For example, after sitting in a chair or driving a car for long, get up and gently do the kicking to relieve stiffness in your lower back and knees. I often get up from my computer and walk into the next room using this kick. When I was a runner, I used to cool down and loosen up by kicking. I still do it when I get off my bicycle to shake out my muscles and bones after riding.

## Kicking the Legs

Standing up, kick each leg once, keeping your foot low as though to brush the floor. As you repeat this light and loose kick, notice several things in your body. Feel the weight of your leg falling down and out of your hip socket. Feel your thigh muscles bounce and your calf and ankle shake. The movement also creates a natural jiggle in your lower back, which you can sense by pressing your fingers on the bony structure of your lumbar area. Don't try to make the bounce happen; the kick is neither deliberate nor strong.

Once your kick is free and easy, start walking with it, as though you were indifferently kicking a tin can. As you walk and kick, become aware of how you feel. If you get tired, stop and rest. If you sense pain, you're exerting too much effort.[16]

sions and regular reviews. They can also elect classes in anatomy, special conditions, movement, physiology, and other subjects. Workshops run from one to six days long.

RESOURCES:

**For instruction, practitioners, video, and publications:** The Trager Institute, 21 Locust, Mill Valley, CA 94941-2806, (415) 388-2688, fax (415) 388-2710, Internet: Tragerd@aol.com.

**Books:** Milton Trager with Cathy Guadagno-Hammond, *Mentastics: Movement as a Way to Agelessness* (Station Hill, 1987).

---

Of all the bodyways I've trained in, I found Trager the most playful to do. My clients and I enjoyed the humorous names taught in the early years for handling different parts of the body—"jelly calf," "playing the bass," "hitchhiking," "around the world"—and we laughed as I rocked their bodies and jiggled their flesh. One child giggled along with me as I made up new names just for her and went "ding dong" with her arms. Her parents and child-care provider later reported a dramatic improvement in her behavior. A woman said that her session felt like a symphony, complete with prelude, exposition, development, recapitulation of themes, and coda. To another woman, it was more like a painting, for she saw different colors. And I loved the sessions I received, too, always feeling lighter and longer when I got off the table.

## Craniosacral Therapy

Today, a wide variety of health-care professionals practice Craniosacral Therapy, but it began as a branch of osteopathy, a medical system of bone manipulation that restores structural integrity to alleviate disease. In the early 1900s Dr. William Sutherland, an osteopathic physician, dispelled the popular notion that the head is one solid, immovable skull when he discovered cranial movement. Twenty-two separate, movable bones are joined to one another by layers of tissue.

Craniosacral Therapy works with the craniosacral system. The cranium, spine, and sacrum (five united vertebrae that form part of the pelvis) are all connected by a continuous membrane of the body's deepest fascia, known as the dura mater, which houses the brain and central nervous system. In a semiclosed hydraulic system, cerebrospinal fluid is pumped through the membranes, creating a pulse of from six to twelve beats per minute. This craniosacral rhythm (CSR) is distinct from that of the heart and blood.

Craniosacral Therapists evaluate dysfunction and distortion in the dura mater and harmonize the primary elements of your craniosacral system. Although they say they can palpate the CSR anywhere on your clothed body—it exists throughout the connective tissue or fascia system—they sense it most easily at the sacrum or the occiput (base of the skull). They look for discrepancies in the rate, amplitude, symmetry, and quality of the CSR. Using gentle compression, therapists help realign the skull bones and stretch the underlying membranes so that the cerebrospinal fluid circulates freely and the CSR is balanced. Once your craniosacral system moves symmetrically and without resistance, your natural, self-adjusting physiological mechanisms can take over and clear up a wide variety of discomforts, including those associated with TMJ disorder, nasal congestion, and dizziness. These and other difficulties may arise from recent or long-ago trauma to the cranial bones or sacrum—anything from insufficient development of facial and jaw bones in utero and jamming of cranial bones during difficult delivery to falls and automobile accidents.

While compressing your head or other body part lightly, therapists will also follow it three-dimensionally in the direction it wants to go for the dura mater or other fascia to "unwind" out of its tension pattern. When your body reaches the exact position it needs to be in for such a release, the CSR will suddenly stop. John Upledger, an osteopathic doctor who has helped further Sutherland's discovery as both an evaluative tool and a corrective one, calls this spontaneous brief cessation the "significance detector." It indicates the possibility of *SomatoEmotional Release* (SER), the term he coined to describe a phenomenon that can, but doesn't always, occur in CST.

At this point, if you feel encouraged and trusting on a subconscious level, your body may assume the position it was in at the time of an accident or trauma, when what Upledger calls the energy of injury entered your tissues in a straight path. According to his theory, in reaction to that blow, your body probably bent away from it. If it couldn't dissipate the energy and thus allow normal healing to ensue, the "energy of injury" compacted into a localized "energy cyst" in the tissues. Whether an energy cyst forms depends on whether you were experiencing negative emotions at the time of injury. As your body unbends into the original position—the straight path of entry—it helps guide therapists to where stored-up emotions are located. These may then be released as shaking, sweating, laughing, or crying. Your whole body goes through an unwinding as energy cysts are freed.

When the memories surface to your awareness, you have the opportunity to resolve the difficulty and let go of symptoms and dysfunction. Upledger believes that we all live with an internal censor that protectively keeps certain memories hidden. However, the cost of such protection can be "pain, disability, unhappiness, chronic anger, irritability, lack of self-esteem and so on," he says.[17] We also live with what he calls an "efficiency expert," who wants to be rid of deeply buried conflicts. In SER,

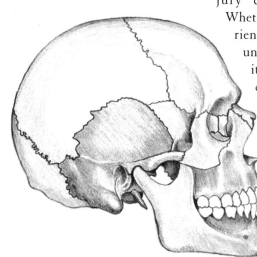

The Skull: Movable Bones Joined by Tissue

# Craniosacral Therapy and TMJ Disorder

John Upledger, D.O., tells the story of a fifty-eight-year-old woman who decided to try Craniosacral Therapy (CST) after suffering disabling episodic headaches, neck pain, and numbness in her arms for about fifteen years. Over the course of ten years she had received treatment from a dentist, a chiropractor, and an internist and, for more than six years, a psychotherapist, in case her headaches were psychosomatic. The woman even used splints in her mouth to prevent her teeth from clamping together too tightly and compressing her temporomandibular joints (TMJ).

After several hours of CST, she no longer had to use a dental appliance, and her aches and pains disappeared. Dr. Upledger surmised that a blow to her head had probably had an impact all the way to the roof of her mouth, which then widened and resulted in malocclusion between her upper and lower teeth and in abnormal wear and tear on her TMJ; his treatment included readjusting the position of her skull and the roof of her mouth.

Eventually the woman remembered that as a teenager on summer vacation at a lake, just as she was coming up from the water next to a raft, a young man had dived into the water and their heads collided. She had nearly drowned and had to be pulled out of the water and given artificial respiration.[18]

therapists align themselves with your unconscious desire to bring things forward to resolution.

Craniosacral Therapy practitioners report that, in addition to freeing accumulated stress, the method has relieved headaches, neck and back pain, eye dysfunctions, dyslexia, chronic middle-ear infections, depression, chronic fatigue, motor coordination difficulties, hyperactivity, and central nervous system disorders, including cerebral palsy. They also indicate success with infant-distress problems such as colic, asthma, and floppy baby syndrome. Dr. Upledger has even treated coma patients. In one case, by increasing the amplitude of her CSR, he successfully brought out a young woman who had been in a coma for three and a half years following a car accident. Although CST is mild, this method is not suitable in cases of acute systemic infections, recent skull fracture, intracranial hemorrhage or aneurysm, and herniation of the medulla oblongata.

Massage therapists, Rolfers, dentists, physical therapists, and other health-care professionals receive their CST training through a series of workshops from beginning to advanced levels. There are two levels of certification. Techniques and Diplomate.

The body often tries to bring our attention back to the "scene of the crime" to help us heal it.

—Christiane Northrup

It may seem strange to think that you can relieve what appears to be a muscular condition by "unwinding" the energy in that part of the body, yet it does happen. I've taken a sprained right arm and a sore left ankle that wouldn't take my full weight to a Craniosacral Therapy practitioner and experienced complete recovery within twenty-four to forty-eight hours. She never massaged or applied any pressure, but merely spiraled my arm or foot to unwind it out of the pattern that held in the energy of the original injury or overuse.

RESOURCES:

**For instruction, practitioners, publications, videos:** The Upledger Institute, 11211 Prosperity Farms Rd., Palm Beach Gardens, FL 33410-3487, (800) 233-5880; Colorado Cranial Institute, 1080 Hawthorn Ave., Boulder, CO 80304, (303) 449-0322; National Institute of Craniosacral Studies, Inc., 7827 No. Armenia Ave., Tampa, FL 33604-3806, (813) 935-0583, fax (813) 933-6355; Myofascial Release Seminars, 10 S. Leopard Rd., Suite 1, Paoli, PA 19301, (800) Fascial, (610) 644-0136.

**Books:** John E. Upledger, D.O., *Your Inner Physician and You: Cranio-Sacral Therapy, SomatoEmotional Release* (North Atlantic/Upledger Institute, 1992) and *SomatoEmotional Release and Beyond* (Upledger Institute, 1990); John F. Barnes, *Myofascial Release: The Search for Excellence* (MFR Seminars, 1990).

# Ortho-Bionomy™

> Given the choice, a body will choose ease over dis-ease.
>
> —Ida Rolf

As a black belt judo instructor in England, Arthur Lincoln Pauls decided to become an osteopathic physician so that he could help his students when they got injured. But because Japanese martial arts had taught him to "move with the energy," he was uncomfortable with the forceful techniques of his new profession and preferred to work by following the line of least resistance. He combined elements from both systems in developing Ortho-Bionomy (O-B) during the early 1970s. It is a gentle, nonintrusive method that works with your body's natural ability to self-regulate and shift toward balance. Loosely translated from its Greek roots, the word *ortho-bionomy* means "a correct application of the natural laws of life." Practitioners sometimes describe it as the "homeopathy of bodywork."

O-B follows the osteopathic principle that structure governs function. ☞ See "Structural Approaches," page 188. But instead of forcing structure into place by manipulation, O-B practitioners use "spontaneous release by positioning," which was discovered by another osteopath, Lawrence Jones. Ortho-Bionomists help guide you into the "preferred posture" or comfortable position, following the direction in which your body wants to move, and where it can spontaneously self-correct. The philosophy behind O-B is that each of us is responsible—has the ability to respond—for our own well-being.

If, for example, you have restricted movement in your head and neck, O-B practitioners first would locate tension points (reflex spots that are tender) in the area that needs attention. ☞ See "Trigger Point Therapy," page 174. Then they would move your head at the correct angle into the comfortable posture and gently add a slight bit of compression. Compression informs your central nervous system that you are needlessly holding certain muscles and that a signal should be sent to let go. Picture this as a knot in a string. If you try to pull the knot out, all you do is tighten it and make it harder to undo. But if you create slack around the knot by pushing both ends together, the knot becomes looser so you can untie it. Ortho-Bionomists wait from a few seconds up to three minutes for a release, which they monitor at your tension point. They also may cradle your neck in the preferred position and rock it gently to integrate the releases between the muscles at the joint. Finally they return your neck to its fully extended position, palpate the tension point for softening and release, and lightly rock your neck muscles. They apply these procedures to various areas of the body, promoting expanded range of motion, increased circulation of blood and lymph, and a greater sense of well-being.

O-B also involves postural reeducation and uses various other techniques to affect organs and balance the endocrine system. There are seven levels in O-B, with one devoted to working entirely with your energy field or aura and freeing mental and emotional fixations. Practitioners give you a homework program of exercises and body awareness as part of a self-care program to reinforce the hands-on sessions. They report that O-B has been helpful in arthritis, whiplash, sports injuries, rheumatic ailments, muscle pain, and emotional stress.

The training program to become a registered basic O-B practitioner consists of approximately 300 course hours and 150 practicum hours; senior practitioners train for an additional 500 hours.

RESOURCES:

**For practitioners and seminars:** Society of Ortho-Bionomy International, P.O. Box 1974-70, Berkeley, CA 94701, (800) 743-4890 or (608) 257-8828.

> Through balance man conserves nervous energy and thus directly benefits all his activities, mental as well as physical.
>
> —Mabel E. Todd

# Body Logic™

Yamuna Zake created Body Logic after various systems—including orthopedics, chiropractic, and acupuncture—proved unsuccessful in relieving acute pain in her left hip after the birth of her daughter. Based on the knowledge she had gained as a Yoga teacher since the age of sixteen, she utilized various postures to release and realign her hip. Within ten days she was back to normal.

Body Logic is a highly organized system of structural therapy, but it works differently than structural approaches that traditionally focus on the fascia. ☞ See "Structural Approaches," page 188. Instead, it seeks realignment by releasing your muscles at their origin and insertion points (where they attach to bones). Through traction of your joints, what Zake calls "muscle spacing" or "space-making," practitioners help elongate muscles and create space in the body. They also rotate joints in every possible position. Both traction and rotation educate the muscles and joints as to how well they can function. By decompressing and removing restrictions, Body Logic enables your body to move more freely, your blood to circulate more easily, and your energy to flow throughout. There's no forcing; rather, you let your body go where it feels safe and comfortable.

That is the body's "logic," "its instinctive knowledge of where it needs to release when given the opportunity," says Zake.[19] Practitioners work with your body's "natural muscle memory" to modify negative postures and painful holding patterns. They act on the principle that once your body "remembers" how good it feels to move effortlessly and painlessly, it quickly corrects itself.

To support your body and facilitate traction, practitioners use their own body for leverage—a hand holds here, an elbow traces a line there, a thigh hooks elsewhere. Because they have to be so physically close to do this, the work is intimate, but it is done neither in an inappropriate manner nor with a sexual overtone.

A session begins with the practitioner stretching your body while you're standing up, to assess where limitations exist. It continues on a padded floor and includes every part of you, even the cranium. Although they work with your physical structure, practitioners also listen to and follow your body's electrical or energy pulses. Zake's understanding of and sensitivity to the body goes beyond the gross physical structure to its energetic nature as well—the chakras and spinal energy channels she learned about in Yoga. ☞ See chakras, page 297. It is common to have a pervading sense of lightness once there is more space in your joints and to fall into a meditative state as your body and energy come into balance.

Body Logic therapists indicate that they deal with a wide range of discomforts and limitations. Dancers, runners, and other athletes especially appreciate this method for enhancing their movement potential and dealing with their injuries. But therapists work with people of any age and occupation, with such conditions as chronic back pain, herniated discs, kyphosis (hunchback curve), migraines, arthritis, strokes, epileptic seizures, and cerebral palsy.

Certified Body Logic practitioners undergo training with Yamuna Zake in intensive sessions that are several weeks long at one- and two-year levels, put in apprentice time, and renew their learning annually.

RESOURCES:

**For practitioners and training:** The Body Logic Studio, 295 W. 11th St., 1F, New York, NY 10014, (212) 633-2143; Philipanthony, 340 W. 87th St., Suite 2-A, New York, NY 10024, (212) 769-6443.

# Structural Approaches

> The minute you lose
> verticality, that minute
> you have lost the
> something plus that is
> available to humans.
>
> —Ida Rolf

As two-legged creatures, we humans experience something unique and distinct from four-legged animals—an upright posture. Our heads lift to the heavens while our feet connect us to the earth. This human reflex to stand is so primary that even in the first months of life, when our muscles are barely developed, we are already exploring how to arch our necks and backs so we can raise our heads and gaze forward while lying on our stomachs.

To remain at ease and function effectively in this upward orientation, according to practitioners of structural bodyways, we need to be in alignment with gravity. That's what such practitioners aim for: to organize or reorganize your structure so that the force of gravity flows through it. As a result, this process may enable you to fulfill whatever psychological, spiritual, and physical potential lies latent but restricted within you. Structural approaches are founded on the belief that the vertical alignment of your body can dramatically influence your health, behavior, and consciousness. In these and other fundamental principles of the field, we hear the echoing voice of Ida Rolf, Ph.D., the creator of Rolfing and the pioneer behind all the structural bodyways available today.

## STANDING UPRIGHT

What practitioners of structural approaches mean by *structure* is not only the skeleton itself, but, more important, the myofascial system. *Myo-* is muscle. *Fascia* is the tough but thin elastic connective tissue that forms an uninterrupted three-dimensional network from head to foot, knitting the body together like one huge sweater.[1] Because fascia ensheathes every muscle, bone, nerve, gland, organ, and blood vessel, it is what allows the body to retain its shape.

Without fascia, our skeletons would fall into a heap of bones and we couldn't maintain our erect carriage. Just underneath the skin, fascia wraps the whole body in a seamless blanket. Then it envelops each individual muscle fiber, bundles the separate muscle fibers, and collects the ends of muscles into tendons, the glistening white fibrous connective tissue that attaches muscles to bones or other body organs. Tough fascial bands or cords called ligaments hold together joints, connecting bone to bone. Fascial membranes called periosteum cover the outside of bone, while those called endosteum line the marrow cavities of bone. Still others, known as synovial membranes, line joint cavities and bursae, small sacs of heavy fluid between muscle and tendon or between bone, muscle, and tendon that reduce friction and facilitate movement.

Fascia also encases each organ, connects one to another, and binds them to the inner walls of the body cavity, so they stay put. Without fascia, your heart, lungs, and stomach could not remain suspended in their places.

Because of its interconnectedness, whatever happens to any part of the fascia can profoundly affect every other part of the body. Hereditary conditions, physical or emotional trauma, poor posture, inflammation, badly learned movement patterns, and other stresses can constrain, twist, or otherwise bind and shorten the fascia. According to physical therapist John F. Barnes, fascial restrictions can exert tremendous tensile forces—more than two thousand pounds of pressure per square inch—on nerves, blood and lymph vessels, bones, muscles, glands, and organs, and can result in various symptoms.[2]

Recall the image of the body as a sweater. If you pull, snag, or turn any part of it, what happens to the rest? Does it keep its integrity, or does it become distorted? If you've ever washed a sweater by hand, you know how important it is to block it afterward; if you don't, it will remain uneven and misshapen. The fascial network is similar, except for

Fascia envelops each individual muscle fiber, bundles the fibers together, and collects the ends of muscles into tendons, which attach muscles to the bones.

# Experience: Examining Fascia

Take a fresh grapefruit or orange. Cut it in half. With your hand, squeeze all the juice out of one half. Look at what's left. The membranous walls that divide sections and the inner lining of the rind are the fruit's connective tissue. If we had all the liquid squeezed out of us, what would remain is the fascia.

Another way to look at it is by peeling a whole grapefruit. Then carefully separate the ball of fruit into its sections. Notice the membrane encasing each piece. Open a section and look at the tiny globules of fruit within it and notice that each one is individually wrapped in a membrane as well. Each muscle and the individual muscle cells within it are similarly wrapped by fascia.[3]

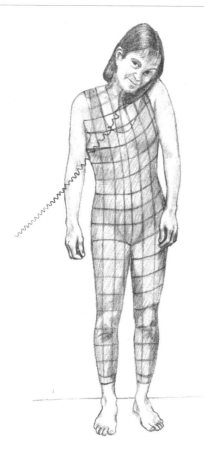

The Body as Fascial Sweater: Imbalanced patterns result in distortion.

its three-dimensionality. In a sense, over a series of sessions, a structural practitioner gradually "blocks" your "body sweater."

## Gravity and Vertical Alignment

Fascia is plastic and highly adaptable. It responds to the shock of any motion and also to the force of gravity. Gravity is one of the most dominant and fundamental powers in the universe. Without it, everything would fly off the surface of our planet. When we are in harmony with gravity, it acts as a support in keeping us vertical. When we're out of balance, it drains our energy as we struggle to hold ourselves up.

The principle of "tensegrity" (a term coined by architect Buckminster Fuller) in the relationship among the skeleton, muscles, and connective tissue explains how we maintain our vertical structure. Picture a tent. Once it's set up, what keeps the fabric from collapsing on the ground or blowing away in a wind? Both the center pole and the cables or ropes pulled to the right tension. Or visualize a radio tower. When the guy wires are equally taut in opposite directions, the tower stands in position and in line with gravity. In the same way, when our fascia and muscles are evenly balanced, they bring the spine in to an appropriate relationship with our center of gravity, efficiently transmitting weight downward and lifting it upward. If the fascia and muscles are too loose or too tight in any direction, the skeleton has to lean accordingly. In this case, gravity will exert a tremendous load on the body's structure instead of sustaining it.

The basic premise of structural bodyways is derived from osteopathy (a medical system of manipulation): The condition of our structure has an enormous effect on how we function. If we are experiencing bodily discomfort, it may be due to structural restriction. The pressure in some area may impede blood from flowing to bring fresh oxygen and nutrients and carry away waste products. It can also block lymph flow. Or it may interfere with information moving through a nerve to reach an organ. Releasing the restriction to balance structure allows the body's self-correcting mechanisms to operate again, alleviating symptoms and restoring proper function.

According to structural practitioners, manual pressure on the fascia changes its intercellular matrix (which it has more of than cells). This material consists of fibers—elastic, reticular, and collagenic—and an amorphous, jellylike ground substance. The polysaccharide gel complex includes highly viscous hyaluronic acid, which lubricates fibers so they can glide over each other, and proteoglycans, peptide chains that make the gel a kind of shock absorber. Because of inflammation, trauma, and chronically poor posture and movements, cross-link restrictions develop in the fibers, and the gel hardens. Manipulation breaks up the cross-links and also induces the ground substance to change from a cementlike solid to a gelatinous consistency, so it is able to absorb the compressive forces of movement or trauma.[4]

Like potters or sculptors working with clay, structural practitioners "tenderize" and lengthen the fascia with their hands, arms, or elbows while you're seated or lying down on a padded table. By manually pressing the tissue, they affect sensory receptors in muscles, tendons, and joints. This information travels as sensory input to your central nervous system, which then translates it into motor output: The fascia softens, and tonus (state of contraction or activity) decreases or increases, according to what would allow the tissue and nervous system to respond in a balanced way. In a sense, structural practitioners are a cross between master architect and master artist. They shape human bodies into stable, supported, yet dynamic forms that can function harmoniously.

> The human body—like the tires on a car or the rug on a floor—wears longest when it wears evenly.
>
> —Hans Selye

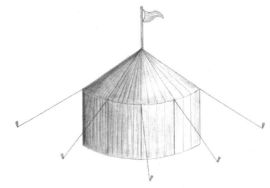

"Tensegrity" at work.

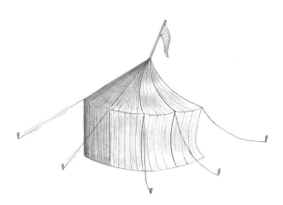

When muscles and fascia are too loose or too tight in any direction, they cause collapse or instability.

# An Experience of Gravity

To feel the powerful and pervasive force of gravity, take a hand weight of between three and five pounds. If you don't have one, fill a jar or plastic container with water, or use a can of food or juice.

Lie on your back, arms resting by your sides. With your eyes shut, take a few deep breaths until you're relaxed. Then, keeping your upper arm down, lift one forearm, bending it at a 90-degree angle to the floor. Let it find the perfect point of balance, where you don't have to make any effort to keep your arm up. When you are at this point with ease, you are harmoniously in line with gravity. Stay there for at least ten breaths.

Next, pick up the weight, jar, or can and put your arm back in the same position of effortless balance. If you find that point again, gravity now is supporting not only your arm, but also the several pounds of liquid or food in the container. Once you feel the easy balance, lower your forearm about halfway to the floor. Hold it here for another ten breaths. Do you notice any difference?

Still holding the weight, lift your whole arm straight up from the floor, seeing if you can find the point of balance again. Hold it there for ten breaths, then lower your arm to a 45-degree angle, also for ten breaths.

What's the difference between being in and out of alignment with gravity? Is one position easier than the other? Are you straining? Do you find yourself breathing harder? Are you getting anxious trying to hold up the weight when it's no longer centered?

Imagine your whole body being off at an angle, whether forward, back, or to the left or right, and having to labor to stay upright. Imagine the difference being upright and aligned with gravity.[5]

## Different Bodyways, Different Ideals

The various structural bodyways share the same basic assumptions: Most of us are not aligned with gravity; we function better when aligned; the body is plastic enough so that we can become realigned. However, there are also differences.

One practitioner may envision the body as a line, while another works in a spiral. The number of sessions may vary, and they may be grouped into a series with specific structural goals or be open-ended. Approaches may differ in where they begin and end in the body and in what is considered the keystone of their work. Movement awareness and attention to personal environment may figure to a greater or lesser degree. Emotional issues may be addressed or referred elsewhere. And the vision of a balanced structure changes from one bodyway to another. For some, there is an ideal to attain. For others, each body has its own appropriate form and no one ideal is suitable for everyone. In fact, ideals of symmetry may not be a true measure of alignment and wholeness.

It's not that ideals are "necessarily a bad thing," says Don Johnson, who left the Jesuits to train with Ida Rolf but later also gave up his Rolfing practice.[6] Indeed, they inspire us to fulfill more of our potential. But, he cautions, ideals can be dangerous if they become an authority used to convince people that they don't know what is best for themselves. The danger lies in one system claiming that *its* ideal shape is the truth, the one that, above all else, embodies the truly human. Thus, other ideals become "more primitive, aberrant, wrong, or even bad."[7] In turn, this can lead to "passivity, authoritarianism, and perverted social values."[8] In fact, says Johnson, there is no ideal symmetry to aspire to or be manipulated into:

> The emphasis on perfect symmetry in the various ideals does not correspond with the design of the body itself. We have three lobes of the lungs on the right side of the chest, two on the left. The organs are asymmetrically arranged. . . . The functions of the brain are asymmetrical. Most manual occupations and sports require us to use our bodies in asymmetrical ways. . . . The designers of somatic ideals, however, would have us try to construct a perfectly symmetrical shell of muscle and bone around

> Mechanically, physiologically, and psychologically, the human body is compelled to struggle for a state of equilibrium.
>
> —Mabel E. Todd

## Experience: Going with the Grain

To get a sense of how Judith Aston, the creator of Aston-Patterning, trains body practitioners to work with their hands, blow up a balloon. Let your hands conform to the shape of the balloon. Lightly move one hand across it in one direction, then in the other. See if you can read the natural direction of the balloon's membrane—clockwise or counterclockwise. Which way is easier to move your hand? Aston teaches body therapists to follow the grain of the tissue so they can glide along the fascia, in the same manner that woodworkers go with the grain of wood. Otherwise, when you go against the grain, you can create resistance and unnecessary pain.

—Courtesy of Ronnie Oliver and Judith Aston.

this core of organic and neurological asymmetry. . . . Moreover, there is no patterned relation between asymmetry and pain. On one hand I have worked with people who are as close to perfect symmetry and alignment as anyone I have ever seen but who still experience intense, debilitating back pain. On the other hand are people like Isaac Stern, who has spent his life playing the violin, a highly asymmetrical use of the body. His body is extremely curved, yet he radiates a grace and bodily pleasure which most of us can envy.[9]

In the same way that we're not inherently symmetrical, neither is posture static. According to Rolf, in its fullest sense posture "implies a dynamic interrelation of body parts in space such that at all times and in all conditions a free interplay exists."[10] There is no perfect posture to achieve and remain in. Rather, the goal is a flexible stature that uses the body's energy aesthetically and economically. Balance is never a fixed position but a fluidly changing movement appropriate to the situation.

## Results

Despite variations from one structural bodyway to another, successful functional results tend to be the same. When physical restrictions release, you feel lighter, easier, taller, younger, more spacious, and alive in your body. Energy that extra effort used to drain is now available. You can move with more coordination and refinement, with greater flexibility and range of motion.

As the body changes, so does the entire person.

—Edward Rosenfeld

You might also notice that initially your new posture feels awkward. But soon you realize that what was "normal" posture before was actually an imprecise organization of your body. Once you adjust to the reorganization, you may find that formerly comfortable furniture, even shoes, no

# Caution: Contraindications

**If you are acutely ill, more than three months pregnant, less than two months postoperative, or suffering a wasting disease (such as AIDS or cancer), structural practitioners should not work in certain areas of your body with particular techniques. Neither is this approach suitable if you have clotting problems, aneurysm, phlebitis, hardening of the arteries, lupus, hernia, severe edema, spondylosis, osteoporosis, or inflammatory arthritis. If in doubt, get a medical doctor's approval before receiving structural work. Generally, practitioners will not work with you if have serious addictions, unless you are in a treatment program, or if you're obese, unless you lose weight first.**

longer feel right. In fact, most chairs and car seats are not designed for true comfort and appropriate posture. We are physical victims of our culture, adjusting and compromising our bodies to the dictates of chairs, rather than the chairs being adapted to our requirements.[11]

As your body changes, so do your attitudes. You may find yourself relaxed, open, and responsive rather than tense, resistant, and reactive, and able to handle stresses with greater equanimity and creativity. In your new balanced structure, you may feel stronger and more secure, willing to experience rather than suppress your feelings, and prepared to face emotional issues you couldn't before. And you may notice that aches, pains, and illnesses diminish or even disappear.

# Rolfing® (Structural Integration)

Rolfing is the tree trunk from which other structural bodyways have branched. Also known as Structural Integration, it is the creation of Ida P. Rolf (1896–1979). It is both a systematic approach to releasing stress patterns and dysfunction in the body's structure and an educational process of understanding the relationship between gravity and the human body.

Rolf viewed the body as an architectural unit made up of several blocks or segments—head, shoulders, chest, pelvis, and legs. The position of each one is relevant to the others and is determined by the length and tone of muscles and fascia. When the segments are out of balance or misaligned, the body is forced to move in a limited or distorted manner. The area that can't respond to a demand for movement has to be compensated for by a part or parts that can. But that kind of adjustment calls for greater effort and energy to overcome the force of gravity, since gravity doesn't properly support and propel disorganized structure. Rolf called this being "at war with gravity."

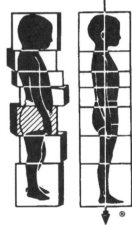

The Rolfing Logo

By manipulating the highly pliant myofascial tissue so that it lengthens and glides instead of shortens and adheres, Rolfers assist your body to reorganize its major segments into vertical alignment. They believe that when these units are balanced around a particular central vertical axis—the Rolf Line—your body can function with the most mechanical efficiency and ease.

Rolfers work from outer superficial layers to deeper ones, which Rolf called respectively "the sleeve" and "the core." You may experience intense discomfort when pressure is applied, but it disappears as soon as the practitioner lifts her fingers, elbow, or forearm. Sometimes there is soreness for a few days, as though you've overexercised; it may be the release of a chronic

# Experience: Checking Your Alignment

Stand in front of a full-length mirror and imagine a plumb line that drops from the center of the head through the level of your ears, shoulders, hips, knees, and ankles. Ideally, the left and right sides of the body are balanced and the pelvis approaches a horizontal position. If you have a three-way mirror, also look at yourself from a side view. Your trunk should fall directly over the pelvis, your head riding above the spine, with the spine's curves shallow, and the legs connecting vertically to support the bottom of the pelvis.

tension that is both physical and emotional. Memories may surface during or after a session. ☞ See "Remembering Through the Body," page 123. In the early years of Rolfing, manipulation was not as refined as it later became, and pain, excruciating enough to evoke cries of distress, was not uncommon. However, through the efforts of various advanced practitioners and instructors, the techniques are now less invasive, more precise, and gentler.

Rolfers work with children and adults, adjusting accordingly. The Rolfing experience consists of a basic series of ten sessions, generally spaced a week or more apart. They follow a particular sequence, but also adapt to the needs of your unique physical structure. Each of the first seven sessions releases restrictions in specific areas of the body and progressively builds upon the results of the previous one. The last three sessions integrate the work of the earlier ones and fine-tune the relationships between segments to bring your body to optimal balance. Many people experience remarkable changes after the series, but how permanent they are varies, depending especially on whether new movement patterns are learned. According to the Rolf Institute, photographs taken of clients years after the Basic Ten show that changes were still present.

Once the Basic Ten are completed, you can reinforce and further the work through a five-session advanced series after waiting six months to a year. In the last ten to fifteen years, advanced Rolfers have progressed beyond the limitations of the original formulistic ten-session series. Instead of following the template of an ideal body—structural symmetry—they aim for functional economy. They also recognize that most myofascial manipulation does not address restricted joints. To free them, they don't "pop" bones into place, the way chiropractors do, but ease them there by working with ligaments and small muscles.

Rolfers also incorporate Rolfing Movement Integration (RMI). Whereas the hands-on sessions are designed to relieve strain in the fascia (structure) the movement sessions eliminate unnecessary encumbrances and tensions in movement patterns (function). Through a combination of touch and verbal communication, RMI teachers help you develop greater awareness of your vertical orientation and habitual patterns. "The premise of Rolfing Movement Integration . . . is that you can restore your structure to balance by changing the movement habits that perpetuate imbalance," says Rolfer and RMI teacher Mary Bond.[12]

How you move—your "movement signature"—often becomes fixed early in life and expresses beliefs, attitudes, and emotions you developed then in relating to the world. Psychological stances appear in physical stances. You can recognize such signatures in the characteristic way people you know walk, stand, sit, and work. In RMI you can learn to release tensions and discover alternative ways to move effectively,

Strength that has effort in it is not what you need; you need the strength that is the result of ease.

—Ida Rolf

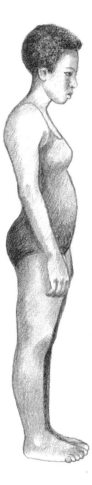
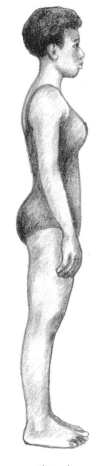

Misaligned                    Aligned

# Ida Rolf

Photographs of Ida Pauline Rolf at eighty portray a kindly-looking, white-haired woman with a flower pinned at the top of her head, soft eyes, and large hands with prominent knuckles—the epitome of a benevolent grandmother. In fact, she was a formidable figure, and this in a time when women were not encouraged to have minds of their own.

Born in 1896 in New York, Rolf grew up in the Bronx, the only child of a successful, domineering electrical engineer and his proper Victorian wife. In 1916 she graduated from Barnard College, and four years later she earned her Ph.D. in biological chemistry from the College of Physicians and Surgeons of Columbia University. Defying her father's injunction against working, Rolf talked her way into a job at the Rockefeller Institute, where she later became an associate in its Department of Organic Chemistry. That same year she also married, eventually giving birth to two sons.

Rolf came to appreciate alternative forms of health care when she saw, through her own experiences, how effective they could be. As a young woman, on a trip to Colorado she received a blow from a horse's hoof and wound up with pneumonialike symptoms. It was the day before her departure for Yellowstone. Stranded alone in a rustic cabin, she was burning up with a temperature of 104°. Eventually Rolf got to a hospital in Montana. Her attending doctor, not satisfied with her rate of recovery, called in an osteopath to treat her. After his manipulations, she was able to breathe well again. Despite a railroad strike, she managed to get back to New York, where her mother took her to a blind osteopath.

When Rolf's father died in 1928, her inheritance allowed her to resign from Rockefeller and continue her pursuit of independent studies. Out of concern for her

Posture is also part of our emotional anatomy: How we hold ourselves somatically is related to how we hold ourselves emotionally and psychologically.

—Clyde Ford

whether driving a car, lifting furniture, playing a flute, sitting at a desk, wielding a hammer, or bouncing a basketball. You see how to modify your environment to suit your needs rather than strain your body to modify it to the environment.

Some instructors also teach Rolfing Rhythms, a series of lively yet relaxed exercises designed to evoke awareness of Rolfing principles of ease, length, balance, and harmony with gravity. The exercises also improve muscle tone and coordination, deepen breathing, and extend flexibility.

People try Rolfing for the same reasons they try other bodyways—to reduce physical or emotional pain, eliminate discomfort, develop greater body awareness, improve athletic abilities, unlock their potential, or otherwise enhance their lives. Research conducted at the University of California-Los Angeles demonstrated that Structural Integration leads to

own health, she studied with a variety of practitioners, including a tantric yogi, somatic pioneer Bess Mensendieck, teachers of F. M. Alexander's technique, homeopaths, naturopaths, chiropractors, and osteopaths. She also explored the teachings of Russian philosopher G. I. Gurdjieff and the work of Alfred Korzybski, the inventor of General Semantics. Through her travels and these various communities, she came in contact with such celebrities as Georgia O'Keeffe and Greta Garbo, who later became her clients.

Osteopathy probably exerted the greatest influence on Rolf's thinking. She developed a close friendship with the blind osteopath and accompanied him to seminars, where she gained an interest in the osteopathic theory that structure determines function. Another of her teachers was Amy Cochran, an osteopath in her sixties who lived in California. Rolf drove back and forth across the country with her two small boys and a big orange cat to learn the exercises Cochran claimed had come to her by psychic perception from Dr. Benjamin Rush, the physician who signed the Declaration of Independence. It was the late years of World War II, a time of shortages, but Rolf convinced the rationing board to let her have enough fuel for her trips.

Rolf built on all the many techniques and theories she investigated, and incorporated what was useful. To the basic osteopathic principle she added the notion that structure in gravity also determines function and behavior. She constantly kept in mind "that bodies had to lengthen" and that the soft tissue had to move "toward the place where it really belongs."

Rolf taught and worked with people around the United States, in Canada, and in England. Then, in the mid-1960s, she went to Esalen Institute on the invitation of Gestalt therapist Fritz Perls. Every summer for years thereafter, Rolf arrived to "hang out her shingle." And there, on the cliffs above the Pacific Ocean, she started teaching Structural Integration, or, as her students affectionately called it, Rolfing.[13]

more efficient use of the muscles, allows the body to conserve energy, and creates more refined patterns of movement. Another study, at the University of Maryland, indicated that the work significantly diminishes chronic stress, transforms body structure (for example, reducing spinal curvature in lordosis or swayback), and improves neurological functioning.[14]

Nevertheless, Rolf herself insisted that her work was not primarily about directly relieving physical symptoms or curing disease. She was more interested in organizing the person into wholeness or integration. To her, the physical body is actually the personality and energy unit we call a human being. An upright body balanced in the field of gravity is a spiritual body: Neuromuscular balance can lead not only to physical grace but also to freedom, love, and wisdom.

In order to become trained as a Rolfer, applicants first must be expe-

# Getting to Know Your Standing and Walking Patterns: An Experience in Rolfing Movement Integration

Choose a room or hallway that is long enough for you to walk twenty paces without having to turn around. Move purposefully, as if you were crossing the room to open a door. Go back and forth until the pace and rhythm of your gait feel ordinary. Tape the questions that follow and play them back or have someone read them to you while you keep walking. Leave room for a pause at the three dots (. . .).

Stand comfortably without wearing shoes. Shift your body around until you are in a position that feels familiar, as though you were waiting on line at the supermarket. What feels more comfortable—letting your body weight settle into your right leg or the left? . . . Do your feet turn outward or inward? . . . Do your knees lock or slightly give? . . . Are you leaning most of your weight on one hip? . . . Shift onto your other hip and notice whether that feels as comfortable. Then return to your familiar position.

What are you doing with your arms? Are they crossed on your chest or akimbo, with your hands on your hips? . . . Does that position make your torso feel stable? . . . Is your rib cage in line with your pelvis? . . . Are your hips forward and your chest caved in . . . or are your buttocks thrust back and your chest forward?

How is your head sitting? . . . Does it balance easily on top of your spine . . . or is your neck tense from holding your head in place? . . . Does your chin jut forward or pull in toward your throat? . . .

Now begin walking and get into a familiar rhythm. Pay attention to the sound your

---

rienced with massage, anatomy, physiology, and kinesiology. The basic certification training itself consists of 700 hours in two phases and covers not only Rolfing theory and practice but also movement education, psychotherapeutic approaches, and other subjects. To become an advanced Rolfer requires 360 additional hours of continuing education.

## RESOURCES:

**For training programs, practitioners, publications, videos, and other information:** Rolf's legacy is carried on by two groups: The Rolf Institute of Structural Integration, P.O. Box 1868, Boulder, CO 80302-1868, (800) 530-8875 or (303) 449-5903, fax (303) 449-5978; and the Guild for Structural Integration, P.O. Box 1559, Boulder, CO 80306-1559, (303) 447-0122 or (800) 447-0150.

feet make on the floor. Continue walking until you know you could recognize that sound on a tape recording. How hard or how lightly do your heels hit the floor? . . . Does one foot strike more strongly than the other? . . . Does one leg take a longer stride than the other?

Notice how far your rib cage is from the ground as you walk. Sense that distance from inside, kinesthetically, not by looking in a mirror or measuring with a yardstick. Does your chest seem far from or close to the ground?

Imagine your body as divided in two, with upper and lower halves. Where is that dividing line? . . . At your hips? Midriff? Upper chest?

Stop walking and stand relaxed. Imagine that you have a motor inside that controls your body's movements. Where is it located? When you take your next step, from where does your impulse to move arise . . . from your body's upper or lower half?

Find the center of your chest. Where is your heart in relation to your knees and feet . . . in front of them or behind? . . . Does it feel as though your heart is reaching to spur you forward . . . or are your hips driving ahead while your trunk lags behind? . . . Does your head stick out in front of your chest?

Just for fun, exaggerate all these details you've just noticed about how you walk. Does the exaggeration feel like something you're accustomed to? Not to worry, says Bond. "Your structure is plastic and its blueprint can change."[15]

**Books:** Rosemary Feitis, ed., *Ida Rolf Talks About Rolfing and Physical Reality* (Rolf Institute, 1978); Ida P. Rolf, *Rolfing: Reestablishing the Natural Alignment and Structural Integration of the Body for Vitality and Well-Being* [originally published as *The Integration of Human Structures*] (Healing Arts, 1989); Brian W. Fahey, *The Power of Balance: A Rolfing View of Health* (Metamorphous, 1989); Don Johnson, *The Protean Body: A Rolfer's View of Human Flexibility* (HarperColophon, 1977); Brian Anson, *Rolfing: Stories of Personal Empowerment* (Heartland Personal Growth Press, 1991); Mary Bond, *Rolfing Movement Integration* (Healing Arts, 1993); Rose Spiegel, *Health and Bodies Consciousness: A Guide to Living Successfully in Your Body Through Rolfing and Yoga* (SRG, 1994).

**Videos:** "Rolfing: Gravity Is the Therapist," Ida Rolf, 25 mins., Rolf Institute, (800) 530-8875; "Rolfing: Dimensions of Change," 23 mins., the Rolf Institute, (800) 530-8875.

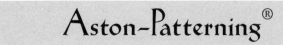

# Aston-Patterning®

Judith Aston was teaching movement education to dancers, actors, and athletes at a college when she found her way to Ida Rolf's hands because of significant injuries she had sustained in two car accidents. Immediate improvement convinced her of the value of Rolf's work. Building on Rolf's postural ideas, Aston created the first full movement education system for Rolfing. In 1971 she began training Rolfers and others in Rolf-Aston Structural Patterning and Movement Analysis, and she assisted them in learning how to use their bodies with greater ease, which resulted in a "softer" Rolfing style.

By 1977 Aston had begun to perceive the body from a perspective that she realized was not compatible with the Rolf Line. She felt that the body should not be shaped into a linear symmetry that was not natural to it. She also believed that the plumb line should fall in front of the maleolus (ankle bone) and on a slight forward incline, which requires a more anteriorly tilted pelvis. Aston left the Rolf Institute to form her own organization. As she gradually evolved her system, she introduced the idea of working in a three-dimensional spiral pattern and added a fitness program and environmental modification to maximize the client's comfort in sitting, sleeping, or engaging in sports.

Aston-Patterning today is an integrated system that also includes a comprehensive formal evaluation process. Three hands-on techniques address functional and structural patterns: 1) Aston Massage reduces everyday tension, calms your body and mind, and enables you to sense and feel your own shape through uniquely three-dimensional, surface-through-to-the-bone spiral strokes; 2) Myokinetics utilizes highly localized three-dimensional spiral strokes that alternately stretch and release the myofascia to remove restrictions and rehydrate the tissue; and 3) Arthrokinetics, the deepest work, affects the joints and junctures of tissue planes in spiral patterns rather than in linear directions.

The movement education component is called Neurokinetics. All the manual techniques serve to create space for or sustain changes produced through movement education. You learn and integrate principles of movement through nine different kinds of units of work with endless varia-

# An Aston-Patterning Experience

Sit on a chair that allows your hips to be lower than your knees. Notice your posture. Does your chest feel shallow and collapsed or full? Is your head sitting forward or back? Is your breathing free or restricted? How much does your rib cage expand when you breathe? Do you feel tension in your neck, shoulders, or lower back? Is your abdomen relaxed or compressed? Move your trunk forward and back. Note how this feels. Raise one arm: Is it light or heavy?

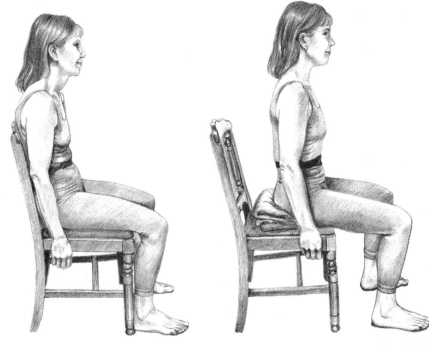

Now, place a folded bath towel or wedge on your chair seat. It should be thick enough so that your hips will be higher than your knees when you sit down. Sit forward on the seat so that the front half of your thighs and your knees are free. Again, notice what's happened to the dimension of your chest, the quality of your breathing, the position of your head, and so on. Does it take more or less work for your neck muscles to hold your head straight? Repeat the earlier instruction to move your trunk forward and back and raise your arm. How does this compare to the first experience?

—Courtesy of Ronnie Oliver, Aston-Patterner.

We will not encounter changes in the body apart from corresponding mental, emotional, and other changes. It seems to be a general rule that an improved condition of the body fosters other improvements.

—Robert Masters and Jean Houston

tions—for example, sitting-to-standing or using the arms in a specific activity, such as reaching.

Aston Fitness, an exercise program, improves proportion, muscle tone, joint resiliency, cardiovascular conditioning, and lightness in movement. It also helps reduce stress, enhance athletic performance, and prevent injuries.

At the core of Aston's system is the Aston Paradigm. It recognizes all movement—physical, emotional, cognitive, and spiritual—as following an asymmetrical, three-dimensional spiral. It respects the whole body and its individual parts as possessing a natural integrity, dimension, and proportion—there is no ideal body type to achieve or conform to. It considers alignment in the body in terms of part to part, part to whole, whole to gravity, and whole to environmental constructs (shoes, chairs, beds, etc.). It defines balance as the negotiation of asymmetrical differences. And it distinguishes between necessary and unnecessary tension.

Unlike Rolfing, there is no set series. Each session is specifically designed for you and can include any component of Aston-Patterning or a combination of several. Although practitioners respect and include an awareness of how cognitive and emotional patterns are related to physical structure and function, when they sense that assistance would be useful to you they may refer you to professional counselors for concurrent verbal psychotherapy.

The certification program to become an Aston-Patterner has a three-level format that includes training in both movement education (Neurokinetics) and soft tissue work (Myokinetics). Coursework takes fifteen months or longer and occurs in blocks of three to six weeks with three- to five-month periods in between for practical application.

RESOURCES:

**For information, practitioners, and training:** Aston-Patterning, P.O. Box 3568, Incline Village, NV 89450, (702) 831-8228.

# Hellerwork

Joseph Heller, a former aerospace engineer, studied with Ida Rolf and Judith Aston and became the first president of the Rolf Institute in 1976. Three years later, he left to found his own system for rebalancing the whole body.

Hellerwork is an integrating process that combines three components. Connective tissue manipulation helps realign your body and release chronic rigidities. Movement reeducation teaches you greater body awareness and stress-free methods of engaging in daily activities. Guided verbal dialogue assists you in recognizing the relationship among your body, emotions, and attitudes, dealing with memories that surface, and discovering new ways to handle stress.

Heller's approach consists of a series of eleven sessions. Each one addresses different physical and psychological themes. Sessions one, two, and three focus on the surface or superficial layers of the fascia and on developmental issues of infancy and childhood—breathing, standing up, and reaching out. Core sessions four through seven work on the deep layers and on adolescent developmental issues—for example, control and surrender. The last four sessions are designed to integrate all the previous ones and look at questions of maturity, such as masculine and feminine styles.

Training to become certified as a Hellerwork practitioner is a 1,250-hour program that includes extensive training in anatomy, psychology, and movement education in addition to theory and practice of the Heller method.

### RESOURCES:

**For training, practitioners, and other information:** Hellerwork, 406 Berry St., Mt. Shasta, CA 96067, (800) 392-3900 or (916) 926-2500, fax (916) 926-6839.

**Books:** Joseph Heller and William A. Henkin, *Bodywise* (Wingbow, 1991).

# Postural Integration

Jack Painter, Ph.D., developed Postural Integration after years of exploring massage, Yoga, Zen, acupuncture, Gestalt and Reichian therapies, and Rolfing. His ten-session system combines deep tissue work, deep breathing, Gestalt, regression, movement awareness, and Acupressure to help loosen rigid postures and habits. While working with the fascia, the practitioner encourages you to simultaneously breathe more freely, express blocked emotions and thoughts, and investigate new physical movements. The first seven sessions release the legs, pelvis, torso, arms, and head and dissolve basic defensive armor—"letting go of the old self." The final three sessions are for integration—"bringing it all together."

Provisional certification as a Postural Integrator requires completion of both theoretical and practical study consisting of two phases in a series of extended weekends over one year as well as an internship at the end of each phase. Full certification is the third phase of training and requires an additional year of working with clients.

RESOURCES:

**For information, newsletter, instruction, practitioners, books, and videos:** International Center for Release and Integration, 450 Hillside Ave., Mill Valley, CA 94941, (415) 383-4017.

**Books:** Jack Painter, *Deep Bodywork and Personal Development: Harmonizing Our Bodies, Emotions, and Thoughts* and *Technical Manual of Deep Wholistic Bodywork: Postural Integration* (Bodymind, 1987).

**Videos:** "Bodymind Transformations," Jack Painter, 45 mins., Bodymind Books, (415) 383-4017; "Deep Tissue and Personal Development: A Review for Bodyworkers," Jack Painter, 4 tapes, Bodymind Books, (415) 383-4017.

# Soma Neuromuscular Integration

Soma Neuromuscular Integration, or Soma Bodywork, also evolved out of Rolf's original work. Bill M. Williams, Ph.D., and his wife, Ellen Gregory Williams, Ph.D., founded the Soma Institute in 1978. One of Rolf's first students, he taught with her and was on the Rolf Institute's founding board of directors. He refined the early style of manipulation by creating easier, less intrusive ways of entering the myofascia.

Soma induces physical, emotional, and perceptual change by structurally balancing your body in gravity and integrating your nervous system. The ten-session series follows the same sequence as in Rolfing. The practitioner directly manipulates your fascia and muscles to remove "blocks" of chronic tension and structural aberration as well as to balance muscular tone. To elevate your level of awareness, Soma incorporates such learning tools as autogenic training (a deep relaxation technique), personal journal-keeping, dialogue, movement education, photographs and/or video.

According to the directors of the Soma Institute, the technique is also based on the three-brain model theory, a way of understanding human consciousness and activity of the nervous system. This model stems in part from neuropsychiatric research that delineates specific functions of the right and left hemispheres of the brain. The third aspect of the model is the "corebrain" of nerve plexi in the abdomen by which the right and left brains translate cognition into activity. It is the "body brain" or source of bodily energy or chi from which arises the coordinated, effortless, fluid movement of dancers and martial artists.

Training is offered in a two-part format. The foundation program of 500 hours teaches the basic educational information required to pass a state board exam in massage. A separate 368-hour course leads to certification as a Soma practitioner.

## Resources:

**For information, instruction, and practitioners:** Soma Institute of Neuromuscular Integration, 730 Klink St., Buckley, WA 98321, (360) 829-1025.

**Videos:** "An Introduction to Soma Bodywork," George Kousaleos, 49 mins., (800) 843-9843.

# CORE Bodywork

George P. Kousaleos was in Bill Williams's charter Soma class. After practicing and teaching the Soma system of structural integration, he founded CORE Bodywork. It is a multiphase educational process in which each phase focuses on balancing progressively deeper layers of connective tissue and musculature. CORE Massage works with the superficial myofascia. CORE Myofascial Therapy is phase one (three sessions) of a ten-session structural integration series; it addresses improvements in breathing, standing postural balance, and pelvic reeducation. CORE Intrinsic Therapy—sessions four through seven—works with the deepest levels of myofascia and emphasizes appropriate organization of the legs, pelvis, thorax, neck, and head. The final three sessions comprise CORE Integration Therapy, for integrating the structure with fluidity, intrinsic balance, and self-reliance.

Certification training in CORE Massage and CORE Myofascial Therapy takes place in four-day workshops each; for CORE Intrinsic Therapy and CORE Integration Therapy there are one-month residential training programs each.

## Resources:

**For information, training, and practitioners:** CORE Institute, 223 W. Carolina St., Tallahassee, FL 32301, (904) 222-8673.

# Myofascial Release

Dr. Robert Ward, an osteopathic physician, coined the term *myofascial release* in the 1960s to describe his contribution to soft-tissue manipulation. It is not a fixed series of sessions; rather, it is one component in a whole group of complementary procedures that evaluate and treat your fascial system. John Barnes, who has been a physical therapist for more than three decades, developed this group of procedures as Myofascial Release (MFR). It is based on aspects of osteopathy, such as Craniosacral Therapy, physical therapy, and Rolfing. The overall intention is to relieve pain, resolve structural dysfunction, restore function and mobility, and release emotional trauma.

To effect these changes, practitioners employ a gentle form of sustained pressing on and stretching of the fascia in conjunction with visual analysis, palpation, soft-tissue mobilization, treatment of trigger points, craniosacral manipulation, and myofascial unwinding. Soft-tissue mobilization techniques break up superficial cross-restrictions of the collagen, whereas myofascial release techniques break down barriers within the deeper layers of fascia by stretching the cross-links and changing the viscosity of the ground substance. Once the fascia unwinds from abnormal twists and turns, structural integrity and better functioning of nerves, organs, vessels, and glands follow.

Health professionals who incorporate MFR include physicians, physical therapists, and massage therapists, among others. They learn the techniques through a series of seminars and use them in hospitals, rehabilitation centers, sports medicine facilities, and in such medical specialties as geriatrics, pediatrics, and dentistry. They report success with acute and chronic pain, neurological and movement dysfunctions, birth trauma, head injuries, headaches, TMJ disorder, and other conditions.

## RESOURCES:

**For information, instruction, and practitioners:** MFR Seminars, 10 S. Leopard Rd., Suite 1, Paoli, PA 19301, (800) Fascial or (610) 644-0136.

**Books:** John F. Barnes, *Myofascial Release: The Search for Excellence* (MFR Seminars, 1990).

**Audiovisual:** Myofascial Release Series, Michael Shea, 5 videotapes with manuals, (407) 627-7372.

# CHAPTER 10

# Functional Approaches

As human beings, we are born with a great capacity for self-determination—the freedom to choose—because we are able to know what we're doing rather than act on instinct alone. This ability to decide for or against one thing over another takes place, at the most fundamental level, in our sensory-motor or neuromuscular system.

"Movement occurs only when the nervous system sends the impulses that contract the necessary muscles in the right patterns or assemblies and in the right sequences in time," said Moshe Feldenkrais, the Israeli physicist turned somatic educator.[1] To carry out any decision—to go forward or hold back—we bend or flex certain muscles (flexors) and extend or straighten others (extensors). In fact, the muscles work in pairs as agonists and antagonists. However, if one side of this equation overcontracts, the opposing side has to overstretch. The result is postural imbalance, weakness, and limited range and quality of movement.

### LEARNING TO MOVE

If we keep repeating a particular pattern of movement or muscular contraction, it will soon become an unconscious reflexive habit—that is, we're no longer aware of what we're doing. What was once voluntary now is involuntary—out of our awareness. After a while, this automatic response even feels "normal." F. M. Alexander, the originator of the Alexander Technique, called this phenomenon "debauched kinesthesia": when what is wrong—that is, an imbalance in musculature—feels right.[2] Habit forma-

> Man is an animal because of his structure. But he is the highest animal and a human being because of the functioning of his nervous system.
>
> —Moshe Feldenkrais

> Habits at first are silken threads, then they become cables.
>
> —Spanish proverb

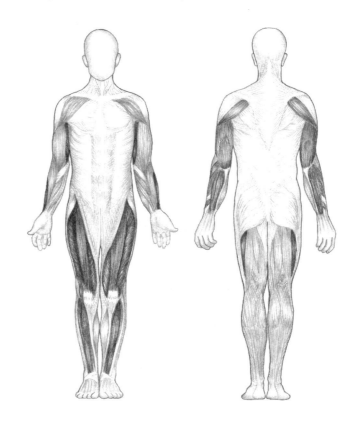

Muscle groups work in pairs.  Flexors (shaded lightly) allow us to bend; extensors (shaded darkly) allow us to straighten.

tion is not in and of itself negative; in fact, it is necessary.[3] Without it, we would have to rethink at each moment how to organize ourselves to move. The problem is that poor body usage can become habitual just as easily as good body usage. And this, unfortunately and too often, is how most of us function.

Whereas structure is about the arrangement or organization of parts and their relationship to one another, function is about how you use that makeup—about how you perform, operate, or move your given structure. In this regard, functional approaches are not techniques for learning a special art, but rather "pre-techniques" that prepare you for mastering particular skills—wielding a hammer, strumming a guitar, mopping a floor, playing tennis, dancing, or chopping wood—with maximal efficiency. Functioning efficiently means using the appropriate or economical—not too much, not too little—amount of effort and energy in any activity, as well as the appropriate organization and choice of body parts and move-

Unlike dogs, human beings form habits of managing their bodies badly, through false notions about "holding" certain parts.

—Mabel E. Todd

ment patterns. This is true even in something as simple as sitting down or bending over and lifting an object.

You wouldn't think you'd need help in knowing how to do the basics. After all, aren't you capable of "doin' what comes naturally"? The originators of the various functional disciplines generally agree that while you probably start out in life moving with natural ease (provided you're not born with a congenital deformity or dysfunction), during the ensuing years your innate movement tendencies get interfered with. A host of physical, social, cultural, and emotional experiences plant the seeds of movement patterns that later lead to a wide range of difficulties. You accumulate poor body habits, including impaired body image and restricted flow of energy, that can distort anything from the way you write to how you reach for things. If, for example, you learned penmanship by sitting hunched over a desk, gripping a pen and pressing hard, your brow furrowed and your jaw set in determination, your stomach and thighs tight, then it's likely that even decades later you'll continue to hold yourself in this tension pattern each time you write. It's your unconscious habit to do so.

Functional bodyways are concerned with helping you come out of such habitual tendencies. Their basic premise is that movement patterns are not permanent because the brain and nervous system are still fully capable of learning: It is possible to reorganize how your body functions and provide new movement options. In turn, this will lead to alternative ways of thinking and feeling.

> Whatever the art you may wish to learn . . . acrobatics or violin playing, mental prayer or golf, acting, singing, dancing . . . there is one thing that every good teacher will always say: Learn to combine relaxation with activity; learn to do what you have to do without straining; work hard, but never under tension.
>
> —Aldous Huxley

## Education, Not Therapy

To help you remove the obstacles that keep you from functioning at your best, practitioners engage you in a learning process that develops your proprioceptive literacy—the ability to read your body's sensations from within. Thus, they call their particular disciplines *psychophysical, physical, neural, physiological,* or *body reeducation,* or *somatic education.* And they consider themselves teachers rather than therapists. You are their student, not client or patient, and their sessions are lessons instead of treatments. Since there is no fixed number of sessions, you may choose never to stop learning how to sense, feel, breathe, move, and live with greater ease and joy. As Robin Powell, a Kinetic Awareness teacher in New York, says, "Awareness work is never finished; it is an ongoing process. It is not a cure."[4]

## Awareness

The most important ingredient in all functional bodyways is sensory awareness—focusing attention on what you're sensing in the body. Moshe

Feldenkrais called awareness the third state of existence, after waking and sleeping: "In this state the individual knows exactly what he is doing while awake, just as we sometimes know when awake what we dreamed while asleep."[5]

> When we truly sense what we are doing, that's when we have a choice, that's where change takes place.
>
> —Sandra Bain Cushman

Without this awareness, you don't fully inhabit your body, and you can't gain control of what you do and how you do it. According to a Tibetan parable recounted by Feldenkrais, each of us is like a carriage with desires as passengers, muscles as horses, and the skeleton as the carriage itself. If the coachman (your awareness) is wide awake and regulates the reins, then the horses will pull the coach and bring every passenger to the proper destination. But if your coachman is asleep—if you are not aware— you will be dragged aimlessly here and there.[6]

This sensory awareness refers to the sensing of actual bodily feelings created by your nervous system as it continuously monitors and relays information about your inner states. To describe these feelings, you would use words such as *cold, tight, numb, heavy, sharp,* or *moist.* These physical qualities differ from the interpretations you make that give your experience meaning, such as *supported, uncomfortable, safe,* and *abandoned.* Sensations are also different from emotions, which include being *angry, elated,* or *sad.* ☞ See also "An Experience of Felt Sense," page 371.

When you focus attention on a part or parts of your body during movement, you can feel what moves and what doesn't; you become aware of the holding or tension pattern. As you systematically explore in this way,

## An Awareness Experience

If you're holding this book in your hands as you're reading, pause to become aware of sensations in your hands. Notice—from inside rather than by looking—how you grasp the book. As soon as you become conscious of what you're feeling, what happens? Do you find yourself making adjustments for greater comfort? Do you relax your grip or alter how your hands are positioned on the book? If you feel the book slipping, do you tighten your hold?

If you're not holding the book, but letting it rest on a desk or table, stop to place your attention on your neck and shoulders. Are you tense and straining forward, or are you comfortable? Notice what happens the moment you beam awareness on this area of your body. What changes do you make? Do the same thing for your stomach, thighs, and breath.

Awareness of kinesthetic or proprioceptive cues—pressure, heaviness, pain, and so on—from sensory receptors induces your muscles to shift to better, easier functioning.

you are engaging your sensory-motor system and establishing communication between your muscles and your brain. Here's how it works.

The central nervous system (CNS) is the functional control center of the body. Motor nerves—nerves that trigger motion—are at the front of the spinal column and spread out to muscular tissues in an efferent (outgoing) network. When electrochemical impulses travel through motor nerves to the muscles they control, the result is muscular contraction. Sensory nerves—nerves that sense what is happening inside and outside of your body—are at the back of the spine and reach out to the same muscles, tendons, and joints. Their job is to report back to the CNS, along afferent (incoming) pathways, such movement information as the degree of contraction, the angle of flexion, and so on. Sensory-motor tracts are similarly arranged in the brain. Information passes back and forth in a constant feedback loop so that you can move. Various sensory receptors let you know where you are in space, how compressed or open your joints are, whether you feel pain, how much pull there is on your tendons, how contracted or relaxed your muscles are, and where your head is in relation to gravity.

## Adding Sensory Information

When muscles remain habitually contracted so that you no longer can relax them, merely telling yourself or having someone tell you to change your posture and movements for the better is inadequate and futile. Unless you vigilantly maintain your attention to "straighten up," despite your good intentions, you collapse back into the old, well-established pattern. Deane Juhan, author of *Job's Body,* explains why:

> Until we have some concrete knowledge about how things are situated, and until we know in what ways and to what degrees they can change, we are generally not motivated to initiate those changes; nor do we know how to make meaningful, helpful changes even if we want to. We are literally feeling our way along the course of our lives, and until we have *felt* something more complete, more harmonious, we don't know how to *be* more complete and harmonious. . . . Sensory input is a primary initiator and organizer of all levels of behavior.[7]

In other words, we need to add new sensory information in order to have new motor control. Body reeducators employ a variety of methods to help you release muscle tension and replace painful and inefficient patterns with

Sensory-Motor Feedback Loop: A tap below the knee triggers the patellar reflex.

# Proprioception: Balance and the Inner Ear

Keeping our balance is a function of the inner ear. In each inner ear, two sensory apparati sense the pull of gravity, and three sense the speeding up and slowing down of the head during movement. Three semicircular canals sit at right angles to each other, all filled with liquid and groups of receptor hair cells. Whenever we tilt our heads, the liquid starts to move, and the hairlike processes pick up its movement and communicate that information to the brain. At the same time, tiny bones suspended in a jellylike substance

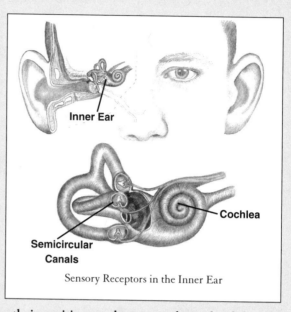

Sensory Receptors in the Inner Ear

in tiny sacs in the inner ear change their positions and press on the ends of the ciliated structures; in turn, they send messages to the brain. Using the information from the kinesthetic receptors, the balance organs in the inner ear and the eyes, and the pressure receptors on the soles of our feet, the brain figures out what changes would help us stay balanced and tells muscles to make the necessary adjustments.

those that are easier and more efficient. They generally use one or a combination of methods—light hands-on work, verbal directions, and movement exercises—on a table or the floor, while you are dressed in comfortable clothes. These teachers do not demonstrate, only provide the instructions and the opportunity for you to make sense of them kinesthetically rather than visually. No aspect of the process is passive; you must be an active, awake, motivated participant.[8]

The objective is not for everyone to attain the same ideal form or posture, but to live in a body that is free from excess muscle tension, with its weight evenly distributed so that there is no strain on muscles and joints and movement is unhampered. Moshe Feldenkrais called this optimal balance between extensors and flexors "the potent posture." F. M. Alexander preferred the word *poise* (equilibrium), and specifically referred to the head's proper poise on the tip of the spine. Feldenkrais or Alexander teachers, for example, may lightly touch and/or lift your muscles to determine where there is holding or jerky movement. They do not forcibly stretch or press, for their task is not to manipulate change but rather to direct you in a process of internalized learning. Guided attention provides the sensory information necessary for your nervous system to begin making changes. Without any muscular effort on your part, their gentle handling helps you become conscious of movements you unconsciously have stopped making, or which you never learned to do.

In a way, the teachers outline a sensory picture of what's there. As they move your limbs and muscles through patterns you no longer perform on your own, they temporarily serve as your motor system. Through the brain's self-balancing, self-correcting mechanisms, this allows your own "frozen" muscles to relax because they realize there's no work for them to do. At the same time, this activates your sensory cells, which now can receive stimuli from the motor system and, in turn, stimulate motor neurons into activity. The result is a new motor pattern on a voluntary level. "Like two knitting needles, the sensory system and motor system are made to intertwine, creating a greater sensory awareness of our internal activities and a greater activity of our internal sensory awareness," said somatic educator Thomas Hanna.[9]

By guiding you through movements, practitioners provide the opportunity for you to sense the difference between what you habitually do and a preferred pattern of action. Once you can feel the difference, you then can gradually replace the old pattern with a new, more efficient pattern.

You can also reeducate your sensory-motor system without the monitoring touch of a teacher, as in Gerda Alexander Eutony, Sensory Awareness, or Kinetic Awareness. While lying down or in other positions, listening to instructions or questions from a teacher, you very slowly move through a particular exercise. By paying close attention—sensing inside—you become aware of where you are limited. That recognition alone can be the gateway to change, helping to eliminate impediments and set you on a new path of movement.

If you're already taking movement classes of one kind or another, keep in mind that many movement teachers incorporate material from the different functional approaches. Somatic pioneers F. M. Alexander, Gerda Alexander, and Elsa Gindler all developed their original methods of body reeducation independently and influenced the creation of diverse systems popular today. Once you become familiar with the functional approaches (as well as the movement arts in Chapter 11), see if you can identify these influences in your class.

Any correction made from without is of little value, and . . . each of us must try to gain understanding for the special nature of our own constitution in order to learn how to take care of ourselves.

—Elsa Gindler

Self-observation is itself the beginning of transformation.

—Dennis Lewis

## Function Before Structure

Neural reeducation systems assume that function modifies structure. In fact, there is no structure unless a function requires it to exist. In this regard, structural and functional approaches are basically two sides of the same coin. Physically, they both deal with our relationship to gravity, posture, and balanced distribution of tension, as well as space and time. But in their aim for significant change, they come from two different perspectives (structure affects function vs. function influences structure) and address two different body systems (myofascial vs. sensory-motor). They also use two different levels of manipulation (deep vs. light—or, in some functional approaches, no manipulation at all). Yet both approaches seek to achieve greater ease in how we function.

## With Ease, Not Effort: Benefits

> Any activity that is learned with excessive tension always will be carried out with excessive tension, and . . . any change predicated on tension can lead only to more tension.
>
> —Judith Leibowitz

If somatic educators were to chant a motto about their work, it would probably be "less effort, more results." Unlike the lessons you learned in school, psychophysical reeducation is not about exerting effort and tension to accomplish fixed goals—F. M. Alexander called this strain "end-gaining." It simply involves you in a process of self-knowledge. You are encouraged to avoid forcing or striving, to let go rather than to overcome. Ultimately, you attain more, and attain it more easily, without hurting yourself or others, if you follow the principle that the body prefers pleasure to pain. It is also important not to react judgmentally—"Oh, how stupid of me to move that way"—for such judgments may actually create even more tension.

According to somatic educators, working with the neuromuscular system to facilitate lighter, easier, smoother movement is vital for more than just dancing gracefully or vacuuming without incurring back pain. For example, when your sensory-motor system adapts to poor body usage, the unnecessary habitual muscular contraction limits your ability to rotate your head. "The head serves as a kind of periscope of the central nervous system in order to bring sensory information into the brain," said Moshe Feldenkrais.[10] Because major sensory organs are located in the head, if you can't turn to see, smell, hear, and balance, you lose your ability to be aware of your environment and respond appropriately to it. In cultures that are less reliant on technology, sensory-motor development and kinesthesia or proprioception tend to be highly developed, for their very survival depends on such faculties. ☞ See "Body Perception," page 52.

The degree of sensory-motor function is also decisive in how you age. Hanna said, "What our culture accepts as the normal effects of aging are, to the contrary, the abnormal effects of our culture."[11] The more efficiently

# A Somatic Experience

To feel in your own body what occurs in a functional approach, try the following exercise. You can do it sitting or standing.

Begin with your head facing forward. Then slowly move it to the right as far as it will go, without forcing or straining. Notice where you start to feel restricted. When you can turn no farther, mark this stopping place in your mind's eye by using the last thing you see as a reference point. Then move your head back to center.

Now take your left hand and grab hold of only your right shoulder muscle, the fleshy trapezius. Let your elbow rest on or in front of your chest. While holding the muscle, slowly turn your head to the right again. How far can you move this time? Did you go past your reference point? Return to center. Then let go of the trapezius and turn to the right again. Did you surpass your previous limitation? Repeat these three steps on the left side, using your right hand to grab your left shoulder.

What happened? Did you notice that you could extend your range of motion? Can you guess why you were able to turn farther? In the second step, when you disengaged the muscle restricting your movement, you sent a signal through your sensory-motor system, telling it, "Tension pattern removed, more movement possible." In the third step, once that wider movement has been performed, the new pattern is now there to be repeated.

---

you function, the more likely you'll be flexible and responsive, vital and capable during your senior decades. Walking stooped over, being limited in your movement, and growing decrepit are not givens. Frozen, folded, failing, forgotten, or feeble parts of the body can reawaken, lengthen, strengthen, and function successfully again. 👉 See "Aging," page 18.

Like structural approaches, functional bodyways offer a wide range of benefits: pain reduction, better health, and greater longevity, as well as relief of rheumatic, neurological, spinal, respiratory, and stress disorders. As habitual patterns of movement disappear, the results are greater range of motion, flexibility, balance, and coordination. And since how you move is how you feel and think, attitudinal and emotional changes also occur.[12] As anxiety diminishes, openness expands. Your self-image and self-esteem improve. You have more of an ability to live in the present moment, to be more receptive to new ideas and experiences, to solve dilemmas, and to tolerate others.

All psychological states, whether healthy or pathological, are always the reflection of the sensorimotor activities going on in the bodily system.

—Thomas Hanna

RESOURCES:

**For ongoing coverage of the field of somatic education, see** *Somatics: Maga-zine-Journal of the Bodily Arts and Sciences,* published biannually by the No-vato Institute for Somatic Research and Training, 1516 Grant Ave., Suite 220, Novato, CA 94945, (415) 897-0336; and *SPPB Newsletter,* edited by Elizabeth A. Behnke, P.O. Box 0-2, Felton, CA 95018 (408) 335-2036.

**For information and referrals:** Contact International Somatic Movement Education and Therapy Association (ISMETA), c/o 148 W. 23rd St., #1H, New York, NY 10011, (212) 242-4962, or c/o 2442A Chestnut St., San Fran-cisco, CA 94123, (415) 567-7121, fax (415) 567-7416.

**For the scientific and philosophical background of the somatic point of view:** See Thomas Hanna, *Bodies in Revolt: A Primer in Somatic Thinking* (Freeperson, 1970). For general theory and practice of somatic education and a survey of somatic pioneers, see Thomas Hanna, *The Body of Life: Creating New Pathways for Sensory Awareness and Fluid Movement* (Healing Arts, 1993). For anatomical and physiological understanding, see Mabel E. Todd, *The Thinking Body: A Study of the Balancing Forces of Dynamic Man* (Dance Horizons/Princeton Book Co., reprint of 1937 ed.). See also Andrea Olsen and Caryn McHose, *BodyStories: A Guide to Experiential Anatomy* (Station Hill, 1991); and Irene Dowd, *Taking Root to Fly: Ten Articles on Functional Anatomy,* 2nd ed. (Contact, 1990).

# The Alexander Technique

The reward for attention is always healing.

—Julia Cameron

Australian-born Frederick Matthias Alexander (1869–1955) discovered his functional approach when doctors couldn't cure him of the recurring loss of his voice. Given his profession as a Shakespearean reciter, this was not an insignificant liability. Through self-observation and self-sensing, he became aware of an unconscious propensity to pull his head back and down. Once he began inhibiting this pattern of exerting pressure on his neck, he healed himself of throat and vocal troubles as well as of respiratory and nasal diffi-culties he had suffered since birth. Alexander concluded that the root of these and other discomforts—such as tennis elbow, fatigue, and shoulder pain—is misuse of the body.

Gradually he organized a method for converting faulty "use" into improved coordination; this method became known as the Alexander Technique. He gave up his own reciting to work with other voice-users and patients in Australia. In 1904 he moved to London, where actors soon flocked to learn his technique and prominent physicians sent him patients. He also established a following in the United States. Among his best-known pupils were George Bernard Shaw, Aldous Huxley, Leonard and Virginia Woolf, an Archbishop of Canterbury, John Dewey, Lewis Mumford, and Nobel prize-winning scientist Nikolaas Tinbergen.[13]

Alexander's work has continued to be popular in the performance world. For example, the late Alexander teacher Judith Leibowitz was a faculty member of the Drama Department at the Juilliard School in New York for twenty years. Laury Christie-Vaughn, a professor of music at the University of South Carolina, incorporates the Alexander Technique in her approach to vocal pedagogy. Although it has been taught as part of the curriculum at various universities, music institutes, theater schools, and drama academies in England and North America, the method has spread around the world beyond theaters and concert halls. People seek it out not only because of professional needs as performers and athletes but also because of back or neck pain, poor postural habits related to occupation (dentistry, carpentry, motherhood), or interest in mind-body efficiency and flexibility.

No matter what your reasons for trying the Alexander Technique, the first step is becoming aware of the interfering habit through your own kinesthetic senses. ☞ See "Proprioception and Kinesthesia," page 57. You do this in one-on-one lessons, or occasionally in a group, in which an Alexander teacher gently uses hands and verbal directions to subtly guide you through movements—bending, sitting, standing up, walking. Although your whole body is involved, the emphasis is on balance in the head-neck relationship, which Alexander called "Primary Control." This is the main objective of the work and also distinguishes it from other functional methods. The teacher lightly steers your head into its proper poise on the tip of the spine, which leads to optimal lengthening of the spine and more fluid movement in general.

By repeatedly experiencing (with the teacher's assistance) correct usage in motion or at rest, you sensitize your internal kinesthetic guide to be a new standard of normal against which to measure your actions. Thus, the intention of each lesson is getting you to recognize what you're doing. Once you're conscious of it, you then can choose whether to continue doing the same thing or not, which is the next procedure in the technique.

The second part of changing a habit is inhibition of the "set"—the old pattern of unnecessary tightening. When you learn to discourage or stop yourself from behaving in the habitual way, you leave your body free to act naturally and easily, allowing the neuromuscular system new

Mastery is the natural result of mindfulness.
—Ron Kurtz

# An Alexander Experience: The Lie Down

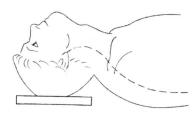

Too Thin

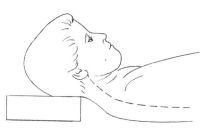

Too Thick

For this experience, you need a book between one and one and a half inches thick. Begin by sitting on the floor. You are going to roll down to a semisupine position, lying on your back. But first widen your attention to include the whole room, the expanse of the floor, the furniture, the windows, the ceiling.

Allow the fingers of one hand to begin extending along the floor. Release the elbow to let the arm follow. Let the shoulder release so that the whole arm can move gently out sideways and you can easily roll onto your side before lying on your back. This will help you avoid lowering yourself onto the floor as you would while doing sit-ups. Resist the temptation to close your eyes or drop your weight onto the floor. Gently allow your torso to follow the guiding arm and it will bring you easily to the floor.

Once you're on the floor, roll onto your back and let your head come onto the book for support. Let your knees bend so that your feet are supported on the ground. (If this causes a lot of tensing at your lower back, put a bolster, pillow, or rolled-up towel under your knees.)

Now, practice doing nothing for ten or fifteen minutes. Leave your eyes open, let your gaze wander around the room, let your back release onto the ground from head to tail, let

freedom. The automatic, tensed responses you have developed are a result of "end-gaining." You rush unconsciously for an immediate result, such as sitting, instead of consciously going through the process—the "means-whereby"—to sit. This (the "means-whereby") is non-doing: There is nothing to force, only muscle tension to give up. Inhibition of the old pattern can lead you out of acting on a habitual impulse and into making intelligent choices during your actions. It involves a clear decision to continue allowing moment-to-moment awareness instead of plunging unreflectively toward an end.

The third element is verbal feedback ("direction"). As you move, you learn the following words from the teacher and incorporate them by repeating to yourself: "Let my neck be free, let my head go forward and up, let my torso lengthen and widen, let my legs release away from my torso, your knees be balanced in one direction by the upper leg and in the other by the contact of your feet. Resist the temptation to position yourself; just practice listening to your body and releasing it. When you are done, let yourself roll to sitting, keeping your eyes alive and your joints easy.

Things to watch for: Notice the thoughts and feelings you have while taking this "time out." Do you tense up when you think of things you should be doing? Do you feel panicky, sad, sleepy, or anxious that someone will catch you goofing off? Do you long to adjust your body so that it feels right—to stretch out a sore shoulder, tighten your legs so they won't fall, press your back flat for good posture? Do you fear failure or not getting the exercise right, or do you have the attitude, "How can this help?"

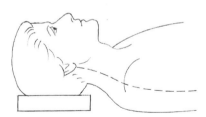

Properly Aligned

The book you rest on should allow you to keep your head easily balanced on the spine, tipping neither back and adding pressure to the spine, nor forward and pinching the larynx.

What the experience can do for you: It helps your back lengthen and widen, lets you break out of old neuromuscular habits, and allows you to practice simply being in your body. The Lie Down lets the discs in the spine recharge with fluid by releasing the surrounding musculature.

—Courtesy of Sandra Bain Cushman, Alexander teacher.

and let my shoulders widen." There is no forcing, only *letting*. These gentle mental reminders lead your awareness, and consequently your movement, toward more expansion and integration.

By working with these three aspects, you can learn to respond with your whole body in a light, easy, simple, and integrated manner that insures appropriate distribution of tension or effort throughout. In turn, you might also find yourself experiencing increased energy and emotional buoyancy. You know you've mastered your Alexander lessons and "graduated" when one day you notice spontaneously that you are *choosing* to "use" yourself well most of the time.

To be eligible for membership in the North American Society of Teachers of the Alexander Technique (NASTAT), teachers must train at least 1,600 hours over a minimum three-year period in NASTAT–recog-

> The body can feel completely at ease and natural every moment. Just let it.
>
> —Eugene Gendlin

nized institutes and centers. Other Alexander societies in America and worldwide have their own requirements.

RESOURCES:

**For teachers, training, and published materials:** North American Society of Teachers of the Alexander Technique (NASTAT), P.O. Box 517, Urbana, IL 61801, (800) 473-0620; Alexander Technique International, Inc., 1692 Massachusetts Ave., Cambridge, MA 02138, (617) 497-2242, fax (617) 876-2709. There are also fine teachers who are not members of these groups.

**Books:** F. M. Alexander, *The Use of the Self* (E. P. Dutton, 1932; Centerline, 1984); Michael Gelb, *Body Learning: An Introduction to the Alexander Technique* (Delilah, 1981); Frank Pierce Jones, *Body Awareness in Action* (Schocken, 1976); Judith Leibowitz and Bill Connington, *The Alexander Technique* (HarperPerennial, 1990).

# Gerda Alexander Eutony™

Gerda Alexander Eutony (GAE), the work of Gerda Alexander (1908–1993), was originally a method of relaxation, which she developed into a sensory-motor learning process or system of mind-body consciousness. Born in Germany, she was not related to F. M. Alexander. She was a teacher of Eurhythmic Education, a system of education based on music and movement that was founded by Jacques Dalcroze.

The word *eutony*—well-balanced tension or tonicity—is derived from the Greek *eu-,* meaning "good" or "harmonious," and the Latin *tonus,* meaning "tension." Central to GAE is working with tonus regulation of all the body's tissues, from the skin and muscles to organs and glands. The purpose is to learn to liberate tonus fixations (for example, when muscle groups keep revving even at rest) and replace them with tonus flexibility, in which every degree of tonicity, from rest to activity, is used with supreme alertness and proficiency. Such flexibility, Alexander theorized, allows creative and spontaneous responses to each new stimulus and demand of life, not only physical but also intellectual and emotional.

To achieve this, GAE teachers instruct you in becoming a master of self-sensing and knowing. The basis of the method is coming into greater sensory awareness and contact with yourself—a state of pres-

> All sanity depends on this: that it should be a delight . . . to stand upright, knowing the bones are moving easily under the flesh.
>
> —Doris Lessing

ence—but in a relational rather than isolated way. For example, while lying on the floor sensing your breath, skin, or body form, you also sense connection with the ground. Maintaining a sensitive, stable presence in

## A Class in Gerda Alexander Eutony

It was my first time taking a class in GAE. Everyone else there had been studying for many years, yet I was able to participate easily, at my own level. Had I arrived on another day, I would have learned something entirely different, for each class is unique and tailored to who shows up.

We began by exploring first, in great detail, the abdominal muscles and diaphragm in anatomical illustrations. Then, to get a tactile understanding, we handled skeleton parts and felt our way along the inside of our own rib cage and pelvic structure. In this manner, we were able to clearly articulate our particular shapes.

In between explorations, we paused by lying on our backs and noticing the contact we made with the floor and the sensations we felt. We shared out loud what results we experienced individually through these investigations.

We also moved our mouths to release any tension—for example, we stretched the upper lip toward the right ear, left ear, nose, and chin, and rotated the tongue 360 degrees. I later learned that the teacher spontaneously included these movements because she noticed that I tend to tighten my mouth while doing something with my hands. The mouth movements gave me the opportunity to become aware of this habit.

We took time to roll across the floor so that it touched every part of our bodies. Then we added a medium-sized rubber ball and massaged our bodies with it, taking note of the curve in our femurs (thigh bones), feeling our abdominal organs, and letting go of any tension.

In addition, the teacher had us feel the changes of form and tension in our skin as it stretches from the feet all the way to the skull and connects to the arms. Through the guided awareness and contact, I felt myself increase in awareness of my "epidermal envelope" and my body image.

No matter what we were doing, the teacher repeatedly reminded us not to let any movement interfere with our breath, to keep our toes and fingers long, and to press at our sit-bones so that movement goes through the spine in a "transport reflex."

Partner work followed. One woman explored my rib cage, pelvis, and shoulder blades as I lay on my back or sides. Then I did the same for her.

Everything we did was gentle and called for awareness and openness. There was no model to follow. By the end of the class, I felt expanded, fuller, as though my body had greater volume. And I knew it better. I realized I'd just had an experience in embodied anatomy.

*The essence of education is the education of the body.*

—Benjamin Disraeli

yourself does not mean shutting out the surroundings, nor does being in touch with the environment make you lose your inner awareness and individuality. Alexander never considered Eutony "a special system to be practiced separately from everyday life."[14] For her, the deepest awareness, and the one that facilitates maturation, is that of the skeleton. Experiencing the bone structure can release your most deeply seated tensions and lead to a feeling of inner solidity and security, along with recovering alignment.

Such involved, detailed, intense sensory exploration takes several years and requires a deep knowledge of anatomy. In fact, GAE is the only somatic method that requires a full-time, four-year training period to become a teacher and therapist. But the result is balance on all levels and the capacity for individual rhythmic expression rather than imitation of movement models. It also stimulates self-autonomy, for teachers hold you responsible for personal development. They invite you, but never push you, to become mindful of yourself. As in other awareness practices, in GAE you develop an observing self, one that does not direct or judge but remains neutrally aware of the present moment. ☞ See "Mindfulness Meditation," page 128, "Kinetic Awareness," page 263, and "Sensory Awareness," page 226. You uncover your individual biorhythms through the setting of tasks for which you must find your own solutions without following a set of patterns.

You can attend group classes or have private lessons, which incorpo-

## An Experience in Gerda Alexander Eutony

"Control positions" in Eutony enable you, alone and within a few minutes, to become aware of the points of tension in your body. If your muscles are of normal length and correct elasticity—essential for optimal movement of your joints and thus for functional posture and movement—you will be able to assume these positions automatically and without difficulty. However, if your muscles are shortened because of tension or overdevelopment, you will probably find the control positions uncomfortable or painful; you might not be able to do them at all.

If you like, try control position #11, which tests the muscles of your vertebral column, back, shoulders, arms, hips, and thighs. Begin by lying down on your left side and sensing your skin. Keep your lower leg long and the knee of your upper leg flexed in front of it on the floor. Let both arms be long in front of your chest. Feel your ribs, the femoral medial condyle (the lower inner prominence of your thigh bone), tibia (shinbone), and the big toe of your upper leg touching the floor. Feel your trochanter (upper prominence of the thigh bone), fibula (bone lateral to the shinbone), and the fifth toe of your lower leg touching the floor. Also feel the direction of the long bones of your upper arm and hand (see figure A).

Now, leading from beyond the tips of your fingers, start making a half-circle above your head with your upper arm and hand. Keep them straight but loose. If you can, during this entire motion keep touching the floor with long easy fingers, your upper knee remaining on the floor, and lengthen your sit bones (see figure B). Observe your breathing. If you cannot touch the floor with your fingertips, do the half-circle in the air until the upper arm is behind you. There again, feel contact with the floor, feel the direction of the long bones in that arm, and observe your breathing. To reverse the motion back to the starting position, first transit through the long bones and lead from beyond your fingertips. If possible, touch the floor, keeping your sit-bones long toward your feet and your upper knee on the floor.

Take a rest, lying on your back, and compare how both sides feel. Then roll onto your other side and repeat the complete procedure. Complete this practice with a final rest and observe how you feel.

—Courtesy of Joyce Riveros, Eutony teacher.

Figure A

Figure B

Control Position #11

rate hands-on therapy as well. There is no restriction as to who can attend and benefit, including paraplegics, quadriplegics, and polio patients. Nor is there a set lesson pattern, because teachers "feel" the people gathered in a class and adapt to you.

Gerda Alexander Eutony is included in conservatories, schools for dance, theater, kindergarten teachers, and physical therapy; Olympic training; physical education departments in major universities; and a wide variety of other educational, commercial, and medical establishments in Western Europe. In 1987, after being observed for two years in clinics and schools in different countries, GAE became the first mind-body discipline accepted by the World Health Organization (WHO) as an alternative health-care technique.

## RESOURCES:

**Instruction:** Monique Nagy, 602 Frankfurt Rd., Monaca, PA 15061, (412) 371-1876; or Joyce Riveros, 1633 Julian Dr., El Cerrito, CA 94530, (510) 234-9362.

**Books:** Gerda Alexander, *Eutony: The Holistic Discovery of the Total Person* (Felix Morrow, 1985), available through Feldenkrais Resources, (800) 765-1907 or (510) 540-7600, fax (510) 540-7683.

# Sensory Awareness

Except for sensations of pain and very general feelings of comfort or discomfort, the sensations from within are like the stars, which only appear when the artificial lights are turned off. When there is quiet enough, they can be very precise.

—Charlotte Selver

The students of somatic pioneer Elsa Gindler, who taught in Germany until her death in 1961, have carried her work to many parts of the world, incorporating it in all kinds of therapies and skills training, from overcoming speech disorders to working with psychiatric patients and teaching music. Charlotte Selver, the best-known Gindler student in the United States, coined the term *Sensory Awareness* for her style of teaching. It has influenced many innovators in the evolution of their own disciplines, such as Fritz Perls with Gestalt Therapy.

Also known as *sensory re-education* or *conscious sensing,* Sensory Awareness (SA) aims at helping you attain clear, direct perception and authentic experience that goes beyond intellectual understanding. Philosopher Alan Watts called SA "living Zen" because of its similarity to meditation and its achievement of a state of mind-body unity.

There is neither a set series of courses to complete in Sensory Awareness nor a recipe of any kind, no guided images, structured movements, specific positions, or anatomical training, just simple inquiry. The teacher

# Elsa Gindler

Elsa Gindler (1885–1961), a Berlin teacher of Harmonische Gymnastik (a kind of physical education), was in her twenties when she contracted tuberculosis. Since at the time the only palliative for the disease was rest and fresh air, her doctor suggested that she take up residence at a sanitorium. In the pure atmosphere of the Alps she could spend her remaining days quietly.

Coming from a working-class family, Gindler was unable to afford such treatment, so she decided to help herself by practicing exercises from a book on breathing. Her doctor told her she would be dead within two weeks if she continued such a program. But she had an intuition that on her own she could find a way to let her infected lung recuperate.

Gindler soon abandoned the book and patiently explored how to breathe with only her healthy lung. After a year of working with great sensitivity and self-awareness, she recovered completely. When she saw her doctor on the street, baffled, he sputtered, "What? You are ... here?"

In fact, Gindler did not die until the age of seventy-six, after a long, productive career in physical reeducation, which she called Arbeit am Menschen, "working with human beings," or Nachentfaltung, "unfolding afterward." Devoted to her humane work, she gave classes even during the bombing of Berlin in World War II. She refused to include the required Nazi indoctrination, but taught practical skills, such as how to endure standing and deal with problems in air-raid shelters. Though she could have been reported and sent to a concentration camp, Gindler gave special classes for her Jewish students, hid some of them in her basement, and fed them with her own meager rations. When a Nazi youth flung a firebomb into her building, it destroyed all of her records. The Nazis discovered and killed the Jewish students. A combination of fear, lack of food, and the loss of friends resulted in Gindler's developing an intestinal ulcer.

Despite her condition, during the last three decades of her life Gindler collaborated intimately with Heinrich Jacoby, a pioneer in human learning and creativity in Zurich. Throughout her teaching years, she was instrumental in the growth of many somatic practitioners. Among the renowned students who perpetuated her work are Carola Speads, who was her assistant for many years, Ilse Middendorf, and Charlotte Selver, the creator of Sensory Awareness.[15]

outlines experiments in which you can become aware of the sensations involved in any movement, from the gross to the subtle, such as changes in the heartbeat or breathing. If the teacher asks, for example, "Where is the movement of breathing felt in you?" you quietly attend to sensing that movement, whether the experiment is about coming to rest or moving into an activity, such as lying, sitting, standing, or walking, picking up a stone, throwing a ball, etc.

An experiment can also be an exploration of a body area, such as the feet, either by touching them with your hands from the outside or by simply attending to the proprioceptive messages from within. In this way, you can wake up the feet, or any other body part, and also *wake up to them.*

In "quiet alertness," you sense how and where you constrict and hinder yourself. And you come out of your previous conditioning to fuller functioning not because a teacher superimposes anything on you, nor because you force anything on yourself. Rather, change occurs when you merely let your body assert its needs. There is no right or wrong, no correct way of standing or breathing according to preestablished criteria, and no models to follow. You simply observe and allow what is natural for your being, shedding whatever amount of strain or effort is unnecessary, such as in raising your arms or brushing your teeth. When formerly bound energy becomes available, you may feel light yet powerful. Your movement can become self-generated and appropriate, rather than mimicked or mechanically repeated. Your breathing can become less restricted, your posture improved, and your coordination, flexibility, and balance enhanced. And you may find your attitude changing—from trying to "get things done" just to be finished, you may switch to approaching each action sensitively, thoughtfully, and joyfully. Such an attitudinal change can also mean that the essential relationship you have with yourself and others can become easier, more honest, and more satisfying.

Only longtime students of Charlotte Selver who have received certification from her are accredited to offer SA. They keep up their practice through continual work with Selver, who in her nineties still leads classes. The Sensory Awareness Leaders Guild is a professional association of such teachers in North America, Europe, and Mexico.

RESOURCES:

**For published materials and workshops:** Sensory Awareness Foundation, 1314 Star Route, Muir Beach, CA 94965. For teachers: Sensory Awareness Leaders Guild, 411 W. 22nd St., New York, NY 10011.

**Books:** Charles Brooks, *Sensory Awareness: The Rediscovery of Experiencing Through Workshops with Charlotte Selver* (Felix Morrow, 1986).

# The Mensendieck System

The Mensendieck System of functional movement techniques originated at the end of the nineteenth century with Bess Mensendieck, a medical doctor. She believed that the postures we assume and the movements we make regularly at work, play, and rest shape and condition our bodies. The results we get—bodies that are slender and lithe or heavy and awkward, vital and strong or weak and racked with pain—depend on whether we use the proper muscles in all our activities. Mensendieck developed a series of "movement schemes" or exercises that require a minimum of physical effort and time for reshaping, rebuilding, and revitalizing.

The Mensendieck System is both corrective and preventive. By first working with a teacher, you can learn to use your conscious will to release tension and improve your body's structural and functional integrity. Once you can move correctly—that is, engage your back, neck, arms, legs, and so on in a beneficial rather than straining way—you can avoid or alleviate aches and pains in your muscles and joints. In addition, instruction in breathing efficiently will have a positive effect on all body functions.

Unique to the Mensendieck training is working undressed or in bikini bottoms in front of mirrors (ideally, one in front of you, another on the side, and a third obliquely placed in the rear). This allows you to observe and feel where a movement originates—for example, in lifting your arm—and which muscles you activate. You correlate what you see with what you feel, getting feedback proprioceptively. You learn to move one part of your body without allowing everything else to compensate or "fall apart." Through correct repetition, you imprint new movement patterns to replace inefficient ones.

Mensendieck teachers begin personalized sessions with the most fundamental Mensendieck technique, the "well-balanced stance." It sets up the correct bottom-to-top alignment and is preparatory for all exercises and walking. There are more than two hundred different exercises to work with. They emphasize correct and graceful body movement throughout everyday activity, such as kneeling down and getting up, lifting and carrying loads, going up and down stairs, sitting and standing up. Teachers explain verbally and with their hands how to assume these stances, but they do not demonstrate, for they don't want to rob you of your own inside-out discovery. The number of sessions you engage in depends on your individual kinesthetic sense and on whether you have a health condition that needs slow and careful guidance. Generally, a session is an hour long, but expert students who want to continue on a regular basis often come for a half-hour once a week.

You can now, in a sense, become a sculptor of your body, helping to shape its limbs and torso almost as though you were working with clay or marble.

—Bess M. Mensendieck

Correction of movements is the best means of self-improvement.

—Moshe Feldenkrais

# Bess Mensendieck

Bess Mensendieck (1861–1957) was born Elizabeth Marguerite de Varel in New York City and spent a good deal of her childhood traveling all over the world with her civil engineer father to sites where he was building bridges. As a sculpture student in Paris in the late 1800s, she became preoccupied with the poor neuromuscular coordination, ungraceful postures, and unbalanced musculature of the studio's models. When Mensendieck realized that she would rather work with human bodies than marble or clay, she became one of the world's first female doctors, graduating from the University of Zurich.

In 1895 she returned to Paris to work at the College of Medicine. Gradually she combined research in kinesiology with the engineering principles she learned from her father to create a new system of functional body education. She lectured throughout Europe and worked with physicians and in hospitals to help restore muscle function in patients suffering paralysis and spasm or recovering from surgery, and in the disabled elderly.

Mensendieck's first famous patron was Kaiser Wilhelm II of Germany. On a visit to Norway with his fleet, he anchored in Hardanger Fjord, near her summer home, and invited her aboard to dine with him. Afterward he summoned Mensendieck to set up her first school of functional exercises. The Kaiser was distressed that the ladies-in-waiting at his Potsdam court had potbellies and looked like beer steins.

In 1905 Mensendieck brought her method to the United States, but she was stymied in publishing her findings. The illustrations of nude bodies, which were indispensable in clarifying the explanation of her work, were prohibited by the Comstock laws then in effect to prevent printing of "immoral" texts. Back in Europe, she found willing, uncensored publishers and established her method. But eventually she returned to New York and, with the Comstock laws repealed, was finally able to publish her books in the United States in the 1930s. During the same period, Yale University's swimming coach adopted Mensendieck training for the physical education department. Before World War II, Mensendieck relocated to Hollywood, where she worked with Greta Garbo, Ingrid Bergman, Frederic March, Jascha Heifetz, and the wives of Fred Astaire, Irving Berlin, and Gary Cooper.

Yet nowhere in her travels did Mensendieck see bodies she considered an exemplary model of harmonious beauty in motion, not even in prima ballerina Anna Pavlova or heavyweight prize fighter Max Schmeling. Finally, on a world tour to study body movements, she found her ideal in Javanese dancers.

The International Mensendieck League, established in 1930 at The Hague, oversees the stringent Mensendieck curriculum. National law in Denmark, Norway, Sweden, and the Netherlands recognizes and regulates the

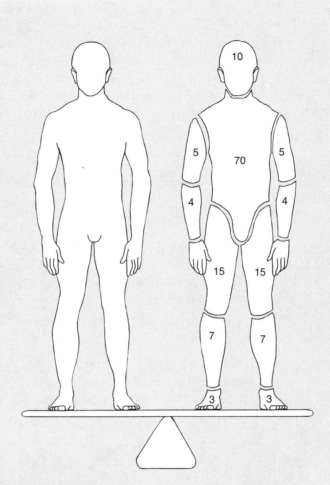

Ideal Body Weight Distribution for a 150-Pound Person

**Bess Mensendieck saw the human body as an assembly of masses rather than as a single mass. When these masses are positioned properly at rest and in motion, their respective weights are supported efficiently so that there is no strain on any muscle group. For example, in a person who weighs 150 pounds, there is the following distribution of weight: head, 10 pounds; trunk, 70 pounds; upper arms, 5 pounds each; forearms, 4 pounds each; hands, 1 pound each; thighs, 15 pounds each; lower legs, 7 pounds each; feet, 3 pounds each.**

—Adapted from Bess Mensendieck, *The Mensendieck System of Functional Exercises* (Southworth-Anthoesen, 1937).

work as a completely separate paramedical profession. In the Netherlands, for example, it is part of the national health-care system and the training program takes three years, including three different full-time internships at teaching hospitals and rehabilitation centers. Therapist-teachers work in private practice as well as in hospitals and rehabilitation centers. They present courses to nurses, factory workers, office employees, store personnel, senior citizens, and pregnant and postpartum women, among others. They report success with many conditions and situations, including low and upper back pain, pre- and post-natal care, post-operative recovery, Parkinson's disease, sports-induced muscle and joint problems, and others arising from improper posture and muscle control, such as fallen arches, knock-knee, and repetitive strain injuries.

RESOURCES:

**For information and a list of instructors in the United States:** Send an SASE (#10 envelope): Mensendieck Academy and Enterprises, P.O. Box 9450, Stanford, CA 94309-9450, (415) 851-8184.

**Books:** Ellen Lagerwerff and Karen Perlroth, *Mensendieck Your Posture and Your Pains* (Doubleday, 1973; Aries, 1982); Jennifer Yoels, *Re-Shape Your Body, Re-Vitalize Your Life* (Prentice-Hall, 1972); Bess M. Mensendieck, *Look Better, Feel Better* (Harper & Row, 1954), *The Mensendieck System of Functional Exercises* (Southworth-Anthoensen, 1937; Kristianstads Boktryckeri, 1989), and *It's Up to You* (J. J. Little & Ives, 1931).

**Audiovisual:** "Freedom from Back Pain: The Mensendieck System," Karen Perlroth, 55-min. video with 40-page booklet, and a 60-min. audio-cassette of the same title, both from Mensendieck Academy (see above)

# The Feldenkrais Method:®
# Functional Integration and
# Awareness through Movement

> The way our movement is organized is a projection of the way our brain is organized, and the way we move organizes our brain.
>
> —Michael Joyce

The Feldenkrais Method is a learning process that brings about new, more efficient, more comfortable, and healthier ways of movement through tapping into the vast potential of the central nervous system. Moshe Feldenkrais, its creator, believed that our human capacity for learning, "incomparably greater than that of any other living creature," provides us with the extraordinary opportunity to build up a mass of learned responses.[16] But along with that gift comes "the special vulnerability" of developing poor behaviors. In contrast, "other animals have their responses to most stimuli wired in to their nervous systems in the form of instinctive patterns of action, [so] they go wrong less frequently unless the environment changes."[17] Despite this liability, according to Feldenkrais, you

# Moshe Feldenkrais

Born in Russian-occupied Poland, Moshe Feldenkrais (1904–1984) immigrated to Palestine in the 1920s. He earned degrees in both mechanical and electrical engineering as well as a doctorate in science at the Sorbonne in Paris. There he spent ten years at the Curie Institute, publishing papers with Nobel prize-winner Frédéric Joliot-Curie.

Feldenkrais was one of the first European black belts in Judo and founder of the Judo Club of Paris; he taught classes to support himself while studying at the university. Engineer and physicist, athlete and Judo master, mathematician and student of acupuncture, he became a functional reeducator after he healed himself of an old knee injury.

As a young man, Feldenkrais had played soccer aggressively and hurt one knee, which never healed. During World War II, while directing antisubmarine research for the British Admiralty, he had to be on a ship every day. The constant pitching to and fro played havoc with his knee. One of the foremost surgeons in England recommended the surgery he'd needed years before but could promise only a fifty-fifty chance of success. Faced with such unappealing odds, Feldenkrais decided to take the matter into his own hands. The doctor warned him that he'd come back in six months begging for an operation.

Undismayed, Feldenkrais studied anything related to human movement: anatomy, biology, physiology, kinesiology, neurology, psychology, and anthropology. His wife, a pediatrician, helped him understand child development. He also explored Yoga, the Gurdjieff philosophy, and the work of F. M. Alexander, and he attended Gerda Alexander's classes in Paris and Israel.

In his efforts to heal his own knee, Feldenkrais developed a unique and comprehensive perspective on sensory-motor function and how it relates to thought, emotion, and action. He taught himself how to walk again without pain and restored function in his knee. The Feldenkrais Method and the Awareness Through Movement group lessons evolved in response to requests from others who wanted to move more freely, too.

can still change. Given the chance, your brain will choose the easiest, most effective way to act, but you have to provide the means for it to do so.

That's what the Feldenkrais Method does. Using physical experiences, not words, it presents your brain with new information and retrains it to accept an improved image, which replaces the old, distorted one. The work accomplishes this by breaking down functional patterns and movements into smaller components to establish new neural connections between the motor cortex of your brain and your muscular system. By going through a movement sequence

> Our ability to learn . . . involves the developing of new responses to familiar stimuli as the result of experience
>
> —Moshe Feldenkrais

# An Experience in Easy Flexibility

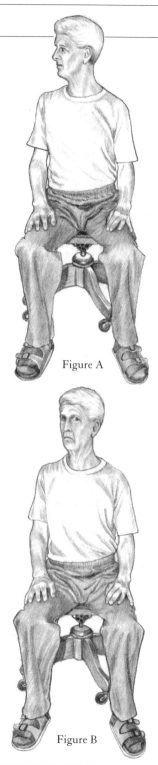

Figure A

Figure B

Try the following instructions to increase flexibility in your neck, chest, and spine and to make your movements lighter and more comfortable.

Sit on the forward part of your chair or seat, your hands resting on your thighs, your feet flat on the floor, shoulder width apart and directly below your knees. Making each movement small, comfortable, and easy, gently turn your upper body as if to look to the right a little (figure A). Slowly face forward again and relax. Mentally note how far you can see without straining. Pause to rest.

Now focus on an object or spot straight ahead. Keeping your eyes still and looking forward, slowly turn your head and upper body to the right as you exhale (figure B). Don't force the movement; keep your neck, shoulders, chest, and legs relaxed. Notice that you don't turn as far to the right because your eyes aren't moving. Pause to rest.

This time, include your eyes as you gently turn your entire upper body to the right. Can you see a little farther? Come back to center. Keep your eyes and head there, facing forward, as you slowly turn only your shoulders and upper body to the right. Notice that your right shoulder moves back and the left moves forward (figure C). Return to center and pause.

Again including your eyes and head, gently turn your entire upper body to the right. Return to the starting position and relax. Is turning to the right becoming easier and more comfortable? Do you notice a difference between your right and left shoulders?

While keeping your foot still and flat on the floor, slightly move your left knee forward. Notice that your lower back, head, and shoulders are turning slightly to the right. Now, as you move your left knee forward slowly, also turn your entire upper body to the right (figure D). Do you feel yourself getting a little taller as you turn? Do you feel your pelvis moving? Do you sense

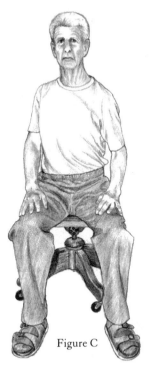

Figure C

how moving your left knee improves your ability to turn?

Pause to rest. Then repeat the entire sequence turning to the left.

Now alternate turning right and left slowly, four to eight times, as one and then the other knee moves slightly forward. Let your hands slide on your thighs as you turn from side to side, keeping your legs relaxed. Move smoothly and continuously.

Continue turning your upper body to the right and left a little, but this time keep your head and eyes still, facing forward. Don't forget to breathe freely. Stop to rest whenever you want. Do you notice how much your flexibility has increased as you move right and left?

Alternate turning your upper body and pelvis to the right and left while turning your head and eyes in the opposite direction. Relax and move slowly and smoothly.

Now, one last time, move your left knee forward as you turn to the right as far as you can without straining (figure E). Then move your right knee forward as you turn to the left. Notice how much your flexibility has improved without stretching or forcing. Do you feel taller? If you're sitting in front of a mirror, do you look taller? Feel your weight evenly balanced on your sit-bones and your lower back slightly arched. Your muscles should be relaxed, allowing your posture to be more upright. When you stand up, notice how light your body feels and how comfortably you move.

—Adapted with permission from David Zemach-Bersin, Kaethe Zemach-Bersin, and Mark Reese, *Relaxercise* (HarperCollins, 1990).

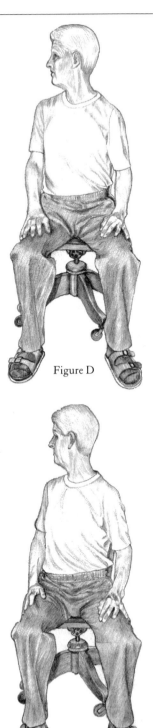

Figure D

Figure E

again and again, you finally experience the new way as "normal" and natural. Repetition is necessary, Feldenkrais believed, because we are so accustomed to how the inefficient habitual pattern feels that our judgment is impaired, and any muscular change will seem abnormal. It's not enough to be conscious of a pattern, he said, for "improvement in action and movement will appear only after a prior change in the brain and the nervous system has occurred."[18]

The Feldenkrais Method subtly "rewires" or reeducates your nervous system in two ways. In Functional Integration, the hands-on table work, the practitioner custom-tailors each movement lesson by using his or her hands slowly and sensitively to communicate new sensory configurations and a new motor organization to your body to meet its unique needs. According to Feldenkrais, this is particularly helpful in cerebral palsy, multiple sclerosis, or similar conditions, including stroke paralysis.

For example, if you have palsylike symptoms, there's no distinct image in your nervous system of what a precise, easy arm movement is like. You may currently not be able to or never have been able to consistently repeat such a pattern to imprint anything but a shaking, jerky action. The Feldenkrais practitioner would carefully take you through the smooth movement, piece by piece, at least twenty times in a row. In this way, a whole new pattern registers in your nervous system. The repeated movements create awareness and then, through that awareness, you can repeat the movement on your own. Several graduate research projects have demonstrated this, particularly in cases of cerebral palsy and brain injury.[19]

Even when we're not physically challenged by a neuromuscular disorder, Feldenkrais believed we can learn to move better and function at a level closer to our human potential. As creatures of habit, don't most of us tend to stand and walk (or sleep, or breathe, or digest) inefficiently as long as we can do it at all? But is getting by really good enough? The problem with such an attitude is that when we don't change muscular patterns, the corresponding motor areas in the brain remain fixed, too. By contrast, Feldenkrais theorized, the more completely we use the muscle system, the more the brain will be activated, and those stimulated regions will in turn activate adjacent areas in control of thinking and feeling.[20] Feldenkrais practitioners notice their clients experience such benefits as fuller breathing, improved digestion, more restful sleep, enhanced mood, better mental alertness, and increased energy, flexibility, and range of motion, as well as fewer headaches and backaches.

Here's where the second aspect of the Feldenkrais Method, Awareness Through Movement, comes in. These group lessons, of which there are in principle thousands, enable you to go beyond "good enough" and function the best you can in daily activities or special performances. Since the "lessons are designed to improve ability . . . to turn the impossible into the possible, the difficult into the easy, and the easy into the pleasant," you never do them with effort.[21] Feldenkrais believed that if activities are hard to carry out and you have to force

Once accustomed to some fault in posture, we no longer feel the superfluous effort.

—Franz Wurm

Pleasure engages our relaxed attentiveness.

—Deane Juhan

yourself to do them, they'll never become a part of your normal daily life. So, to teach the brain without tiring the muscles, lessons most often have you lie down or sit on the floor to relieve the extensor and flexor muscles that hold your body up in habitual standing patterns. ☞ See figures on page 210.

A Feldenkrais practitioner verbally leads the group through highly sophisticated, structured movement experiences. (You can also do this with tapes at home.) With the curiosity of an infant, you make your own discoveries of what is right for your body, rather than comparing it to anyone else's or imitating a teacher's. Only when *you* know what *you're* doing can you choose what you want to do. For Feldenkrais, that choice, not an imposed external standard, is what "correct" movement is all about. He saw the body as a flexible functional unit rather than something to be molded into some rigid mechanical fit. He said it "should be so organized that it can start any movement—forward, backward, right, left, down, up, or turning right and left without previous arrangement of the segments of the body, without any sudden change in the rhythm of breathing, without clenching the lower jaw or tensing the tongue, and without any perceptible tensing of the neck muscles or fixation of the eyes. . . . If these conditions are maintained during an action, then even lifting the entire body is not sensed as an effort."[22] Feldenkrais practitioners do not see what you do as incorrect and then attempt to correct it. Rather, they create conditions that enable you to have more choices.

Although each lesson concentrates on a particular body area or joint, other parts will experience positive change as well because of integrated neuromuscular linkages. The result, say Feldenkrais practitioners, is that by the end of a session, you may feel refreshed, your whole body hanging lightly from your head and gliding gracefully as you move. And, over time, you may find yourself establishing a more complete body image. There is no established number of hands-on sessions. You can take group lessons as long as you like, enabling you to constantly improve how you function, whether you suffer no major dysfunction and just want to enhance your performance skills or whether you're dealing with a limitation such as a cervical condition or rheumatoid arthritis.[23]

To become certified in the Feldenkrais Method, over a four-year period practitioners undergo between 1,600 and 1,800 hours of training, as well as logging many hours of practice. To maintain proficiency, they must attend additional classes or workshops each year.

## RESOURCES:

**For a list of certified practitioners, training programs, and published and audiovisual materials:** The Feldenkrais Guild, P.O. Box 489, Albany, OR 97321-0143, (800) 775-2118, (503) 926-0981, fax (503) 926-0572. For a catalogue of books and audio and video materials: Feldenkrais Resources, 830 Bancroft Way, Suite 112, Berkeley, CA 94710, (800) 765-1907, (510) 540-7600.

**Books:** Moshe Feldenkrais, *Awareness Through Movement* (Harper & Row, 1972), *The Case of Nora* (Harper & Row, 1977); Ruthy Alon, *Mindful Spontaneity: Moving in Tune with Nature: Lessons in the Feldenkrais Method* (Prism/Avery, 1990); David and Kaethe Zemach-Bersin and Mark Reese, *Relaxercise* (HarperCollins, 1990); Yochanan Rywerant, *The Feldenkrais Method* (Keats, 1991).

**Audiovisual:** To receive a catalogue of a wide variety of audiocassettes and videotapes that feature Moshe Feldenkrais or the practitioners he trained, contact the Feldenkrais Guild or Feldenkrais Resources, above.

---

# Hanna Somatic Education®

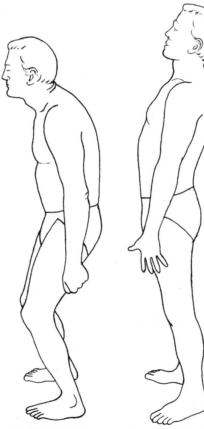

Red Light Reflex     Green Light Reflex

Thomas Hanna (1928–1990) was a philosophy professor before he turned to somatic education. After directing the first Feldenkrais training program in the United States in 1975, he founded the Novato Institute for Somatic Research and Training and started *Somatics: Magazine-Journal of the Bodily Arts and Sciences,* of which he was editor.

Hanna Somatic Education (HSE) is based on the original ideas of Hans Selye, the endocrinologist who recognized stress as a cause of disease, and of physicist Moshe Feldenkrais. Hanna noted that in response to the unending stresses and traumas to which we are subjected, the sensory-motor system reacts with specific muscular reflexes. He called them *Red Light reflex* (startle response), *Green Light reflex* (Landau arousal response), and *trauma reflex.*

The first two are basic adaptive reflexes that are deeply wired into the central nervous system because they're essential to survival. In the Red Light reflex, when you feel threatened and experience fear, you withdraw by closing your eyes, tensing your jaw and face, pulling your neck forward, lifting your shoulders, flexing your elbows, tightening abdominal muscles, contracting your diaphragm and holding your breath, and so on, all the way down to your feet. In the Green Light reflex, when circumstances demand that you act (the phone rings or someone knocks on the door), you prepare to move forward by opening your eyes and jaw, pulling your neck

## Louise's "Frozen" Shoulder

Louise went to see Thomas Hanna when she was fifty-six years old. Two years earlier she had broken her upper right arm, but despite several surgeries and physical therapy, she found herself in intense chronic pain and with restricted mobility. Despondent over returning to normal functioning, she decided, though only in midlife, "I guess I'm just over the hill."

Louise's bone structure had healed normally, but Hanna noticed that certain muscles in her back, chest, and abdomen remained in constant powerful contraction, pulling her arm down and preventing her from lifting it, as though she had a crippled wing. Because Louise did not even sense these rigidities, she could not relax them. Hanna's task was to help her become aware of the contractions from within her own central nervous system. He placed his hands on different areas of her body and moved them simultaneously so that she could perceive their connection—for example, between her right shoulder and lower back. He also had Louise contract one of her back muscles as hard as she could, making her shoulder even tighter, while he pulled her arm firmly so that she would contract even harder. Hanna did this to provide sensory feedback that would make her conscious of tightening her own shoulder into a frozen position. He repeated the action with all the muscles involved.

As Louise practiced voluntarily contracting and releasing her shoulder, the muscles released their spasms, becoming soft and loose, and finally allowed her shoulder to move freely again. With Hanna's help, she was able to "defrost" her "frozen" shoulder and relearn how to use her muscles efficiently. He also taught her a somatic exercise to rehearse her newly found sensory-motor ability before going to bed and upon waking.

Exultant over the transformation, Louise wept as she realized she had regained control of herself and her life. Her shoulder restriction never returned, and she remained comfortable, supple, and active, forgetting her age and acting like a much younger, confident, and vibrant woman.[24]

# An Experience in Somatics

The following movement series communicates to the extensor muscles of the back, which can be activated by the Green Light reflex, and to the flexor muscles of the abdomen, which are involved in the Red Light reflex. ☞ See figures on page 238.

Rest on your back, knees bent, feet flat on the floor. Be aware of the tip of your tailbone and press it down to the surface you're lying on as you inhale. Move gradually and only to the degree that is comfortable. Breathe in and allow your lower back to arch in response. As you exhale press your lower back down, then inhale and arch, take note of what occurs elsewhere in your body. For example, is your skull moving in response to the movement of the spine, pelvis, and tailbone? Instead of muscling this action, let your skeleton be the means of taking you through the motion. Learn to move without great effort or force.

Do the same movement, only this time interlace the fingers of both hands beneath the back of your head. Inhale and let your lower back arch in response to the pressing of the bottom tip of the spine to the floor. Simultaneously press your elbows down to the floor. Notice that your shoulder blades want to draw in toward the spine. Exhale, pressing your belly button toward your spine and flattening your lower back as you lift your arms and head high enough to look at your knees. Continue this arch and curl, sensing how everything is lengthening from the back of the skull to your pelvis as you curl. As you exhale and curl, lift your head with the strength of your center.

This movement is similar to a flower opening and closing. By doing it, you are creating a healthy spine while reeducating your muscles not to be stuck in a habitual reflexive pattern.

Repeat this series six times, slowly and easily. Let your breath determine when you move. Let your sensitivity lead the way in knowing what's enough. Sense how you can use this movement to adjust tension and bring more relaxation to the lower back.

—Courtesy of Carol Welch, BioSomatics teacher.

back and shoulders down, extending your elbows, opening your hands, lifting your chest, and so on.[25] The trauma reflex can occur anywhere in your body when you need to guard against severe injury and pain, as in accidents and surgery. For example, when you receive a blow, you cringe and set off an imbalance to one side.

When everyday life repeatedly triggers these reactions, the result is habitual muscular contractions that are so deeply unconscious that you can no longer voluntarily relax them, nor can you remember how to move about freely. Instead, you function with stiffness, soreness, and within only a limited range of movement, because "what we do not sense, we cannot move: what we cannot move, we cannot sense."[26]

Hanna called this habituated state of forgetfulness *sensory-motor amnesia* (SMA). This kind of amnesia has nothing to do with brain damage; it is "a memory loss of how certain muscle groups feel and how to control them."[27] With it comes a variety of chronic conditions and limitations. Hanna estimated that as many as 50 percent of chronic pain cases are a result of SMA. That's because muscles that never get a chance to relax become sore, painful, and/or weak due to constant exertion. In turn, that causes clumsiness, an energy drain on the body, postural distortions, and poor weight distribution. These difficulties "will cause secondary pain typically mistaken for arthritis, bursitis, herniated disks, and so on," said Hanna.[28] He was emphatic that reeducation could reverse these and other so-called inevitable symptoms of aging, as well as overcome or help avert many other physical conditions that plague us in a high-stress technologized environment.

Hanna favored reeducation because SMA is a learned adaptation to stress and trauma, which means it also can be unlearned. HSE reprograms your nervous system through hands-on table work and movement lessons. The Pandicular Response is the primary method used to "wake up" the sensory-motor cortex. Instead of providing sensory feedback by their own manipulations, practitioners invite you to make a strong voluntary contraction of the amnesic muscles and create your own sensory information, which simultaneously restores the action of the motor neurons. According to Hanna, muscle groups in contraction for years release and, eventually, with some help and movement reinforcement, stay relaxed. As your body gives up restricted physical patterns, rigid psychological habits are also cut loose.

## RESOURCES:

**For information, practitioners, books, and tapes:** Somatics Educational Resources, 1516 Grant Ave., Suite 220, Novato, CA 94945; BioSomatics (in the tradition of Thomas Hanna), Box 206, Grand Junction, CO 81502, (970) 245-8903.

**Books:** Thomas Hanna, *Somatics: Reawakening the Mind's Control of Movement, Flexibility, and Health* (Addison-Wesley, 1988), and *The Body of Life* (Healing Arts, 1993); Jim Dreaver, D.C., *Somatic Therapy: A Neuromuscular Approach to Pain and Stiffness* (Jim Dreaver, 1991).

**Audiovisual:** "Unlocking Your Body—Regaining Youth Through Somatic Awareness," Thomas Hanna, 90-min. video, Somatic Educational Resources (see above); "BioSomatics Developmental Movement Re-Education," 76-min. video, Carol Welch (program based on Hanna's work), Grand Junction, CO 81501, (970) 245-8903; "Somatic Exercise," Thomas Hanna, 39 audiocassette tapes, Somatics Educational Resources (see above).

# Body-Mind Centering®

Where does the body end and the mind begin? Where does the mind end and the spirit begin? They cannot be divided as they are interrelated and but different aspects of the same all-pervading divine consciousness.

—B.K.S. Iyengar

Body-Mind Centering (BMC) is Bonnie Bainbridge Cohen's comprehensive educational and therapeutic approach to movement to help release the stress, fear, aches and pains, and restrictive habits and perceptions that keep you from functioning at your best. Through a special kind of awareness— "active focusing"—you can open to new options in thinking, feeling, and moving with greater ease, coordination, balance, and integration. In turn, this enables you to prevent injuries, face challenges, and expand your creativity.

Bainbridge Cohen's influences in movement came early and in an unusual way. Growing up in the Ringling Brothers and Barnum and Bailey Circus, she watched a wide variety of human and animal performers. Her mother was a trapeze artist who also rode two horses while balancing one foot on each. In developing her original perspective, Bainbridge Cohen studied and practiced widely—dance, Yoga, Aikido, voice, dance therapy, Laban Movement Analysis, Kestenberg Movement Profile, neuromuscular reeducation, occupational therapy, Craniosacral Therapy, neurodevelopmental therapy, Zero Balancing, Zen, and *Katsugen Undo,* a Japanese system. She founded the School for Body-Mind Centering in 1973.

BMC is not a technique but a study of movement. It is an experiential and cognitive journey for understanding how your mind expresses itself through your body in motion. At the core of BMC is the intimate experience of your own anatomy and physiology from within—that is, being able to sense each body system and tissue separately and to initiate action from it. Unlike bodyways that are primarily concerned with the musculoskeletal system, BMC expands your sensory awareness of ligaments, nerves, fascia, glands, skin, organs, fat, and fluids (blood, lymph, synovial, and craniosacral). According to BMC teachers, just as you can feel yourself moving your toes, so too can you develop the ability to sense any tissue or organ, and to move and change it at need.

BMC associates a particular state of mind or qualities with each tissue. Thus, when you alter the quality of your movements, you also create physiological, psychological, and even spiritual changes. For example, the organ system is related to feelings, expression, and sense of volume; the nervous system governs alertness, thought, precision, and perception; the endocrine system underlies intuition, energy flow, and internal chaos or balance. Through such an exploration, you can learn to access any part of yourself.

Because BMC is a body-based language with an experiential vocabulary, practitioners are able to apply it broadly: in movement, speech therapy, physical and occupational therapy, perceptual-motor development, education, dance, psychotherapy, Yoga, voice and music, athletics, meditation, visual arts, and other bodyways. They work with all ages from infancy on.

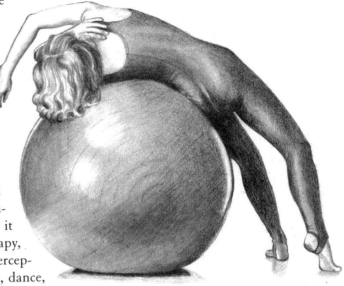

Working with a Large Ball in Body-Mind Centering

BMC practitioners customize sessions to meet your individual needs. They combine hands-on work, movement, guided imagery, developmental repatterning, pictures, dialogue, and playful props, including large balls, stretch bands, springers, music, and videos.[29] Practitioners first make contact with an aspect of their own bodies, such as the lymph, before contacting it in you and then inviting it to shift to a more organized or coherent pattern of movement. Through their hands, they provide sensory feedback so you can become aware of the particular system, recognize what state it's in, and activate the state in which it could function best. In the process, you release excess tension. When practitioners facilitate a gentle experience of moving with greater efficiency and awareness, you can drop limiting patterns and gain new strength and flexibility.

BMC is unique in not only fostering consciousness of every major body system but also working with developmental patterns of movement. Bainbridge Cohen has identified sixteen basic patterns that evolve as human beings progress from fetal movement through creeping, crawling, and walking. This ontogenic or individual development closely parallels phylogenetic or group development in the animal kingdom, from one-celled creatures through the primates. Each pattern gives rise to and supports successive stages, like overlapping waves.

According to Bainbridge Cohen, underdevelopment or inefficiency in any pattern affects all the others and can lead to postural or movement dif-

# A Body-Mind Centering Experience

Invertebrate patterns underlie vertebrate patterns in the developmental process of movement. One such pattern is Mouthing. As an infant, you use your mouth as a kind of first "limb" with which to reach, grasp, and release. The Mouthing pattern takes over immediately at birth, when the umbilical cord is no longer your means of survival and your main concern is getting fed. Your nose and mouth, not your eyes or ears, instinctively search for food. Your sense of smell tracks where milk will come from and your mouth reaches like a hand for the nipple. Your earliest movement into the environment arises from this primal desire, which starts deep in your internal organs. You're like a sea squirt, an organism attached to the ocean floor that is a mouth waiting for nourishment.

To experience leading from your mouth, cover your eyes with something you can tie around your head, for you don't want vision to guide you. Then lie down curled up on your side. Turn your head the way you usually do. Notice how you do that. Are you moving from your skeleton—your skull and the vertebrae in your neck? Come back to center.

Now contrast this with initiating movement from a different place. Explore your mouth area. Lick your lips. Swallow. Move around inside with your tongue. Observe any sensations that might arise: Does your stomach gurgle? Are you suddenly hungry?

The area around your mouth is highly sensitive to touch, so, with your fingertips, gently and lightly stroke around your lips and cheeks. Wait until you feel a place of stimulation that motivates you to move in one direction or another—from your mouth, not your skeleton. Let your mouth find your thumb. Don't put your thumb into your mouth, but let your mouth take it in. Notice the difference. What happens when your lips reach? Can you feel how that sets up the rotation of your head, neck, throat, esophagus, and eventually your entire digestive tract all the way to the anus? It is this "soft spine" that acts as a source of internal support. Explore this movement of your torso as though you had no bones in your head, neck, shoulders, and chest, and as if the only way you could move is from the tube that goes from your lips all the way to your stomach and beyond.

As you lead with your mouth, find yourself beginning to roll onto your back, keeping your knees bent and feet off the floor, arms flexed close to your body, just like a baby. Continue to play with your mouth and let it take you to the other side and back again. If you like, keep exploring the environment with your mouth. See where it leads you.

—Courtesy of Lisa Clark and David Beadle, Body-Mind Centering practitioners.

ficulties; obstacles in perception, organization, memory, and creativity; learning disabilities; brain dysfunction; and social and psychological obstacles. For example, if, as a child, you failed to establish certain reflexes for catching yourself when falling, you may have found yourself clumsy and uncoordinated and thus were reluctant to engage in physical activities as well as fearful of falling, even as an adult. By establishing a good developmental base early in life, you can help prevent difficulties from occurring in later years. Even as an adult, through a process of repatterning, you can fill in the missing pieces of your development and correct limitations at the root level.

Bainbridge Cohen explains that the more neurological pathways you lay down in your body—new patterns—and the more basic integration your body has, the greater, wider, deeper, and broader are your possibilities for expression and understanding. "If the body is the instrument through which the mind is expressed, then one can just play more kinds of melodies, or different kinds of verse, kinds of timbre," she says.[30]

BMC training attracts a wide variety of professionals, including dancers, massage and other somatic therapists, and psychotherapists. The Practitioner Certification Program involves four terms of study over the course of four years, plus fulfillment of outside requirements. The Teacher Certification Program also offers advanced training for certified practitioners with a minimum of two years' experience.

## RESOURCES:

**For information, practitioners, training, books, and videos:** The School for Body-Mind Centering, 189 Pondview Dr., Amherst, MA 01002, (413) 256-8615, fax (413) 256-8239.

**Books:** Bonnie Bainbridge Cohen, *Sensing, Feeling, and Action: The Experiential Anatomy of Body-Mind Centering* [collected articles from *Contact Quarterly* dance journal, 1980–92] (Contact Editions, 1993); Linda Hartley, *Wisdom of the Body Moving: An Introduction to Body-Mind Centering* (North Atlantic, 1995); Beth Goren, *Rapids* (North Atlantic, 1995).

For the functional and movement-education aspects of two structural approaches, ☞ see "Rolfing Movement Integration," pages 196–198, 200–201, and "Neurokinetics in Aston-Patterning," page 202. See also Chapter 11: "Western Movement Arts."

# Western Movement Arts

*Life is movement,*
*movement is life.*
*To live is to move, to*
*move is to be alive.*

—MK

Eastern movement arts, such as T'ai Chi Chuan, Yoga, or Aikido, began in relation to self-defense and/or spiritual practice and evolved as healing arts. Western movement arts had a different beginning—in the world of dance. And although you can use some Eastern and Western movement arts as exercise, that's not their purpose. Mindlessly repeating movements does not help you break into new territory, whereas unpredictability in movement can awaken you. Aerobics may add years to your life, but it won't necessarily add life to your years.

## STARTING FROM DANCE

*Movement is the uni-*
*fying bond between the*
*mind and the body.*

—Deane Juhan

Since how we move is how we function, many Western movement arts have a lot in common with functional approaches. In both the objective is to enhance all of you, whereas in exercise, for the most part, the intention is to improve your figure or condition your cardiovascular system. Instead of aiming at losing weight, for example, movement arts and functional body-ways focus on losing habitual patterns that limit your movement and thinking. Both are an educational process, another means of getting to know yourself and expand your possibilities. Movement complements hands-on work by providing the experience of power, balance, confidence, energy, strength, coordination, and capability in action. It gives your body a chance to go from receiving information passively to practicing it actively. The two groups are also similar in using a high degree of kinesthetic awareness or self-sensing.

But unlike the functional bodyways, the movement arts originated with dance and choreography professionals, or established a foothold first among them, to help elevate performance levels. Even so, the scope of their practice has extended far beyond the dance community to individuals with a wide variety of physical and emotional needs. Most of the movement arts in this chapter could also appear easily in the one that covers functional approaches and some could fit in the chapter on convergence therapies.

As in functional bodyways, movement arts address our movement skills. We first explore and acquire these skills as infants and children. If nothing or no one interferes with our development, the movement abilities that are wired into our system will unfold naturally. If not, we experience difficulties later in life. "There are no shortcuts: no child can afford to miss any part of the learning process. If one never learns to crawl as a child, something will be missing as an adult," says Ted Kaptchuk, a doctor of Oriental medicine at Beth Israel Hospital in Boston.[1] Those missing pieces in the developmental process translate into unused movement potential.

During our early years, we explore endlessly, twisting and turning, rolling, reaching, climbing, and falling in the process. But as adults, generally we stop delving into new possibilities and become fixed in the way we move, think, and express our thoughts. We move through life in familiar ways because when we step outside of our usual limitations, we tend to experience confusion and anxiety. We don't realize that we can also experience enrichment. Restricted movement goes hand in hand with a restricted mind. When we free our movement, we also free our personality. Emotional and mental liveliness accompanies effortless movement.

Like the functional approaches, movement arts are excellent vehicles for filling in the pieces that were missing earlier in life. These bodyways can bring forth what is intrinsically there but may never have developed fully. They can take your nervous system into unfamiliar or "forgotten" terrain by breaking movement down into small messages. Your nervous system then can assimilate and eventually synthesize them into functional patterns of movement.

In teaching new movement possibilities, the movement arts may help you gain a new ease in your body and expand not only how you move but also how you feel and think. You can learn to move from within your own body rather than from an external image, and you can discover how to move at your own pace, without pushing and causing tension. You can use these arts as a tool for exploring who you are.

If you are already engaged in movement classes, you may recognize elements in them from the movement arts I describe below or from various functional bodyways. Depending on their own training background, movement teachers often combine diverse features from different approaches.

Children and primate man have both a natural gift for bodily movement and a natural love for it. In later periods . . . man becomes cautious, suspicious, and sometimes even hostile to movement. He forgets that it is the basic experience of existence.

—Rudolf Laban

If life means movement and death means non-movement, then . . . more movement means more life and . . . less movement means less life. . . . A diminished capacity for movement is equivalent to diminished life.

—Thomas Hanna

RESOURCES:

**For information and referrals:** Contact the International Somatic Movement Education and Therapy Association (ISMETA), c/o 148 W. 23rd St., #14, New York, NY 10011, (212) 242-4962. There are movement schools and institutes across the country where you can take classes and find therapists to work with; check your local resources, including dance studios.

# Laban-Bartenieff

*If we accept that the way people sit, walk and make gestures has any relevance to how they are thinking and feeling, then it is only a short step towards the idea that a more subtle and deep analysis of the composition of the movement can lead towards a greater understanding of the personality.*

*—Marion North*

"Actions speak louder than words," a universal proverb tells us. Do you know what your movements reflect about you—your personality, your interaction with others, the culture that socialized you? How aware are you of the unique way you move? Do you show a preference for light, quick movements or heavy, slow ones? What parts of your body do you use most? Where do your movements originate from? How do you move through the space around you—at an angle or in a circle? How delicate or vigorous are your movements? Labanalysis and Bartenieff Fundamentals$_{sm}$ address these questions.

Rudolf Laban (1879–1958) was a Czech choreographer, dancer, and teacher who worked with great figures in European modern dance. He studied the movement process not only in dance (folk and modern) but also in martial arts, factory assembly lines, and everyday actions. While exploring the basic principles of movement structure and purpose, Laban developed an internationally used system of movement notation: Labanotation records body movement like a score records music. He also evolved the system of movement analysis that now bears his name—Labanalysis.

Laban's student Irmgard Bartenieff (1900–1981), a German dancer and choreographer, applied his work to physical therapy, particularly with polio patients. Acutely aware of the psychological implications of movement, she also helped found the American Dance Therapy Association. Both Laban and Bartenieff abhorred a mechanistic approach to movement, which they considered not only inefficient but also harmful for an individual's self-image.

Formerly known as Effort-Shape, Labanalysis or Laban Movement Analysis (LMA) is a comprehensive system for discriminating among, describing, analyzing, and categorizing the patterns and variations of how we move—anything from a conversational hand gesture to a complex action. Because its standardized terminology makes possible precise communication about nuances of movement, LMA can be applied in a wide variety of profes-

# Dance Therapy

Dance or movement therapy is a form of psychotherapy that uses movement rather than words as the primary medium for assessment, insight, and change. A basic premise underlying this practice is that there is no division between the workings of the mind or psyche and the behavior of the body; how people feel is visible in their movement. Most dance/movement therapists work in mental-health settings, both psychiatric hospitals and outpatient programs; their clients include autistic, brain-injured, and learning-disabled children, the elderly, the developmentally disabled, the blind, and the hearing-impaired. Other therapists work privately with clients interested in personal growth and deal with the same issues as those in verbal psychotherapy—self-identity, assertiveness, self-acceptance, boundaries, communication, relationships, and so on. Although several dancers in the twentieth century made pioneering contributions before her, Marian Chace is credited as the mother of dance therapy.

RESOURCES:

**For information and registered therapists:** Contact American Dance Therapy Association (ADTA), 2000 Century Plaza, Suite 108, Columbia, MD 21044-3263, (410) 997-4040. For a book on Marian Chace and the development of dance therapy, see Susan Sandel et al., *Foundations of Dance/Movement Therapy: The Life and Work of Marian Chace* (Marian Chace Memorial Fund of ADTA, 1993).

sions: dance, choreography, athletic coaching, fitness, body disciplines and therapies, psychotherapies, acting and directing, teaching, even ethnology.

Certified Movement Analysts can observe recurring patterns, note movement preferences, assess physical blocks and dysfunctional movement patterns, and then suggest new possibilities. While still valuing the uniqueness of your patterns, they can offer movement experiences to guide you through expressive and functional changes that improve everyday life, enhance performance in dance and athletics, or mitigate disability.[2]

There are four major components of LMA. Each one deals with a different aspect of movement and all of them provide pathways to neuromuscular repatterning. Although *Effort* (in German, *Antrieb,* "impulse toward motion") sounds as though it is about exertion, it is not. In Laban's system, it describes the dynamic qualities of movement and inner attitudes toward four physical dimensions of energy—flow (free or bound), weight (strong or light), time (sudden or sustained), and space (direct or indirect). Everyone moves in and out of all four, but each of us has individual prefer-

# Experience in Bartenieff Fundamentals: Arm Circles

Arm Circles can help you establish a clear diagonal connection between the upper and lower parts of your body—right upper to left lower, left upper to right lower. Maintaining that diagonal connection continuously is key to efficiency of motion in manipulating tools, such as felling a tree with an axe, and in dance and other expressive movement.

As you do the circles, move gradually, as smoothly and easily as possible, without locking your elbow or jerking so that the circle is not lopsided.

Part 1: Lie on your back, with your knees bent and your feet flat on the floor. Let your arms rest straight out on the floor at shoulder level. Let your knees drop comfortably to the right, without holding them tightly together, and rest a moment. Extend your left arm at a diagonal from your shoulder (figure A). Sense how that movement also pulls your right hip. Move your left arm, palm up, in a large counterclockwise circle overhead and around on the ground, as though you were drawing a circle on the floor and over your hips. Allow your eyes to follow your left hand, moving your head slightly as you need to (figure B). Keep your pelvis anchored to the floor. Be aware of changes in arm rotation at the top and bottom of the circle. When your hand returns to where you started, rest a moment. Then reverse the direction of the circling and move your arm clockwise. Rest again. Then drop your knees to the left and repeat all the steps to make a circle with your right arm.

Part 2: Return to the starting position, with your knees up, arms horizontal, and palms down. Drop your knees to the right and rest a moment. Repeat the counterclockwise circle with your left arm, but this time as you come around and reach toward your left knee, gradually increase the energy of the movement so that it brings you into a twisted sitting position. Notice how the drive of the circular arm sweeping causes a shift in lower body weight from right to left, allowing you to sit. Don't stop here but finish the

ences. And, whether we're aware of them or not, we make choices in life according to these preferences. For example, a predilection toward control is reflected in flow, while one toward assertion is reflected in weight. LMA helps you become aware of these predispositions.

The second component, *Space,* describes the pathways in space through which the body moves. The third, *Shape,* focuses on the body's changing forms. The last, *Body,* has to do with body usage: initiating movement from different parts of your body, mobilizing your body efficiently in its environment, and preparing it to perform the widest range of movement qualities and shapes possible.

Bartenieff Fundamentals (BF) carries this analysis further, outlining

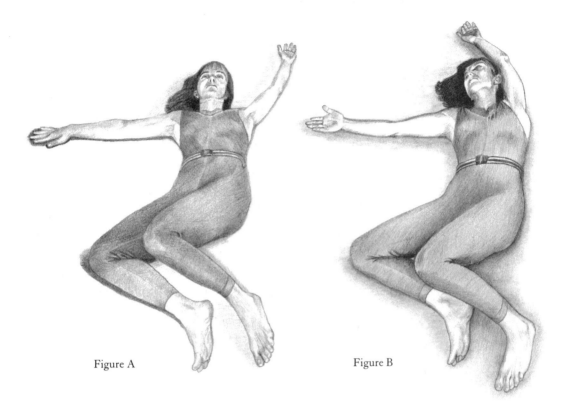

Figure A                                    Figure B

**cycle. Keeping your arm movement continuous, sink diagonally back into the knee-drop position on the floor. Notice how your lower body weight now shifts from left to right. Repeat from the opposite side.**

—Adapted with permission from Irmgard Bartenieff and Dori Lewis,
*Body Movement: Coping with the Environment* (Gordon and Breach, 1980).

six basic movement patterns into which any movement can be broken down. As a system of body training or body reeducation, BF emphasizes the functional aspect of movement—how you use intention, weight shift, initiation, spatial awareness, muscular sequencing, breath rhythm, and body-part relationships. It is a means of improving your alignment and increasing ease, efficiency, and expressivity. BF includes specific exercises you can practice lying on the floor, sitting, or standing. These are designed to help you achieve more efficient use of your deeper muscles (because we generally tend to rely on our superficial muscles) so that you can engage in a wider range of movements. BF also integrates body awareness with spatial awareness. You accomplish these intentions by working with simple movements in a relaxed way, feeling your whole body move in all directions, and experiencing the importance of fluid breathing in all activities. When you can do the Fundamentals correctly, you can move easily, getting your right and left sides or upper and lower parts of your body to work both separately and in concert.

The idea behind Bartenieff's work is that it confirms what is fundamental within you and repatterns less-efficient movement. The system also addresses a cultural phenomenon in the West, that of overidentifying with the upper body and disidentifying with, even deadening, the lower body. Like Eastern martial arts, BF is a way of healing this split by rediscovering your relationship to the center of your weight and your grounding, and by getting your lower body to move. The basic premise is that once you have the physical foundation of your life working, then it's easier to express complexity and richness on emotional and intellectual levels as well.

Becoming a Certified Movement Analyst (CMA) involves the study of Laban Movement Analysis, Bartenieff Fundamentals, observation training, and seminar study, with more than five hundred in-class hours, after completing anatomy, kinesiology, and other prerequisite courses. CMAs work as performance coaches, fitness directors, athletic coaches, and personal trainers, as well as with patients in medical settings for rehabilitation and postural and neuromuscular reeducation. For example, Ellen Goldman, who helped found the Laban/Bartenieff Institute of Movement Studies, calls her work Integrated Movement; it focuses on movement in the context of communication in our daily lives. Her book *As Others See Us: Body Movement and the Art of Successful Communication* (Gordon and Breach, 1994) teaches you how to build awareness of your continuous body movements and how to experience the subtleties of body language.

## RESOURCES:

**For training, practitioners, and published materials:** Laban/Bartenieff Institute of Movement Studies, 11 E. 4th St., 3rd floor, New York, NY 10003-6902, (212) 477-4299, fax (212) 477-3702.

**Books:** Irmgard Bartenieff with Dori Lewis, *Body Movement: Coping with the Environment* (Gordon & Breach, 1980).

---

> Movement and a willingness to perceive the movement brings access to bodily knowledge, or embodiment. In this way, the feeling component of thought is brought to life, enabling one to experience the feeling that connects thoughts.
>
> —Peggy Hackney

# The Pilates or Physicalmind Method

For most of this century, the Pilates (pronounced "pill-ah-tees") Physicalmind Method was virtually unknown outside of the performance community, especially dancers, where it produced lithe and lean bodies without aerobics or weight lifting. Now it's also gently conditioning people of all shapes and sizes—amateur athletes, women before and after childbirth, teenagers, senior citizens—as well as helping others recover and rehabilitate from injuries. The strengthening and stretching movements, which are stress-free and non-impact, are showing up in sports medicine clinics, physical therapy units, spas, fitness centers, martial arts studios, and dance schools.

Physicalmind is concerned with economical movement. It relies on kinesthetic monitoring in developing balanced muscle use for ease of motion. As an inside-out approach that combines sensory awareness with physical training, Pilates can lead to mental equilibrium as well. Joseph Pilates, the method's originator, believed that ideal fitness is "the attainment and maintenance of a uniformly developed body with a sound mind fully capable of naturally, easily and satisfactorily performing our many and varied daily tasks with spontaneous zest and pleasure."[3]

A Physicalmind instructor first will analyze your movement patterns for any functional or structural problems and then design a program for your particular needs. The principal intention is learning how to move from a stable, central core, whether you're walking or shaking someone's hand. You begin by working with the three primary control centers of your torso—the lower and deeper abdominals and the midback muscles—and then your arms and legs. Exercising the core muscles develops a "girdle of strength" that supports the entire spine and stabilizes the pelvis. Instead of tucking or arching your pelvis, you become able to maintain it in a neutral position.

To achieve strength and flexibility, you work with a variety of equipment invented by Joseph Pilates, including the Universal Reformer, Trapeze Table or Cadillac, Wunda Chair, Spine Corrector, Ped-O-Pul, and Magic Circle. Even though you could easily mistake these unusual-looking contraptions for medieval torture devices, they can help you increase range of motion, correct misalignment and weight distribution, and control muscles and expenditure of energy. There are also workouts (not in the aerobic, cardiovascular sense) you can do without the equipment on a floor mat.

The main apparatus is the Universal Reformer. It resembles a single-bed frame, but has a padded carriage that slides back and forth and ad-

> The key to all life experience is movement. . . .
>
> —Ida Rolf

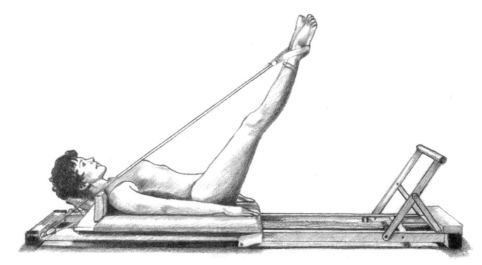

Working on the Universal Reformer

justable springs that regulate tension and resistance. Cables, pulleys, bars, and padded straps allow you to push or pull with your hands or feet while lying on your back, sitting, kneeling, or standing. It's crucial that you don't mindlessly repeat the movements fifty or a hundred times, but instead execute only five to ten repetitions slowly, carefully, and patiently so that they are rhythmic and smooth. You focus on *eccentric* contraction, which elongates the muscles, rather than on *concentric* contraction, which shortens and hardens muscles. The instructor supervises your movements, of which there are hundreds, for specific placement, precise rhythm, and systematic breathing. Control and concentration are key.

Through the emphasis on correct usage, you become aware of which muscles will enable you to move in a balanced way. For example, when walking, you engage not only your quadriceps muscles (front of the thigh) but the hamstrings (back of the thigh) as well. Physicalmind is geared so that you work with multiple muscle groups simultaneously—you can't rely on only your stronger muscles to the detriment of your weaker muscles. Rather than focus just on the site of injury or difficulty, each routine takes into consideration the whole body as a single, integrated unit. Although it is strength-oriented, Physicalmind also increases flexibility; instead of bulking up your muscles, the movements elongate them. The combination of strength, flexibility, and balanced muscle use helps support your structure and prevent injuries.

Instructors vary in their background. Some start out as physical therapists or practitioners of various bodyways, including Yoga and Body-Mind Centering, and integrate Physicalmind. Others may have benefited from it as injured dancers and gone on to become trainers themselves. Once you learn Physicalmind from an instructor, generally in one-on-one lessons, you can do it on your own at home with a training video and/or home-use equipment.

In order to qualify for certification in the Pilates or Physicalmind Method, students must know the entire repertoire in their own bodies first. The teacher training program at Physicalmind Institute™ is 204 hours. A separate clinical training program which focuses on rehabilitation is offered at St. Francis Hospital in San Francisco.

## Joseph Pilates

Joseph Pilates was born in 1880 near Dusseldorf, Germany. A frail child afflicted with rheumatic fever, rickets, and asthma, he was taunted by classmates. But he was so determined to overcome his weakness that by the age of fourteen he was posing for anatomical charts. He worked diligently at building his body and mind with both Eastern and Western practices, including Yoga, Zen, and ancient Greek and Roman regimens. Pilates also became a gymnast, diver, and skier.

In 1912 he left for England to train as a boxer. When World War I broke out, because he was a German national, Pilates was interned as an "enemy alien." In a Lancaster camp he taught wrestling and self-defense to other inmates; on the Isle of Man he invented devices to help rehabilitate disabled people. Once the war ended, he returned to Germany and continued to create new machines. Rudolf Laban watched his work and incorporated some of Pilates's methods into his own movement teaching. ☞ See "Laban-Bartenieff," page 248. But when the German government took notice and invited Pilates to train the army, he left the country.

On the ship headed for New York in 1926, he met the woman who would become his wife, Clara, a nurse. Together they established a Pilates studio in the city and later at Jacob's Pillow in Massachusetts, where dance legends George Balanchine, Martha Graham, Ruth St. Denis, Ted Shawn, Hanya Holm, Alvin Ailey, Jerome Robbins, and their protégés flocked to heal, reshape, align, and condition their bodies. A long list of screen stars and professional athletes followed suit, working with Joe and Clara or second- and third-generation instructors who carried their method across the country and to big cities in Europe and Asia. Among them are Gary Cooper, Katharine Hepburn, Glenn Close, Sigourney Weaver, Jessica Lange, Candice Bergen, members of the San Francisco 49ers and Cincinnati Bengals football teams, Ben Vereen, Chris Evert, Martina Navratilova, and Kristi Yamaguchi.

Pilates worked until the day he died in 1967, when a fire in his studio forced him to hang from the rafters for more than an hour—he inhaled too much smoke. A stocky, muscled, but trim man, people had always thought him twenty to thirty years younger than his age.

RESOURCES:

**For information, instructor referrals, and training programs:** Physical Mind Institute, 1807 Second St., #28129, Santa Fe, NM 87505, (505) 988-1990 or (800) 505-1990; and Center for Sports Medicine, St. Francis Hospital, 900 Hyde St., San Francisco, CA 94109, (415) 353-6410. To obtain equipment for home use, contact Ken Endelman, Current Concepts, 7500 14th Ave., #23, Sacramento, CA 95820, (800) 240-FLEX, or Physicalmind Institute. You can also contact local dance companies and the dance departments of colleges in your area for referrals.

**Audiovisual:** "Full Body Workout I," "Working Out the Pilates Way," "Working Out the Pilates Way, II," and "The Eve Gentry Technique," Physicalmind Institute, (800) 505-1990; "Pilates Conditioning Techniques on the Mat and Apparatus," Elizabeth Larkham, Director, Center for Sports Medicine, St. Francis Hospital, 900 Hyde St., San Francisco, CA 94109, (415) 353-6410.

# Ideokinesis

Lulu E. Sweigard, Ph.D., coined the term *Ideokinesis* to describe her particular approach to neuromuscular reeducation. Taken from the Greek, *ideo-* means "idea" and *kinesis* means "motion." Ideokinesis is thus a process of using mental imagery to change motor patterns. Sweigard based it on the pioneering work of her own teacher, Mabel Elsworth Todd, who taught at Columbia University in the 1920s and 1930s.[4] Before her death, in 1974, Sweigard spent many years teaching in the dance department of the Juilliard School in New York. Especially in Todd's and Sweigard's time, using imagery was a radical departure from the long-established method of exerting conscious, voluntary effort to "put" and "hold" parts of your body in better alignment.

The premise of Ideokinesis is that the nervous system directs and coordinates all postural alignment patterns, muscle use, and skeletal movement. In order to change your posture or movement patterns, you first have to change neurological activity. Sweigard also believed that imbalanced muscle usage might be a factor in joint and muscle pain and in limited range and vocabulary of movement. To enhance balance in standing, she taught people to visualize "lines of movement" traveling through their bodies. She had them do this first while lying down in the "constructive rest position," before performing a desired movement.

In creating the lines of movement, Sweigard sought to bring the various weights of the axial skeleton (skull, vertebral column, and rib cage) as close as possible to the line of gravity and also lower the center of gravity. In turn, this would minimize overall muscle activity in maintaining an upright posture. She also wanted to balance muscle usage around the joints to allow freedom of movement in any direction.

Sweigard neither codified her work nor taught it as a method. Thus, there are no Ideokinesis teachers as such, but there are individuals who use Ideokinetic imagery in the process of teaching movement. They use words and touch to instruct you in the lines of movement. Each has a specific location and directional pathway and must be described in a way that suits your express needs. By visualizing a particular set of images that constitute a line of movement through your body, you initiate impulses along certain neural routes to various muscles. In effect, you train or prepare your nervous system to stimulate muscles appropriately for the intended movement. You unlearn one motor pattern and replace it with another one. If you continue to give your nervous system a clear mental picture of the movement you intend, it will automatically take care of the "how" and select the most efficient coordination to perform the movement. This will minimize physical stress and maintain more balanced alignment of your bones. Athletes who use ideokinetic imagery, for example, might improve their performance because they become more efficient in how they use their bodies.

Daily attention also eventually can transform your body's shape. Those muscles that you once overcontracted become more flexible; those you hardly used develop better tone, strength, and endurance. However, although you can effect these changes without working up a sweat, it takes constant vigilance to repattern a habit, approximately three months of practicing every day. Ideokinesis does not build bulk or stretch muscles; it is a complement to, not a substitute for, other conditioning or training modalities.

Sweigard maintained that Ideokinesis is strictly a facilitator of the learning process and deals neither with diagnosing structural pathology nor with medically treating difficulties. Instead, it gives you useful tools to enable you to move more effectively and, in this way, remove those habits that might be causing troublesome conditions. It is necessary in this work to be familiar with your own anatomy and understand the biomechanics of the musculoskeletal system.

> Relaxation does not mean going limp or collapsing. . . . [It] means moving efficiently. It means resting while you are moving.
>
> —Anna Halprin

# RESOURCES:

**For instruction and referrals:** Send a SASE to Irene Dowd, 14 E. 4th St., #606, New York, NY 10012, or inquire at the dance department of your local college.

**Books:** Lulu E. Sweigard, *Human Movement Potential: Its Ideokinetic Facilitation* (Dodd, Mead, 1975); Irene Dowd, *Taking Root to Fly: Articles on Functional Anatomy,* 3rd ed. (Irene Dowd, 1995).

# Contact Improvisation

The living body is a moving body—indeed, it is a constantly moving body.

—Thomas Hanna

In the early 1970s modern dancer Steve Paxton began experimenting with the rolling, falling, and partnering skills of the Japanese martial art Aikido. Contact Improvisation evolved out of these explorations as a play between the body and the physical forces that rule its motion—momentum, gravity, inertia. Contact is a movement form, an unstructured dance, or "art-sport" that unfolds spontaneously—you improvise in the moment rather than follow a formal series of steps.

To engage in Contact is to carry on a physical dialogue with another person, often in silence and always in motion. You must stay focused not only on your own movement (perceiving movement in your body through the sense of kinesthesia), but also on your partner's. You do this more through touch than vision by maintaining a constant awareness of gravity, simultaneously sensing the internal space of your body and shaping/moving it in space.

In a Contact duet, you each take and give weight-rolling, sliding, inverting, lifting, leaning, falling. You use momentum to move in concert with your partner rather than exert strength to control him or her. Because of this, people of radically different sizes and weights can do Contact together. You generate ongoing movement by constantly changing points of contact between your body and your partner's.

The most basic skills in Contact are sensitizing yourself to weight and touch and learning to be disoriented, to be turned upside down or sideways and to move through space in spiraling or curving motions.[5] However, although Paxton didn't plan it, other skills emerge as well: nonverbal communication, self-responsibility, immediate responsiveness, and the ability to give and trustingly receive support and to let things "happen."

Contact Improvisation provides a mirror in which to see and feel yourself physically, emotionally, and spiritually. If you've always considered yourself as *not* a dancer, Contact may change your self-image, enhance your self-esteem, and loosen your inhibitions about moving and relating. As a fun activity, it affords the opportunity to become more playful and respond to creative urges. Because of the close contact, you may learn how to experience sensual contact that is not sexual and to establish boundaries within the sense of connectedness to others. You may become aware of your per-

Movement is a medicine for creating change in a person's physical, emotional, and mental states.

—Carol Welch

# A Contact Improvisation Experience

Stand side by side with a partner, your shoulders touching lightly. Maintaining that contact, begin to walk. Come to moments of stillness so you can explore how much pressure with which you lean into each other. Notice what you have to do to increase the pressure. How different is the contact when you're only at the skin-to-skin level? Try pressing muscle to muscle, bone to bone.

Now try rolling off your partner's shoulder and across his or her back with yours till you make contact with the other shoulder. Do it lightly or with heavy pressure. Practice making a smooth transition. Now add walking again to this movement of contact, allowing your direction in space to vary.

—Courtesy of Leigh Hollowell, Contact Improvisation teacher.

sonality patterns—that you never take the initiative but always follow, or vice versa; that you're afraid of risks, or you're a risk-taker.

Contact is also a form of movement reeducation. For example, if, early in your development, you experienced falling or hanging upside down without support, you may have developed fear and an unwillingness to risk these movements.[6] Contact offers you a chance to learn how to release your weight in order to fall or be supported in a relaxed and safe manner. Supporting other people's weight can help you strengthen multiple body parts simultaneously. Through its emphasis on balance and the unexpected, Contact also stimulates lower brain functions. And because it calls for hand support, it reinforces the early developmental patterning of locomotion.

Although some dancers perform Contact Improvisation and others use it to develop choreography, you don't have to be a dancer to enjoy its exhilarating pleasure or experience its benefits. Since there is a whole continuum of movement with which to work—from touching lightly to flying through the air—Contact teachers use it with a variety of populations, including octogenarians, the blind, hemiplegics, and paraplegics (in or out of a wheelchair). People meet to do Contact in workshops and "jams," working with one partner or several. Classes are more structured, with warm-ups and a process for dropping into a reflective place and body awareness, as well as instruction in how to safely roll, fall, lie down, and get up.

There is no certification process in Contact Improvisation. The Contact community regulates teachers informally.

We do not know very much about our body unless we move it.

—Paul Schilder

RESOURCES:

For the best source of information about Contact Improvisation, its uses, teachers, and location of jams, workshops, and festivals worldwide, see *Contact Quarterly,* a journal devoted to the contemporary movement arts. To subscribe: *Contact Quarterly,* P.O. Box 603, Northampton, MA 01061. For an illustrated study, see Cynthia J. Novack, *Sharing the Dance: Contact Improvisation and American Culture* (University of Wisconsin, 1990).

# Continuum

> Awareness changes how we physically move. As we become more fluid and resilient so do the mental, emotional, and spiritual movements of our lives.
>
> —Emilie Conrad Da'oud

Emilie Conrad Da'oud studied ballet and non-Western dance in New York before spending five years as a choreographer with a folklore company in Haiti. Through her experiences there, she realized that how we move, talk, and think is primarily a cultural construct, but that beneath culture are essential biomorphic movements common to all life forms. In 1967 Conrad began teaching this primary movement process as Continuum.

"Movement is something we are rather than something we do," she says. "We are verbs, not nouns."[7] But we use only a fraction of our movement vocabulary. In our neuromuscular developmental process as fetuses and infants, we experience movement stages that resemble the action of a snake (head to tail, tail to head), frog (both arms together, both legs together), lizard (left arm and leg together, right arm and leg together), salamander (left arm and right leg together, right arm and left leg together), and so on. Then, as we're socialized to move in the ways our culture expects, we may "forget" some of these earlier movements.

> A living body is not a fixed thing but a flowing event, like a flame or a whirlpool.
>
> —Alan Watts

Continuum offers you an opportunity to let go of fixed cultural imprints and move spontaneously, from an inner impulse and more in accord with what your body is biologically capable of. For example, a basic premise of Continuum is that wave motion is fundamental to all living creatures and reflects our evolutionary origins in an aquatic environment. We carry the movement of water in every cell of our body. Deep within us a dance is always going on. We are always moving, even if we appear paralyzed (Conrad prefers to call it "hypnotized"). There are micromovements at an internal level that we can't easily observe externally.

Continuum workshops are an invitation to identify and live as movement, rather than as a form or parts, and to sense yourself as a liquid presence that flows in and through other streams of movement. In a safe environment, you have a chance to explore the creative flux that you call your "body" so that you can enliven yourself from the inside out. In turn, that will translate into greater dynamic expression in the world.

Continuum exercises help you develop sensitivity to movement at all levels, from the subtlest breath to rapport with others. When you learn specific sounds—such as HU, AW, SSS, Dragon, or Wind in the Cave—and let your body uninhibitedly move with them, they often evoke an experience of "being" the very animal the sounds and movements reflect. As you

## At a Continuum Workshop with Emilie Conrad Da'oud

In a large room, I wait expectantly in a group of about fifty women and men. I have no idea what we're going to do. I don't know yet what Continuum is.

First we learn how to do the HU breath, the centerpiece of this work. It is a way of stoking our internal fire, Conrad explains, of warming our vessel. Immediately I notice I've now got a pump going in my diaphragm and it sends heat out into the rest of my body. As I breathe in this unaccustomed fiery, percussive style, suddenly I'm a chimpanzee. My lower jaw protrudes forward, then I pull it back and bare my teeth. I flail my arms and legs loosely up and down. I'm not thinking about being simianlike, I'm just being an ape. Conrad clarifies that doing the HU breath excites the limbic system, the primitive part of the brain that still remembers how to be a creature.

When I learn the AW breath, I feel as though my spinal fluid is moving one drop at a time, and I begin to cool off. I'm no longer a chimpanzee but a lizard, making reptilian movements with my head and neck. Then my shoulders flutter as though they were fins. My spine reverses its curve as it undulates and my head bobs at the end of it.

From the AW we move to the Dragon, and at once I am a prehistoric monster. I'm not imitating anything I've seen in the movies—I'm being it.

We move in and out of these breaths and the states they evoke. It's a challenge to be so flexible, so versatile, so fluent. But once I get the hang of it, I love shuttling back and forth between these realms.

On the evening of the last day of the workshop, I go to dinner with two old friends from the area. I'm amazed when one of them launches into an attack against me, dredging up resentments from seventeen years ago. But even more surprising is how easily I handle the scene, slipping in and out of being a participant who responds calmly and an observer who can evaluate the situation and remain detached. After the woman spews the last of her venom and leaves the restaurant, I realize I'm not bent out of shape. I have moved as fluidly as I did all weekend in the workshop.

# An Experience in Continuum

Sit in a chair and make yourself comfortable. Become aware of the space between your head and one of your shoulders. Think of that space as being alive. When you move, consider that you're narrowing the space rather than moving your body and bringing your ear to your shoulder. Be sure to go slowly. When you feel ready, reverse the movement by thinking of enlarging the space. Notice how it feels to change your referent point from your body to the space around your body. This is extremely important. There should be a definite change in sensation when you shift your referent point in this way. You may suddenly feel very light or experience a deep relaxation of your head and neck and reverberations in your spine. Since each one of us is unique, your response will vary. Use this simple exercise as a guide. You may have to do it several times on each side before you perceive the change in sensation.

Once you have gotten the feel of moving in this way, you can widen your experimentation by lying on the floor on your back or side. This time move from the space between your arms or legs. If you think of them as tentacles, this will give you a greater fluency of movement. When you think in conventional terms about your body—for example, "I am moving my head" or "I am moving my arm"—you create a sense of mass and density. Many ideas about what the body is and is not are ruled by how you relate yourself to movement. Relating to space, rather than to an object, has an enormous effect on orientation. What is remarkable in this simple experiment is that it is quite easy to experience a change in mass and density by simply shifting your referent point for movement. The less mass and density there are, the more capable your body is of healing.

—Courtesy of Emilie Conrad Da'oud and Linda Chrisman.

move in and out of these different combinations, your self-image breaks up and allows you to feel a wider range of possibilities for who you inherently are and can be. There is an emphasis on round, spiral, unpredictable movements rather than a set linear routine.

Conrad prefers unpredictable movements in multiple rhythms because they're much more stimulating to the brain. In contrast, the repetitive motions of conventional fitness, developed according to the tenets of the Industrial Revolution, have a dulling effect on intelligence and creativity. "It is in the fluid world that our connection to intelligence takes place," she says.[8] In this watery place it is also easier to give, recognize, and receive love, which rigidity hinders.

Her ultimate objective in Continuum is to shake us out of our hardened minds and get us to dive deeply into our bodies and into an ocean of love.

To teach Continuum, instructors must undergo extensive training with Conrad or with Susan Harper and receive their approval. To continue as teachers, they are expected to engage in ongoing study.

RESOURCES:

**For information on workshops:** Continuum, 1629 18th St., #7, Santa Monica, CA 90404, (310) 453-4402, fax (310) 453-8775.

**Books:** Emilie Conrad Da'oud, *Life on Land* (Tilbury, 1996).

# Kinetic Awareness®

Dancer-choreographer Elaine Summers was born in Australia in 1925 and raised in Boston. When she was only twenty-seven years old, orthopedic physicians diagnosed her as having osteoarthritis and said that in five years she would be unable to walk. Summers decided to find a way to forestall the doctors' dire predictions. She studied with Elsa Gindler's students Carola Speads and Charlotte Selver and experimented on her own. ☞ See "Sensory Awareness," page 226. Kinetic Awareness (KA), Summers's method of body reeducation, evolved out of her response to her own need for healing. Instead of becoming a wheelchair-bound invalid, she resumed her dance career.

KA, also known as "ball work," is concerned with releasing what Summers calls "frozen tension." Tension itself is not negative—it is a necessary and positive force for movement. However, when you hold tension unconsciously, your muscles become rigid and immobile, and you distort your alignment and constrain your movement, leaving you susceptible to strain and injury. KA is not interested in ridding the body of all tension, but in working with and using *appropriate* tension.

You can do KA privately or in a group. In an introductory class, you examine each specific body part in depth, usually in a series of eight to twelve weekly sessions. The KA teacher sets up situations in which you can learn at your own pace to make individual discoveries and investigate possible causes of pain or movement restriction. You practice how to use rubber balls of various sizes as tools to focus your attention inward, support part of your body in a stretched position, and massage that area of your body. Moving slowly over the ball encourages elasticity and responsiveness of the muscles and joints. After working in this way, you may notice in-

> When you lie down and are quiet you can feel the fact that your body is never still.
>
> —Elaine Summers

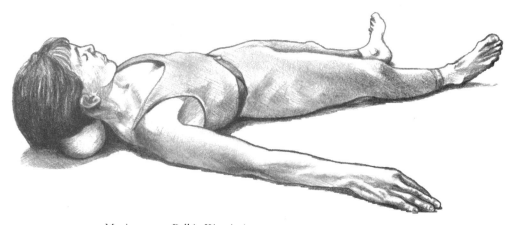

Moving over a Ball in Kinetic Awareness to
Stretch and Massage the Neck and Back of the Head

creased sensation, greater movement range, and a pleasurable ease in the area where you used the ball.

There are five phases to KA. In the first phase, you learn to move each body part separately and slowly in all directions, with the least amount of effort, while also noticing feelings and sensations. Summers believes that if you move every part of your body all the ways it is capable of moving, often and without pain, then your body will be able to find its own dynamic center. Moving extremely slowly allows you to feel more clearly any limitations and holding and to experiment with new ways of moving.

Sessions in phase one may include some massage by the practitioner, usually of the area worked. The introductory class incorporates anatomy lessons to help you understand the musculoskeletal system. KA teachers may also use them in private work to enhance your study of your own body. Since Summers was influenced by Wilhelm Reich, ☞ see "Psychological Dimensions of Bodyways," page 117. KA emphasizes not only physical but also emotional inquiry. Teachers invite you to share your feelings during the session and in group discussion.

The subsequent phases of KA are cumulative, utilizing and integrating the knowledge and consciousness gained from the previous phase. In the second phase, you can move more than one part at a time while being aware of your total body systems, such as breathing and circulation. Phase three involves exploring your body's ability to move at varying speeds. In the fourth phase you develop the ability to change tension levels consciously. In the fifth you are able to combine all the knowledge and understanding gained in the first four while relating to another person or performing.

You may also choose to work in phase one for a long time, since it emphasizes learning to monitor everyday tension levels and helps you live your life with greater awareness. Once learned, KA is yours to use and adapt. The balls provide a portable and practical tool to help release muscular tension and increase well-being.

## An Experience in Kinetic Awareness

Choose a quiet, clear space where you can lie down, preferably on a carpeted floor or thin exercise mat. Lie quietly for several minutes to check in with your body (as you have in other Experiences) and begin to deepen your awareness of your breathing, contact with the floor, and how different parts of your body feel. Then focus attention on your pelvis. Can you feel the bones? The muscles? The organs? The skin? How does your breath relate to your pelvis?

Bend your knees and place your feet flat on the floor. Begin to move your pelvis very slowly and gently in any direction: Tilt forward or back, shift to one side or the other, stretch one hip down or up, and so on. Try not to push your pelvis with some other part of your body, but find even the smallest impulse to move in the pelvis itself. Move with as little effort as possible. Feel the process of moving and all the sensations that come while you move. Continue to breathe normally, taking a deeper breath any time you like. Once in a while, stop to rest completely. Check to see if you can release any unnecessary effort anywhere else in your body.

If you have hollow rubber balls on hand, you can stay in this same position or prop your lower legs up on a couch, chair, or pillows so that your calves rest horizontally. Using balls the size of a grapefruit, place one under the center of each buttock. Rest for a few breaths, then begin to move slowly, as before, in any direction. Try to initiate movement from where you feel contact with the balls, and allow your body to glide slowly over them. Very small movements are best. It's also good to stop occasionally to check for extraneous tension.

You can move the balls to a different place under your buttocks and repeat in the same way, slowly and gently moving in all directions. When you're ready to stop, remove the balls slowly and lie flat on the floor, feeling the effects on your back, breath, and anything else.

—Courtesy of Ellen Saltonstall, Kinetic Awareness teacher.

Although KA is popular especially among dancers and other performance artists, it holds appeal for individuals in other walks of life as well. According to KA teachers, the work helps you not only to gain more energy, flexibility, coordination, lightness, and comfort, but also to articulate movement fully, deal with chronic pain, and move easily again after injuries. As a method of nonjudgmental mindfulness, KA eases the way for a quiet alertness of the mind to develop. In turn, such a state allows you greater access to creativity and an enhanced ability to handle stress.

Certified KA teachers have undergone a 500-hour training program with Elaine Summers and other master instructors.

RESOURCES:

**For teachers and instruction:** The Kinetic Awareness Center, P.O. Box 1050, Cooper Station, New York, NY 10276.

**Books:** Ellen Saltonstall, *Kinetic Awareness* (Kinetic Awareness Center, 1988).

# Authentic Movement

Movement, to be experienced, has to be found in the body, not put on like a dress or a coat.

—Mary Starks Whitehouse

Mary Starks Whitehouse trained with dancers Mary Wigman and Martha Graham before developing, in the 1950s, a process she called "movement in depth." It was an outgrowth of her understanding of dance, movement, and depth psychology. Some of Whitehouse's students developed the work for use in personal analysis, performance and choreography, dance therapy, education, and ethnology. One of them, Janet Adler, established the Mary Starks Whitehouse Institute in 1981 to further her mentor's discipline after her death two years earlier. The work is now commonly known as Authentic Movement (AM).

At the core of AM is the bodily felt sensation of moving and being moved—the conscious awareness of what is happening in your body. That experience is in contrast to everyday habitual, unconscious movements, done automatically for utilitarian ends—for example, reaching to open a door. In an AM session, you suspend that kind of purposeful "doing it" in favor of "letting it happen." This allows you the possibility of perceiving where movement comes from inside you—the unconscious impulses and images that move you—and what it reveals about yourself. For Whitehouse, the "body is the physical aspect of the personality, and movement is the personality made visible."[9]

AM is simple. There are movers who move and witnesses who witness them move. This takes place between two persons or in a group. Movement is self-directed: No one imposes anything on anyone and there is no ideal or preconceived way to move.

As the mover, you begin in any part of the studio space by closing your eyes in a standing, sitting, or lying-down position. You can engage in AM even if you are in a wheelchair. You then wait and "listen" for a sensation, impulse, or energy to arise uncensored from deeper levels within you, rather than from your conscious will. It's not unlike how a dream appears unbidden with unexpected characters and scenes. A feeling, sound, thought, picture, or memory may emerge that leads you into movement. In other words, you surrender to movement instead of controlling it. In doing so, you may also discover how your body prefers to move, which may be unlike how you habitually move. This can allow you to shift naturally out of old, less effective patterns.

Your spontaneous movement response can deal with anything—a difficulty in your body, joy or ecstasy, trauma or pain. The movements you make may be "visible or invisible to the witness."[10]

If you're the witness, you observe the mover with "a special quality of attention or presence" rather than merely looking at the person moving.[11] Simultaneously you become aware of what a particular movement quality or form in the mover awakens in you. As a witness, ideally you are compassionate, nonjudgmental, and understanding. After the agreed-upon time has passed, the witness announces the close of the session. Both witness and mover then engage in a verbal dialogue (or write or draw) about the experience.

In a group session, you may also come into physical contact with others. You always have the choice whether to move with another person or not. What's important is that you stay true to your own inner impulses even in the presence of others rather than take care of anyone else, that you present yourself as you are rather than as you imagine someone wants you to be. It is an opportunity to feel seen and heard and, through that experience, also to become able to see and hear others.

You can use AM as a vehicle for personal development in a way similar to meditation. You learn to become a noncritical witness or observer of yourself: You see what arises and face it without condemnation, and you come to accept yourself just as you are. AM gives you access to the richness of your inner world, to the messages your body wants to communicate. Like dreams, the movements make conscious what was unconscious, whether that be preverbal memories, creative ideas, or habitual movement patterns. Some choreographers also integrate AM into performance pieces.

> Loss of soul is a "stuck" condition in which the flow has stopped . . . when "the currents" no longer run . . . an absence of movement. Medicines that treat the soul must therefore have a kinetic nature.
>
> —Shaun McNiff

> All the pirouettes in the world, all the spectacular feats cannot impress me as much as a simple movement that originates from a deep feeling of aliveness and understanding of the miracle of the human body.
>
> —Frances Becker

For individuals to work with, contact the Authentic Movement Institute, c/o Neala Haze, P.O. Box 11410, Oakland, CA 94611, (510) 237-7297, and the Center for Authentic Movement, c/o Zoe Avstreih, 4 Channing Rd., Eastchester, NY 10709, (914) 337-0494. For a quarterly publication, see *A Moving Journal*, c/o Annie Geissinger, 168 4th St., Providence, RI 02906, (401) 274-2765.

# Skinner Releasing Technique

Joan Skinner, a professor of dance at the University of Washington in Seattle, has been dancing since she was a young child. After college, she became a member of the Martha Graham and Merce Cunningham dance companies. One night, during a grueling four-month bus tour, she ruptured a spinal disc in the middle of a performance. As long as she rested, it would heal, but as soon as she went back to class, it would break down. Working with an Alexander teacher enabled her to dance again.

Combining the Alexander Technique's principles of alignment and movement with imagery, in the 1960s she began evolving the Skinner Releasing Technique (SRT) into a system of kinesthetic training. It employs two categories of images: *specific,* which deals with experiencing effortless movement of specific body parts, and *totality* or *image cluster,* which cultivates an overall state of multidimensional awareness, such as effortlessness. In such a state, you may feel a loss of orientation, but it also can be the opportunity for a fresh, unconditioned response to arise, one that allows new kinesthetic patterns of muscle use to emerge.

SRT has four primary goals: 1) multidirectional skeletal alignment, 2) multidimensional balancing, 3) autonomy of body parts in movement, and 4) economy of movement, that is, movement with a minimal expenditure of energy. Skinner views proper alignment and balance not as a static position you consciously hold, but as a dynamic process of continual adjustments as your weight changes in space. SRT teaches such alignment through a checklist of suggestions, which are reminiscent of F. M. Alexander's advice. For example: "Let your head float off the top of the spine while your shoulders drop and ease open to the sides, your ribs drop toward your feet, and your back expands backward in all directions."

In an introductory class, Skinner's checklist techniques help you to focus on different areas of your body and let go of excess tension in each of

*Our human movement is the interplay of energy and structure in time and space for the purpose of expression.*

—Darrell Sanchez

# An Experience in Skinner Releasing Technique

This experience should be done as one continuous session. It will be smoother if you tape-record it first or have someone read it to you. Be sure to pause frequently, as indicated by three dots in the instructions (...). If you like, have music playing in the background.

### Relaxation Checklist:

Lie on the floor. Gather your focus to the breath for a moment ... just listening to and feeling it ... allowing it to move of its own volition. And with the movement of the breath, all your tissues can begin to soften ... melting along the bones. Tissues of the face seem to melt along the bones ... from the forehead ... over the cheekbones ... and along the jaw. Tissues of the throat and along the back of the neck soften into melting ... tissues along the shoulders melting into the upper arms ... tissues of the arms melting along those long bones to the fingers ... tissues along the ribs in front melting along those bones ... tissues of the upper back melting into the middle back ... tissues of the middle back melting into the lower back ... tissues of the legs melting along those long bones ... toward the feet ... and the breath continues to move of its own volition, deepening in the torso, and deepening in the back.

### Totality Image:

Now take a moment to imagine yourself lying in an enormous hammock ... larger than anything you've ever seen. Perhaps you see the hammock out over an open field, caught between two very tall trees ... or two clouds. You're lying in the deepest part of the hammock as it swings in its slow ... deep ... arcs. Spend a few minutes in this hammock. ... Then the hammock lets go of the trees or clouds and begins to drift slowly to earth ... landing ... perhaps, with a soft ... whisper. You can still lie in the hammock, even as it's on the earth.

### Specific Image:

Continue to cultivate the feeling of lying in the hammock. Gently flex your knees so that your feet rest on the hammock. Notice that your back can melt easily into the hammock when your knees are bent, and the back can spread backward in all directions. And as the breath moves, it can deepen in the torso and deepen into the back.

Then, out of nowhere, marionette strings appear. They attach themselves to the very center of your knees, even as you continue to melt into the hammock. Those strings begin to move your legs. They create a delicious autonomy of your legs as your back continues to melt into the hammock . . . your back melting backward. Your knees float as the marionette strings move them. Delicious autonomy of legs . . . knees floating . . . legs free . . . back melting and expanding . . . spreading in all directions.

And then, gently, the strings evaporate. But other strings appear out of nowhere, wrapping around the middle finger of each hand, bringing your arms into play. Your shoulders are easy, allowing the strings to move . . . your arms . . . delicious autonomy.

Then, just as those strings evaporate, yet another marionette string appears out of nowhere, attaching itself to the center of the top of your skull. Floating and suspending your skull for a moment . . . and then . . . that string disappears. All those marionette strings seem to appear and disappear somehow . . . the knee strings . . . the string wrapped around the middle finger of each hand . . . and . . . the head string. This then becomes the string dance . . . appearing and disappearing string dance.

—Courtesy of Joan Skinner.

Releasing is waiting, emptying, opening, falling, soaring, telescoping, rattling, ripple spasms, spinning, wonder, play.

—Joan Skinner

them. Once you relax into a deeper level of consciousness, you're ready for image work. You may also engage in what Skinner calls "graphics," exercises for developing awareness of your tension patterns. Or a partner can assist you with a light touch in relinquishing control of a certain area of your body—for example, releasing tissues around your hip joint so that your leg can dangle freely. A partner might also trace three-dimensional energy patterns along the surface of your body. In addition to the experiential work, SRT includes seminars and journal-keeping.

Although SRT is a dance technique for developing optimal alignment, strength, and flexibility, Skinner says it can be applied to healing, sports skills, psychotherapy, and voice training. Ultimately, SRT is a process of discovery; it is about cultivating an awareness of yourself as a vital, creative, moving being. Training to teach this process is with Skinner herself.

RESOURCES:

For information about programs and teachers: Joan Skinner, Dance Program, Meany Hall, A-B-10, University of Washington, Seattle, WA 98195, (206) 543-9843.

# Wetzig Coordination Patterns

In the 1930s Jennifer Rathbone at Columbia University developed a Manual Tension Test to evaluate neuromuscular tension. She found four distinct patterns: assistance, resistance, posturing, and perseveration.[12] In the 1960s and 1970s, New York choreographer and movement researcher Betsy Wetzig investigated the effects of these patterns on the styles of creativity and communication in the Wetzig Dance Company and Sound Shapes, her improvisational group. She noted that each neuromuscular pattern uses a different set and order of muscular contractions to create a specific kind or quality of movement—which she calls *Thrust, Shape, Swing,* and *Hang*—as well as a trigger center or initiating group of muscles, and an alignment of the body.

These four basic patterns designate the four ways our muscles, nervous system, and brain organize themselves. Thus, each pattern also simultaneously includes a quality and type of mental processing. That's because the way we move and how our brain processes information are the same neurological event: Each pattern is both mental and physical.

*Thrust* movements tend to be asymmetrical, with sharp, straight lines that are often diagonal and have a push motion. This is the dominant pattern of the Martha Graham technique in dance and of sprinting. The ability to be in Thrust gives assertive power, contraction and release, and the extension reflex. Karate, Shiatsu, Pilates, and Rolfing are examples of the Thrust pattern.

*Shape* is the dominant movement pattern of classical ballet. It has the effect of making a clear shape. It holds and places weight, generally moving the body vertically through space. It gives balance, posture, and lift. Movements tend to be symmetrical or balanced. Shape is necessary in shooting a basketball and having good form in figure skating and dressage. Yoga, Mensendieck, and Laban exemplify the Shape pattern.

*Swing* has the effect of swinging, swaying, bouncing, or rocking. A movement you do on one side is generally repeated on the other; the same is true for moving with the upper and lower parts of the body. This is the dominant movement pattern of belly dancing, hula, swing jazz, and José Limon's style of dance. It loosens the joints, gives endurance, and tends to be playful and interactive. It's what you need in jumping, swinging bats and golf clubs, long-distance running, and dribbling a ball. Trager reflects Swing.

*Hang* is a going-with, sequential activity with a tendency toward random movement or a falling, flowing, hanging motion. It was the dominant movement pattern of dancers Isadora Duncan and Doris Humphrey. Its

To understand life means to understand the ways in which individual beings move.

—Thomas Hanna

Movement continually demonstrates and affirms the transcendence of the contrived categories: body and mind.

—Seymour Kleinman

ease, grace, and connectedness are necessary in tumbling, sliding into base, rolling with a fall, and moving evasively. T'ai Chi Chuan and Contact Improvisation demonstrate Hang.

Although we use all four patterns, each of us is born predisposed to a dominant or "home pattern," the one of lowest tension level. This is our pattern for relaxation, alpha brain wave activity, and creativity. Our particular style is made up of our home base and one other pattern. When we are competent in a variety of styles and use these patterns properly, they can lead to good alignment, spinal support, flexibility, and full movement potential and range. If we override a pattern, it can cause misalignment and injury as well as blockages in energy, feelings, and mental processes. Trauma, cultural and family styles, or bad sports or dance training can cause a weak pattern or an override. According to Wetzig, Coordination Pattern Training to achieve what she calls "Full Potential Movement" can help prevent injury or heal a chronic condition or dysfunction because it restores balance between muscles and thus proper alignment.

In a private session or Coordination Training class, she uses and teaches a simple neurological test to determine the four neuromuscular patterns. Through a series of simple and easy exercises, you can learn to access and apply all of them correctly while developing an awareness of how each one functions in your life. You also can apply the training to creativity, learning, and business styles.

RESOURCES:

**For information, classes, and workshops:** Betsy Wetzig, 1335 Russet Dr., Allentown, PA 18104, (610) 398-9652.

> Nothing happens until something moves.
>
> —Albert Einstein

## More Movement Bodyways

**In addition to the Western movement arts described above and the functional bodyways in Chapter 10, there are movement components in some structural bodyways.** ☞ **See "Rolfing Movement Integration," page 200–201, and "Neurokinetics of Aston-Patterning," page 202. For additional Western practices, see "Trager Mentastics," page 180, and "Rosen Method of Movement," page 355–356.**[13]

## CHAPTER 12

# Eastern Energy

In Western scientific parlance, energy is the capacity to do work, to be active; it is also usable power, such as heat or electricity, and the resources for producing such power. But in Eastern understanding, it is the "life force" or "vital energy" called *chi* (*qi* in Chinese or *ki* in Japanese). It is the element or quality that distinguishes life from death, the animate from the inanimate. One traditional Chinese doctor has said, "To live is to have Qi in every part of your body. To die is to be a body without Qi. For health to be maintained, there must be a balance of Qi, neither too much nor too little."[1]

### THE LIFE FORCE

This concept of a life force or energy has appeared in cultures around the world since ancient times. It goes by a variety of names: *élan vital, pneuma, ruah, mana, ha, prana, ether, orgone, odic force, vital fluid, archaeus, x-force, bio-cosmic energy,* and *bioplasmic energy,* among others. Belief in such a force presupposes a particular worldview, one long held by traditional peoples: that life is an all-pervading unity of the physical, mental, and spiritual, endowed with a special energy that vitalizes it.

All of us share in the same energy that comprises the universe—from petroleum, sunshine, and electricity to animals, plants, and human beings. Without it, nothing would function. Without it, we could not overcome disease and heal our wounds. Hippocrates, the father of Western medicine, called the body's natural ability to recuperate *vis medicatrix naturae*—the healing power of nature. Energy-based healing systems stimulate or activate movement of this life force.

To understand how this works, we'll look at several energy-oriented

It's said that when we die, the four elements—earth, air, fire, water—dissolve one by one, each into the other, and finally just dissolve into space. But while we're living, we share the energy that makes everything, from a blade of grass to an elephant, grow and live and then inevitably wear out and die. This energy, this life force, creates the whole world.

—Pema Chödron

systems—the Chinese, Japanese, and Indian traditions, as well as such Western offshoots as Polarity Therapy, Therapeutic Touch, Reflexology, and Zero Balancing. Even a simple understanding of the traditional Asian medical systems will help you get a better sense of what's behind such bodyways as Acupressure and Shiatsu, which are needleless versions of acupuncture, and later derivatives, for example, Jin Shin Jyutsu. It will also help clarify Asian movement arts, including Chi Kung, T'ai Chi Chuan, Karate, and Aikido, and other Asian bodyways, including Thai Massage and Kurdish Breema.

## THE CHINESE TRADITION

Traditional Chinese medicine is the best-known system predicated on energy. The first written record of it is in *The Yellow Emperor's Classic of Internal Medicine.* Although attributed to the mythical emperor Huang Ti, (2696–2598 B.C.E.), modern Chinese scholars now believe it was written by three different authors and initially published between 200 and 100 B.C.E. The major components of the Chinese system are chi, yin and yang, the Five Elements, meridians, and acu-points. In treating patients, doctors try to affect these aspects by means of herbs, needles, and massage as well as lifestyle recommendations—diet, movement arts, and breathing exercises.

## *Chi*

*The universe really is motion and nothing else.*

*—Socrates*

Western medicine deals with what's visible, palpable, and measurable—the anatomy and physiology of our bodies. What moves through the body can be tracked along pathways: blood, lymph, and nerve impulses all travel through vast charted networks of vessels. Chinese medicine also deals with what moves through the body, but the structure and function are invisible, impalpable, and immeasurable to untrained eyes and hands. There's no bright red fluid we can follow on its journey around the body. Instead, there is chi, a different kind of "substance," which flows in an altogether different kind of circulatory system.

## *Yin and Yang*

According to the ancient Chinese philosophy of Taoism, the universe emerged from the Great Void, a formless, indivisible whole made up of chi. Everything arises from this energy and everything returns to it once dead. This original unchanging unity, with no distinction between day and night or birth and death, then split into two separate but complementary aspects called *yin* and *yang*. You've probably seen the symbol that represents this principle: a circle divided into teardrop-shaped black and white halves, each with a dot of the color of the opposite half to indicate that each of these two ways is always in the process of becoming the other in a constant ebb and flow, contraction and expansion. Each not only opposes the other but also contains its opposite.

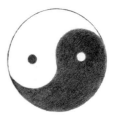

To understand this, picture a mountain. Yin and yang are its sunny and shaded slopes. In the morning, one side becomes bright and warm (yang) as the sun ascends in the sky, while the other side remains dark and cold (yin). However, by afternoon, the yang side turns cool and shady (yin) while the opposite slope is now sunny (yang). In the same way, day (yang) becomes night (yin) becomes day becomes night . . . This ever-changing relationship between opposites influences all natural events, for each aspect controls, balances, and harmonizes the other. Equilibrium between the two forces constitutes health; disharmony between them leads to disease.

Balance, whether between yin and yang or between excessive and deficient chi, is a central concept that pervades traditional Chinese medicine and philosophy. The objective of various healing arts (both hands-on and movement-oriented) and spiritual practices is to find the middle way among physical, emotional, and mental extremes. If you're too agitated and fast, the system strives to calm and slow you down; if you're too dispirited and lethargic, it aims to stimulate you. Balance means an unimpeded flow of chi. Treatment is not directed at symptoms per se—for example, a cough or insomnia—but at the underlying imbalance that produces them. The definition of health, then, is to be in complete harmony internally, as well as externally with nature.

## The Five Elements

Yin and yang further divide into five elements or phases of energy—wood, fire, earth, metal, water—of which everything in the universe consists. Each element has a corresponding flavor, sound, season, organ, emotion, color, direction, and weather condition. The Chinese refer to these elements not as actual physical objects but as qualities or ideas. They represent forces of influence. Thus, if you burn *wood,* you create *fire,* which will result in ashes, or *earth,* from which you can mine *metal,* which when heated, becomes molten, like *water,* which is necessary for the growth of plants and *wood*—coming full circle. Similarly, wood controls earth, which prevents water from flowing, and water controls fire, which melts metal, which then cuts wood.

With respect to organs, the same pattern applies: If you tonify (strengthen or stimulate) the liver, which is associated with wood and the emotion anger, then you automatically tonify the heart as well, which corresponds to fire and joy. This chain-reaction effect works in a negative way

The source wherefrom the sun, moon, and stars derive their light, the thunder, rain, wind, and cloud their being, the four seasons and the myriad things their birth, growth, gathering, and storing: all this is brought about by Qi. Man's possession of life is completely dependent upon this Qi.

—Zhangshi Leijing

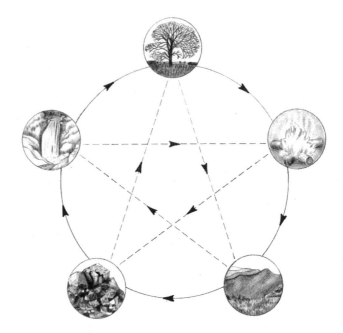

The Five Elements in Traditional Chinese Medicine

as well. I had a chance to experience this in my own life while revising this book and dealing with multiple crises. My acupuncturist said that my kidney pulse showed a deficiency of yin and yang. (In Chinese medicine, the chi concept of kidneys also includes the adrenal glands, which are anatomically located on top of the kidneys.) Since the water element of kidney is supposed to support and nourish the wood element of liver but couldn't, I also had liver stagnation. In turn, the liver commonly affects or controls the spleen (earth element) and, under further stress, could have led to various digestive problems. In other words, indigestion, heartburn, irritable bowel syndrome, constipation, Crohn's disease, or diarrhea all could have started from exhausted kidneys and adrenals.

## Source of Chi

The chi we each possess comes to us through two different sources. We inherit our original, genetic, or prenatal chi from our parents; this is the ancestral life force over which we have no control, and it determines everything from eye and hair color to body shape. We also have an acquired postnatal chi, which comes from the food, water, and air we take in; it is this force that we can regulate by our dietary, sleeping, exercise, and behavioral habits. In both cases, chi exists before physical structure and causes it.

Chi exists in all parts of the body. It causes blood to circulate and other fluids to be disseminated and eventually excreted as urine and sweat. It transforms the food we eat and activates our organs. There is nothing that chi doesn't affect.

## Meridians

Chi flows through specific, though invisible, conduits or channels called *meridians,* which are distributed throughout the body. They're like inter-

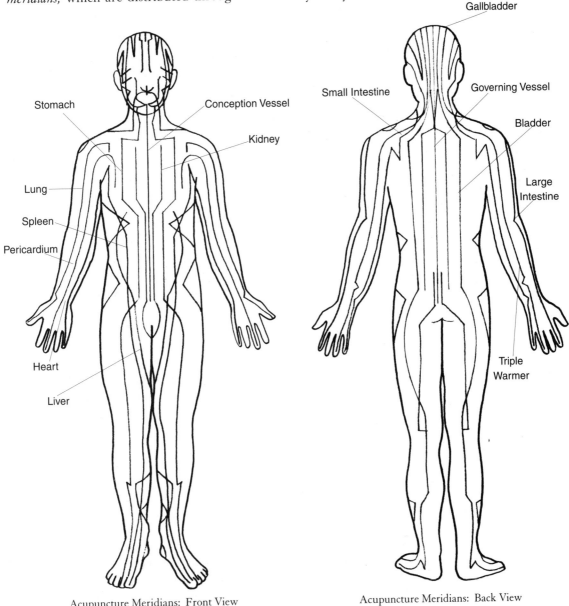

Acupuncture Meridians:  Front View

Acupuncture Meridians:  Back View

state highways that connect cities and towns from coast to coast. As one channel terminates, another one begins. Although there is a network of more than fifty meridians, the most important are the twelve major channels associated with twelve major organ systems, plus two extraordinary vessels (called the governing and conception vessels), which oversee all the others.

## Acu-points

According to traditional Chinese medical theory, when chi either stagnates and becomes depleted or accumulates in excess along a channel, stimulation of certain points close to the surface of the body can unblock and regulate the chi flow. These points—as many as a thousand—are small energy centers that are generally sensitive to pressure. There are several methods to either drain excess chi or activate deficient chi: insertion of hair-thin needles (acupuncture), application of pressure (Acupressure), or slow burning of an herb (mugwort) to produce heat (moxabustion).

Activation of these points leads to reflex responses in other parts of the body because specific points correspond to particular areas and functions of the body. As a result, pressure or needling of points can prevent illness, reduce specific symptoms such as cough, nausea, or itching, and diminish pain (because it triggers the release of the body's own morphinelike substances called endorphins or enkephalins). It can also relieve or eliminate the condition afflicting particular organs, even though they may lie far from the point itself. That's because the organ is not considered a separate unit; rather, it is an energy subsystem within the overall energy system.

Consider, for example, the kidney channel. This meridian starts under each big toe, ascends up the inside of each leg, connects with the kidney, then moves upward to end near the collarbone. A second branch of the channel begins in the kidney and ends at the base of the tongue. The kidney is said to store reproductive energy and also manage maintenance of the body's bones. When chi does not flow properly in this channel, such difficulties as backache, chronic ear conditions, or chronic asthma can result.

## Self-Responsibility

Diet, environment, behavior, and emotions (anger, sadness, joy, rumination, grief, fear, and fright) can all contribute to an imbalance of chi flow through any of the organs, which in turn affects the meridians. According to traditional Chinese theory, your health and longevity depend not only on genetics but also on how you live, what you think, and how you feel. You are responsible for your own well-being. In ancient China, the primary role

> The healer's job has always been to release something not understood, to remove obstructions (demons, germs, despair) between the sick patient and the force of life driving obscurely toward wholeness.
>
> —Robert O. Becker

of a physician was to guide and assist individuals as they quested for their own physical and mental balance. Traditional doctors were not only practiced medical technicians but also scholars and masters of martial arts. They treated each patient individually. Richard Chin, M.D., who is trained in both Western and Oriental medicine, points out that even if you and your partner both have a bout of the common cold, you won't necessarily receive exactly the same treatment from a Chinese practitioner. That's because "no two people's energy systems are alike, no two illnesses are alike, no matter how similar the symptoms may be."[2]

RESOURCES:

For further discussion of the concepts and practices of traditional Chinese medicine, see Felix Mann, *Acupuncture: The Ancient Chinese Art of Healing and How It Works Scientifically* (Vintage, 1973); Richard Chin, *The Energy Within: The Science Behind Every Oriental Therapy from Acupuncture to Yoga* (Paragon, 1992); David Eisenberg, with Thomas Lee Wright, *Encounters with Qi: Exploring Chinese Medicine* (W. W. Norton, 1985); Ted J. Kaptchuk, *The Web That Has No Weaver: Understanding Chinese Medicine* (Congdon & Weed, 1983); Manfred Porkert, with Christian Ullman, *Chinese Medicine: Its History, Philosophy and Practice* (Henry Holt & Company, 1982); and Harriet Beinfield and Efrem Korngold, *Between Heaven and Earth: A Guide to Chinese Medicine* (Ballantine, 1991).

## INVISIBLE YET VISIBLE: THE BODY ELECTRIC

Thousands of years of observation and practice have led the Chinese to believe in and rely on the efficacy of their medical system. But most Western physicians and scientists exposed to it have been unable to agree that a distinct energy system even exists within the body. And that's despite the fact that modern physics has proved that everything in the universe is energy in one of its forms—wave or particle. Atoms and molecules are held together by electromagnetic forces to form matter.

It's curious that the West has had such difficulty accepting "invisible" energy. To a practitioner of traditional Chinese medicine, this energy *is* palpable. One of the ways a physician determines the state of chi in your body is by feeling a series of six pulses (three superficial and three deep positions, which together cover the twelve meridians) at the radial artery of each wrist. The feel of the pulse—there are twenty-eight qualities, from floating and sunken to scattered and slippery—indicates which energy channel needs toning up and which needs sedating. The doctor also looks at your face and tongue, and takes into account your smell, behavior, and emotions

From galaxies to atoms, from bodies to thoughts, all things are energy fields of varying degrees of permanence, power and clarity.

—Mike Sayama

for what internal condition they might reflect. ☞ See the story of Yeshi Dhonden, page 104. Practitioners of Acupressure will feel which points along the meridians are sensitive, like Western trigger points. Although you can't get an X ray of chi and the meridians, the way you can of your bones, that doesn't mean they don't exist. When you use a portable telephone, you see no wires, no visible source of power, yet you experience that it works, and you don't doubt it. Consider that the same may be true in energy-based healing.

Gradually Western scientists are making inroads into the mystery of chi. For example, American orthopedist Robert O. Becker, M.D., has scientifically documented the presence of an underlying electromagnetic life force that animates the body and causes it to grow and heal. As the Chinese have known since ancient times, but in different terms, we are a complex web of electrical currents. Becker's research suggests that the acupuncture meridians are electrical conductors that carry a message of injury and pain to the brain, which responds by sending back an appropriate level of direct current to stimulate healing in the troubled area and reduce pain. Since a current grows weaker with distance, amplifiers are needed along the line to boost the signal. Located only a few inches apart, "acupuncture points [may] serve as 'booster' electrical amplifiers for the very small DC electrical currents flowing along the meridian," says Becker.[3] He describes them as "hundreds of little DC generators like dark stars sending their electricity along the meridians, an interior galaxy that the Chinese had somehow found and explored by trial and error over two thousand years ago."[4]

Although the meridians and acu-points have been invisible to the eye, two French medical doctors, Jean-Claude Darras and Pierre de Vernejoul, offer evidence that they do exist. They conducted experiments at the nuclear medicine section of Necker Hospital in Paris to test the validity of the theory that energy is being transported along acupuncture meridians. After injecting a solution of isotopes into various acu-points of patients, they traced the isotopes' uptake with gamma-camera imaging. They also injected isotopes into random points on the skin in a control group of patients. In the first group, the isotopes moved along the classical Chinese energy pathways; in the control group, there were no such results. The physicians also demonstrated that the movement was not through the blood or lymph vessels.[5]

We are more than a biochemical factory, with hormones, blood, lymph, enzymes, and amino acids constantly in production and circulation. And we are more than a mechanism of pulleys and levers, with muscles lifting and placing bones. We are also an electrical plant and, in Becker's words, "a self-mending electrical net." Our entire nervous system works on the basis of electrical currents. Even the heart is an electric pump. Every contraction it makes is accompanied by an electrical charge called an

*Movement is the index of life, its outstanding expression.*

—Ida Rolf

"action current." These currents are strong enough to be recorded by an electrocardiograph to produce an EKG (electrocardiogram), which is used in diagnosing abnormalities of heart action.

Bodyways practitioners have long described the body as more than flesh and bones. But to the scientific world, their experiences of the body as a "swirling dynamic ball of electromagnetic energy," as one massage therapist put it, are only anecdotal evidence.[6] Now laboratory equipment is measuring the validity of these practitioners' perceptions and of the energy approaches the Chinese have practiced for five thousand years.

## Experience: Feeling Energy

**You don't need laboratory equipment to feel energy. Here's a simple way to get a sense of it with your own hands.**

Sit comfortably, with both feet on the floor, or if you prefer, stand. Close your eyes and take a few deep breaths to slow yourself down. When you feel relaxed but alert, begin. You can keep your eyes open if you want to, but you'll probably be able to concentrate better and feel more when not looking at anything.

Keeping your elbows and forearms away from your body, hold your palms so that they face each other. Bring them close together without actually touching. Then separate your palms about two inches. Slowly move them back toward each other. Separate them again, only now increase to about four inches before going back to the original close position. Repeat this with a separation of six inches.

Move gradually and steadily each time. As you go back and forth, do you notice any pressure between your hands? Do you feel any other sensations—tingling, pulsing, coolness, warmth? What happens the closer your hands get to each other?

Finally, separate your palms so that they're eight inches apart. This time, as you bring them together, stop every two inches to experience the energy field between your hands. What do you sense as you "bounce" back and forth with your hands?

If the energy still isn't palpable to you, just try again after shaking out your hands, taking a few breaths, and closing your eyes. And make sure you're not holding your arms and elbows close to your body.

—Adapted from Dolores Krieger, *Accepting Your Power to Heal: The Personal Practice of Therapeutic Touch* (Bear & Co., 1993).

RESOURCES:

For a Western scientific explanation of the body as electromagnetic energy, see Robert O. Becker and Gary Selden, *Body Electric: Electromagnetism and the Foundation of Life* (William Morrow, 1985); and Robert O. Becker, *Cross Currents: The Perils of Electropollution, the Promise of Electromedicine* (Jeremy P. Tarcher, 1990).

## CHINESE BODYWAYS

The principles of Chinese traditional medicine lie at the core of every Chinese bodyway. Chi is central to all of them, including Acupressure massage, Chi Kung, and T'ai Chi Chuan.

# Chinese Massage/Acupressure

Chinese massage is a combination of what in the West we call Acupressure (pressure applied to acu-points on the surface of the body), meridian treatment, and neuromuscular therapy. But in China it is known as *anmo* ("press and stroke") and *tuina* ("lift and press") and involves a whole range of techniques. In addition to pressing, massage therapists knuckle-roll, rub, squeeze, knead, grasp, push, stretch, dig, drag, pluck, tweak, hammer, vibrate, and knock, as well as manipulate joints and tread on your body with their feet. Although many of these methods look similar to Western techniques, the chief difference between the two systems is in the diagnosis of symptoms and application of treatment according to traditional Chinese medicine theory. The purpose of these methods is to stimulate the body's natural self-healing capacity and to get the chi flowing again.

In Chinese clinics and hospitals, massage therapists use these various techniques to treat an extensive array of medical conditions, from rheumatoid spondylitis, chronic lumbar pains, sprains, and fractures to paraplegia, infantile paralysis, hypertension, peptic ulcer, and pneumonia. But in the West, most practitioners mainly use Acupressure. They too report relief of many difficulties, from acne, allergies, anxiety, arthritis, and asthma to hiccups, insomnia, PMS, and wrist pain. It is useful as well in increasing body awareness and total relaxation. And when Acupressure is performed on children with learning difficulties, teachers have noticed that acupressure improves balance, coordination, language, and social skills.[7] ☞ See also "Improvement of Skills," page 17.

# An Acupressure Experience

It's not often that working with only one place in your body can afford relief for many different pains in other areas. But such a point does exist in Acupressure. Located in the web between your thumb and index finger (on the large intestine meridian, LI4), *hoku,* or Joining the Valley, is the most widely used acu-point for relieving general pain, particularly in the upper body. Among other things, it can alleviate arthritis, headaches, tooth- aches, and shoulder and neck pain. (However, if you are pregnant, do not do this Experience.)

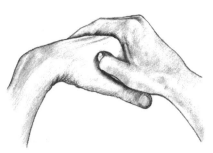

The Hoku Point

To get the greatest benefit from working with hoku, combine it with movement. First, find the sorest spot at the top of the muscle between the thumb and index fin- ger. Then press firmly on it, getting underneath the bone that connects with your index finger. This should produce a mild hurt. While you're pressing there, simultaneously move the joint closest to that part of your body that's in pain. For example, if your neck aches, move your head up and down. Hold for a minute or two, then switch and repeat the same thing on the other hand.

—Adapted from Michael Reed Gach, *Acupressure's Potent Points: A Guide to Self-Care for Common Ailments* (Bantam, 1990).

---

There are various theories as to how Acupressure works. Like acupuncture, it may stimulate the production of endorphins, the body's nat- ural opiates, to control pain. The release of endorphins also leads to the release of cortisol, the body's own anti-inflammatory chemical. Similarly, the reflex or referred action of acupuncture is what also operates in Acupressure, regulating nerve function, strengthening resistance to disease, and even making joints more flexible. In addition, the actual pressing applied to the body increases blood and lymph circulation, removing metabolic wastes and bringing fresh nutrients to the muscles while relieving tension.

Because practitioners do not use oil, you can receive Acupressure while fully dressed. It's best to wear comfortable clothing and avoid tight collars, belts, ties, foundation garments, or shoes that might restrict your

# Caution: Contraindications

Whether the practice is Acupressure, Shiatsu, or another Asian pressure therapy, certain precautions are necessary.

During pregnancy, finger pressure should be gradual and moderate. It should be avoided in the abdominal area as well as at acu-points LI4 (in the outer web between thumb and index finger), K3 (midway between the inside ankle bone and the Achilles' tendon), and Sp6 (four fingers' width above the inner anklebone) because strong stimulation might induce uterine contractions and increase the risk of miscarriage or otherwise harm the fetus. Pressure is discouraged in patients who are susceptible to internal bleeding from external stimulation, such as those suffering from ulcers, aneurysms, or hemophilia. Practitioners also do not work directly on a serious burn, infected or ulcerous area, recently formed scar, or fractured bone. In lymph areas (groin, below the ears, etc.), only a light touch—no pressing—is recommended. Neither are they supposed to apply any pressure in the abdominal area in conditions such as intestinal cancer, tuberculosis, and leukemia. Other times to avoid pressure-point massage include after a stroke or heart attack and in cases of contagious skin diseases, sexually transmitted diseases, acute infections, fevers, and arteriosclerosis.

circulation. You may lie down on a padded table or a floor mat, or sit in a chair. Practitioners may press in a sequential pattern over your entire body for a general treatment or focus only on certain areas according to the complaints you present. You may feel some discomfort when pressure is applied to sensitive points, but the overall effect can be relaxing, as well as providing relief of symptoms.

Western practitioners of Acupressure generally do not receive the same kind of extensive training as massage therapists in China, which may include pulse diagnosis, moxabustion, ear seed acupuncture, hot cupping, cutaneous tapping needles, and herbal remedies during three years of study at a traditional-medicine college followed by an internship. A few Westerners go abroad to take special courses set up for them in Chinese clinics. Most study Acupressure in massage schools in North America. Several institutes specialize in teaching Acupressure and/or other Asian bodyways. For membership in the American Oriental Bodywork Therapy Association, a certified practitioner must graduate from a program of at least 500 hours; an associate member must complete a 150-hour training.

Resources:

**For practitioner referrals and educational programs:** American Oriental Bodywork Therapy Association, Suite 510, Glendale Executive Park, 1000 White Horse Rd., Voorhees, NJ 08043, (609) 782-1616, fax (609) 782-1653.

**Books:** Anhui Medical School Hospital (China), *Chinese Massage Therapy: A Handbook of Therapeutic Massage,* trans. by Hor Ming Lee and Gregory Whincup (Shambhala, 1983); Kuan Hin et al., *Chinese Massage and Acupressure* (Bergh, 1990); Sun Chengnan, ed., *Chinese Bodywork: A Complete Manual of Chinese Therapeutic Massage* (Pacific View, 1994); Michael Reed Gach, *Acupressure's Potent Points: A Guide to Self-Care for Common Ailments* (Bantam, 1990); Michael Blate, *The Natural Healer's Acupressure Handbook, Vol. 1: Basic G-Jo,* rev. ed., and *Vol. 2: Advanced G-Jo* (Falkynor, 1982); Chris Jarmey and John Tindall, *Acupressure for Common Ailments: A Gaia Original* (Simon & Schuster, 1991); Julian Kenyon, *Acupressure Techniques* (Inner Traditions, 1987).

# Chi Nei Tsang

Chi Nei Tsang (CNT)—"transforming energy of the internal organs"—is also known as Internal Organs Chi Massage or Internal Organs Integrated Massage. Mantak Chia, born in 1944 into a Chinese family in Thailand, has been instrumental in bringing this practice to the West. He studied with Chinese masters residing in different parts of Asia after they left communist China. CNT is one part of the Healing Tao System, Chia's synthesis of all those teachings.

CNT focuses on the region of the navel, which the Chinese consider the most powerful energy and communication center of the body, and on the internal organs (liver, kidneys, bladder, spleen, and so on) in the abdominal cavity. In Taoist thinking, everything in your body had its beginning in the umbilicus—it is where you first breathed, took in nutrition, and removed wastes as a fetus. If this area is out of balance, tight, or twisted, that will affect everything else. The circulatory, lymphatic, and nervous systems, acupuncture meridians, and organs of digestion, assimilation, and elimination all cross paths in the abdomen, which acts as their seat of control.

According to Chia, if you look at the body as an electrical system, the meridians are like the wiring, the acu-points are like the light bulbs, and the organs and navel are the energy generators. Instead of trying to replace

# Chi Nei Tsang Experience

Lie on your back, using a pad or blanket on the floor. Bend your knees enough so that your lower back and abdomen can relax, or place a pillow or two behind your knees.

Take long, deep, yet gentle breaths in three parts: first, fill up your abdomen, then move the air down to the pelvic floor, and finally expand into your chest. Exhale, emptying your chest first, then the abdomen. Breathe like this throughout the massage.

Expose your abdomen. Using the fingertips of both hands, feel the thickness and quality of the skin around the rim of your navel. With one finger, one spot at a time, massage firmly, but gently stimulating the skin, especially wherever it is hard or tight. If you feel discomfort, press more gently. If you do this massage for five to ten minutes daily for a week, you may notice that your digestion and elimination improve, that you retain less water, and that back and neck pains disappear.

To end, lay your hands flat on your abdomen and send heat from your hands inside. Absorb the heat into your body and breathe softly as long as you like.

—Courtesy of Gilles Marin, Chi Nei Tsang practitioner.

---

the bulbs each time they go out—that is, working on peripheral points—CNT concentrates on the energy generators—in other words, working in the center. This direct manipulation of the organs is what differentiates CNT from acupuncture and Shiatsu, systems that work indirectly on the periphery in order to affect the internal organs.

CNT practitioners use massage, Acupressure, and guided breathing to clear unhealthy energies and waste products from these organs, tissues, and bone, and transform them to promote health on all levels—physical, emotional, spiritual. For the Taoists, the organs contain the essence of our spirit and soul. When that essence gets blocked or weak, too hot or too cold, we have imbalances in all areas of our lives. They originated CNT to help maintain the smooth and abundant flow of chi necessary for esoteric spiritual practices.

According to Taoist teachings, the internal organs also generate and store emotions. For instance, the liver is associated with anger and arrogance as well as kindness; the kidneys hold fear and nervousness along with gentleness. None of the emotions is wrong or bad except when they become tensions and obstructions that upset the overall balance and flow of chi and set off a chain reaction of adjustments and compensations—in your attitudes, emotions, behavior, physical structure, and spiritual life. This can result from traumas, overwhelming stress or negativity, overwork, poor diet, improper breathing, environmental poisons, injuries, and other factors.

CNT practitioners first observe your abdomen by noting the shape and position of your belly button. If it pulls in one direction or another, that indicates the organ in which there might be difficulties. They may also read your pulses or analyze your tongue for further signs. With their hands, they feel for any stiff or tense areas, which show up as knots, tangles, or lumps, and they sense heat or cold, expansion or contraction. Then, in a procedure called "skin detoxification," they release surface tension and relax the tissues by spiraling with their fingertips around the navel (the hub), gradually moving outward to the organs. The action on the skin, transmitted to the underlying fascia, suspensory ligaments, and interstitial tissues, also releases the affected organs, improving their circulation and lubrication and increasing metabolic rates.

CNT practitioners use a variety of other hand and elbow techniques to scoop, pat, rock, press, rub, or penetrate in order to train the different organs to function better. They also soften tensions seated close to the spine and the psoas muscles to help correct certain postural conditions and improve your immune system. Although practitioners directly manipulate your abdominal organs, it is not an invasive method, for they work with "soft hands." In addition to the hands-on work, they may teach you to intone the Six Healing Sounds, to support each organ and promote self-awareness through the visual, auditory, and kinesthetic senses.

CNT is taught in weekend workshops or ongoing classes at fundamental, intermediate, and professional levels.

RESOURCES:

**For training programs and practitioners:** Healing Tao, 1205 O'Neill Hwy., Dunmore, PA, 18512, (717) 348-4310, fax (717) 348-4313; Gilles Marin, Chi Nei Tsang Institute, 2315 Prince St., Berkeley, CA 94705, (510) 848-9558.

**Books:** Mantak and Maneewan Chia, *Chi Nei Tsang: Internal Organs Chi Massage* (Healing Tao, 1990).

## THE JAPANESE TRADITION

# Anma

Many centuries ago, the principles and practices of Chinese medicine, meditation, and martial arts immigrated to Japan, where they took on their own distinctive forms. Chinese anmo became *anma* or *amma,* Japanese traditional massage. This was not a simple relaxation massage but a therapy that also included diagnosis. By the first decade of the eighth century, the medical college at Nara gave regular courses in anma.

During feudal times, the fifth Tokugawa shogun, Lord Tsunayoshi, in gratitude to blind practitioner Waichi Sugiyama for curing him of an abdominal illness, helped establish dozens of medical schools for the blind and made anma their special bailiwick. So much a part of Japanese daily life were these blind massage therapists that they appear as characters in tales about that period. They have shown up even in English-language novels. In James Clavell's *Shogun,* the European sailor Blackthorne, new to the Japanese ritual of bath and massage, at first resists the treatment, but then grows to yearn for "that old blind man with the steel fingers" who attended to his bruises and made him feel new again.[8]

The blind masseurs enjoyed certain rights and privileges and formed one immense guild under the direction of two provosts who governed from Kyoto and Edo (now Tokyo,) respectively. After undergoing vigorous training, the therapists had to pass examinations and pay fees before receiving a license to practice, and were ranked according to proficiency. The introduction of Western medicine after the Meiji Restoration in 1868, which returned authority to the Japanese emperor and forced the shogun to abdicate, spelled changes. While some blind massage therapists were still steeped in the traditional medical system, others were trained in no more than a simplified version for relaxation.[9]

Nevertheless, into the twentieth century, the itinerant blind anma practitioners remained familiar figures in inns and households, and they were depicted in woodblock prints of the time. As they walked through a neighborhood, they announced their availability by stamping their ringed iron staff, blowing a double-barreled whistle, and calling out, *"Kami-shimo"* ("from top to bottom," meaning an entire body massage). But there were complaints that traditional anma "had degenerated into a pleasurable indulgence for the rich and powerful."[10] To dissociate themselves from this "corruption" and to avoid licensing laws for anma massage, practitioners of *koho anma* ("ancient way") began to create new names for their therapeutic work, such as *Shiatsu.*

# Shiatsu

Early in the twentieth century, *Shiatsu* (Japanese for "finger pressure") developed as a therapy form distinct from anma. New information provided by Western medicine stimulated revolutionary thinking in traditional practice. By 1919, Tamai Tempaku brought together a system that blended Western anatomy and physiology with koho anma, *ampuku* (hara treatment or abdominal massage), acu-point therapy, Do-In (breathing practices and physical exercises to stimulate chi), and Buddhist philosophy.[11] The Japanese teachers later responsible for spreading Shiatsu to the West were among his students or influenced by them—for example, Toshiko Phipps, Katsusuke Serizawa, Tokujiro Namikoshi, and Shizuto Masunaga.

In 1925 these and other practitioners formed the Shiatsu Therapists Association. That year, Namikoshi also established his first clinic on Hokkaido, which became the Institute of Shiatsu Therapy. Fifteen years later, he founded the Nippon Shiatsu Institute in Tokyo, then the only one in Japan devoted exclusively to Shiatsu.[12] Various other clinics and schools followed, so that by 1955 the Japanese Ministry of Health and Welfare formally recognized Shiatsu as a valid treatment. It was included in a general category with anma and Western-style massage; to become licensed, practitioners were required to train for two years. Eventually, major industries jumped on the bandwagon and provided Shiatsu therapy free to their employees because of its preventative effects, which reduced work absences.

Different schools of Shiatsu developed according to the emphasis of each teacher. For example, the style derived from Katsusuke Serizawa focuses on *tsubo,* the Japanese term for the traditional acu-points. There are 360 tsubo along the meridians on each side of the body, for a total of 720 points, plus 300 extra points.

Tokujiro Namikoshi's technique is concerned with the neuromuscular system. He organized the tsubo according to Western physiology and pathology. Anatomically, many of the tsubo are where blood and lymph vessels, nerves, and endocrine glands concentrate or branch. Pressing on these points, according to Toru Namikoshi, Tokujiro's eldest son, invigorates the skin, stimulates circulation of body fluids, promotes supple muscles, corrects skeletal misalignments, harmonizes the nervous system, regulates endocrine function, and activates normal functioning of internal organs.[13] Carl Dubitsky, an American Shiatsu teacher, relates that it was Tokujiro's success in treating Marilyn Monroe in 1953, when she was acutely ill during her honeymoon with Joe DiMaggio in Japan, that finally led to governmental recognition of Shiatsu.[14]

Zen Shiatsu, created by Shizuto Masunaga, who taught at the Nippon

# Experience: Shiatsu Thumb Pressure

Although Shiatsu therapists use their palms and fingers, they work mostly with their thumbs, singly or together. The thumbs may be held side by side or, for concentrated pressure, one on top of the other. To get a sense of what that feels like, while seated, apply pressure vertically to the front of one of your thighs with the ball of either thumb. Don't bend your thumb. Now apply pressure with the tip of your thumb, provided you don't have long fingernails. Can you feel the difference? One way, you're applying firm pressure, as if you're resting your body weight into your thumb. The other way, you're jabbing your thumb into the flesh.

Apply pressure again, holding for three to five seconds. Gently release, without lifting your thumb, then renew the pressure. Repeat two to three times. Now shift placement of your thumb after each pressure hold so that you move up or down your thigh. You can also progress along your thigh with two thumbs next to each other or with one thumb overlapping the other. Now try the other thigh. Do you sense any difference between the two? How comfortable or painful this feels will depend on how much pressure you apply and whether you have any underlying condition that might sensitize the tsubo. According to Toru Namikoshi, Shiatsu on the front of the thighs regulates the functioning of the stomach and intestines as well as relieves knee ailments.

Apply pressure with the ball of the thumb.

Shiatsu Institute, emphasizes the meridian lines rather than specific points and does not adhere to a fixed sequence. Also unique to his style is a complex system of abdominal and back diagnosis and an extended set of meridians.[15]

Shiatsu came to North America in 1950. The first qualified Japanese Shiatsu therapist was Toshiko Phipps, who practices and teaches Integrative Eclectic Shiatsu. Three years later, Toru Namikoshi began teaching his father's system at Palmer Chiropractic College. Other Namikoshi-trained teachers as well as those of other lineages followed to the United States and Canada.

Additional styles of Shiatsu therapy available in America include Macrobiotic Shiatsu, founded by Shizuko Yamamoto, which involves hand and barefoot techniques and stretches. It also embraces lifestyle treatment: corrective exercises, postural rebalancing, self-Shiatsu, dietary guidance, medicinal plant foods, breathing techniques, and Chi Kung. Integrative Eclectic Shiatsu combines Japanese Shiatsu with traditional Chinese medical theory and Western methods of soft-tissue manipulation, along with dietary and herbal methods. Five Element Shiatsu uses the five-element paradigm in tonifying, sedating, or controlling patterns of disharmony. Still other derivative practices are ANMA Therapy, a Korean form invented by Tina Sohn; Shiatsu/Anma Therapy, introduced by DoAnn Kaneko, and OhaShiatsu, developed by Wataru Ohashi.

The diverse systems are all based on the approximately one hundred hand techniques of anma.[16] Only the Namikoshi neuromuscular style, grounded in Western anatomy and physiology, is officially considered the "pure and correct Shiatsu system" in Japan.[17] The main objective of all the anma-based practices is to stimulate the chi so that it flows unimpeded through the meridians. As Masunaga, founder of the Royal Medicine Institute in Tokyo, said: "The basic and most important principle underlying health is the balancing of the life force and reliance on our body's own natural healing power."[18]

Some people turn to Shiatsu for relief of common difficulties. In fact, popular Shiatsu books outline which points to press for a long list of conditions, including constipation, high blood pressure, fatigue, menopausal symptoms, motion sickness, cramps, numbness, constipation, diarrhea, headache, asthma, stiff shoulders, sinusitis, nasal congestion, and even sexual dysfunction. Other people use Shiatsu in a preventive way; they see a practitioner once or twice a month to maintain their health with a "tune-up." Although the acu-points in Shiatsu and Acupressure are the same, the treatment protocol varies according to each teacher's system.

To achieve good effect, Shiatsu practitioners press your body with fingers, hands, elbows, knees, and sometimes feet, holding points for only a few seconds. A session may also include range-of-motion manipulations and gentle stretching. You can remain dressed, wearing soft cotton clothing, or be clad only in underwear and draped. If the practitioner strictly adheres to Japanese custom, you will lie on a futon or mat on the floor; otherwise, you will rest on a padded table.

*The pressure of the hands causes the springs of life to flow.*

*—Tokujiro Namikoshi*

# Do-In Experience

Figure A

Introduced to the United States from Japan by macrobiotic proponent Michio Kushi in the late 1960s, Do-In (pronounced "dough-in") is a form of self-massage. It means "to lead with the breath." A cross between exercise and Shiatsu, it combines yogalike postures with firm pressure on acu-points along the twelve major organ meridians and two extraordinary vessels to promote physical health as well as spiritual harmony. As in Acupressure and Shiatsu, it discharges blocked energy so that chi can circulate freely throughout the body.

If you practice Do-In in the morning, you can invigorate yourself for the day, stimulate your circulation, and help prevent difficulties before they arise. A

Shiatsu training varies according to the particular school, ranging from 100 to 2,200 hours. A few Shiatsu therapists have studied in Japan. For membership in the American Oriental Bodywork Therapy Association, certified practitioners have to graduate from a program of at least 500 hours; associate members require only 150 hours.

## RESOURCES:

For practitioner referrals, educational programs, and other information on twelve different styles of Eastern body therapy: American Oriental Bodywork Therapy Association, Suite 510, Glendale Executive Park, 1000 White Horse Rd., Voorhees, NJ 08043, (609) 782-1616, fax (609) 782-1653.

Books: The following books represent a variety of styles: Carl Dubitsky, *Oriental Bodywork Therapy* (Inner Traditions, 1996); Yukiko Irwin, *Shiatzu Acupuncture Without a Needle* (Lippincott, 1976); Toru Namikoshi, *The Complete Book of Shiatsu Therapy: Health and Vitality at Your Fingertips* (Japan Publications, 1981), and *The Shiatsu Way to Health: Relaxation and Relief at a Touch* (Kodansha, 1988); Katsusuke Serizawa, *Tsubo: Vital Points*

morning series can include everything from rubbing your feet to tapping your head. Here's one of the exercises.

Kneel, resting on your heels. Use your fists to gently pound on your back, beginning as high as you can reach (figure A) and moving downward to your hips and buttocks as you lift up slightly from your heels (figure B). Don't pummel your spine, only the muscles alongside it. Go up and down several times. When you stop, close your eyes and notice the sensations you feel. If you have a slump during the day, try this again and see if it takes the tiredness out of your back.[19]

Figure B

for Oriental Therapy (Japan Publications, 1976); Shizuko Yamamoto, Barefoot Shiatsu: Whole-Body Approach to Health (Japan Publications, 1979); Shizuko Yamamoto with Patrick McCarty, Whole Health Shiatsu: Health and Vitality for Everyone (Japan Publications, 1992); Tina Sohn, Anma: The Ancient Art of Oriental Healing (Inner Traditions, 1996).

**Videos:** "Shiatsu-Anma Therapy—Level I," DoAnn T. Kaneko, 60 mins., (916) 757-6033; "The Art of Pressure," David Palmer, Anma Institute, 2 hrs., (800) 999-5026; "Barefoot Shiatsu," Shizuko Yamamoto, Turning Point Publications, 1122 M St., Eureka, CA 95501-2442, (707) 445-2290; "Meridian Shiatsu," Kaz Kamiya, Shiatsu School of Canada, (800) 263-1703, fax (416) 323-1681.

# Hoshino Therapy

Hoshino Therapy is a pressure-point system developed by Tomezo Hoshino, who was born in 1910 into a Japanese family that had practiced acupuncture and traditional medicine for generations. Blinded in a motor-cycle accident as a teenager, he learned anma massage to earn a living. Another accident eighteen months later knocked him unconscious and restored his vision.

It took many years for Hoshino to evolve his system. During that time, he immigrated to Argentina, where he began to suffer from neuralgia, returned to Japan for treatment from his acupuncturist uncle, studied acupuncture himself, went back to Argentina, and returned to Japan again, this time because of bursitis. When acupuncture could not relieve his condition, he finally healed himself, using only the warmth and pressure of his own hands. Back in Buenos Aires, Hoshino put his new method into practice. In 1952 the Argentine government officially recognized it as a medical therapy; it became a postgraduate program for physical therapists and kinesiologists. In 1980 he established a clinic in Florida as well.

According to Hoshino, arthrosis, a degenerative joint condition which results from the hardening and shortening of muscles, tendons, and ligaments, is the cause of various musculoskeletal conditions, including arthritis, tendinitis, frozen shoulder, tennis elbow, back and neck pain, and hip difficulties. What brings it on is a lack of exercise or an overuse of muscles, poor posture and movement habits, and age.

To reverse this hardening of the soft tissue, Hoshino therapists apply digital pressure and cross-fiber friction to 250 acupuncture points that relate directly to biomechanical functioning. Differing from Shiatsu practitioners, they use the first joint of the thumb with full hand contact. Although the pressure and friction may cause discomfort, even pain, they help loosen the muscle. As circulation increases, waste products leave the cells and the tissue becomes softer, moister, and more elastic, flexible, and resilient. The overall effect can be both relaxing and stimulating.

Therapists train for two years, with programs available at Hoshino clinic-schools in both Buenos Aires and Miami. In addition to the hands-on therapy, they learn evaluative procedures to detect presymptomatic problems in children and adults.[20]

### RESOURCES:

**For information, instruction, and practitioners:** Hoshino Therapy Clinic of Miami, Inc., 430 South Dixie Highway, Miami, FL 33146, (305) 666-2243.

## THE INDIAN TRADITION

The Chinese were not the only culture to create a whole health-care system based on an energetic model. In fact, some historians believe that the principle may have originated in India. About three thousand years ago in India, *Ayurveda* (Sanskrit, *Ayur,* life, and *veda,* knowledge, meaning "knowledge of life" or "science of longevity") became established as the traditional Hindu system of medicine. From there it spread to Sri Lanka, Tibet, and China, where it took on modified or entirely different forms.

## AYURVEDA

The origins of Ayurveda are shrouded in Hindu mythology. They are attributed to Brahma, the Great Creator, from whom arise all consciousness and *prana* (life energy). Each of us is a creation of that consciousness consisting of both female and male energies. But unlike the similar Chinese yin and yang, in Ayurvedic thinking, the female energy is the active form, while the male is passive.

Prana animates every aspect of life. According to Swami Vishnu-devananda, who originated the Sivananda Yoga approach, "*Prana* is in the air, but is not the oxygen, nor any of its chemical constituents. It is in food, water, and in the sunlight, yet it is not vitamin, heat, or light-rays. Food, water, air, etc., are only the media through which the *prana* is carried."[21]

Prana manifests materially in five primary states or forces known as the *pancha maha bhutas:* earth, water, fire, air, and ether. As in Chinese theory, these are not literal but metaphorical elements. Water, or the liquid condition, is associated with bodily fluids, the kidneys, and genitals; air, or gas energy, enables the body to move and is connected to the nervous system; earth, or the solid state, is related to the body's waste materials; and so on. Each element also creates the senses and oversees their functions: for example, ether with hearing and the ear, and fire with the eyes and seeing.

*Tridosha,* the three biological humors or forces, called *vata, kapha,* and *pitta,* unite these elements and explain how the body works. Vata initiates and promotes all movements in the body; pitta is responsible for the generation of body heat, digestion, and metabolism; and kapha provides nutrition to the bodily tissues. The particular blend of doshas in each of us creates our unique birth-given constitution, or *prakruti,* of which there are seven. Some people are predominantly one of the doshas; others are a combination of two; and a few have equal amounts of all three.

Keeping the individual doshas in balance results in health. Any disharmony—too much or too little of a dosha—can cause all kinds of disturbances. For example, since vata's main responsibility is control of the

# India's Love Affair with Oil Massage

There is a proverb in Tamil (a language spoken in southern India) that says, "The money that you pay to the physician may as well be paid to the oilman." This means that if you apply oil profusely to your body, you will be able to prevent many diseases. In fact, everywhere I traveled in India, that is what I saw and experienced—massage with lots of oil and all kinds of oil.

India's appreciation for massage goes far back in time. According to an ancient Ayurvedic text, there are great benefits to be derived from oil massage. When performed daily on the head, it is said to prevent headache, baldness, gray hair, and loss of hair. The hair becomes firmly rooted, flowing, and very black, while the cranial bones become stronger. The sense organs are toned up and facial skin grows beautiful. Good sleep and happiness are other reputed results. In short, an oily head massage can help avoid the effects of aging.

In a similar way, daily massage of the body is supposed to act not only as a tonic to the skin, leading to comeliness, strength, and smoothness, but also as a preventive measure against serious injury of the limbs and as a palliative for vata disorders. This is true also of foot massage, which has the added merit of eliminating roughness, stiffness, fatigue, achieving bright eyes, and dryness of your feet, and preventing sciatica.

Until modern times in India, those who could afford it had a masseur come every day to the home. It was customary for such men to go from house to house at night to massage the limbs of the elders before they retired. Some households retained female domestic servants to massage the women and children. In the home of friends I stayed with in New Delhi, the patriarch of the family still had a man come to massage him regularly.

I visited many Ayurvedic clinics and hospitals in different Indian states as well as in Sri Lanka. There I saw patients receive special massage treatments for all manner of ailments—everything from paralysis, hemiplegia, and neuralgia to fractures, rheumatism, and arthritis. At one center in Sri Lanka, massage was even part of a detoxification program for drug addicts.

Not content to stand by and watch, I indulged in several massages myself. I received some by hand, others by foot, as I lay on the floor or on a table or sat in a chair. All were administered with copious amounts of oil, so copious that on one occasion I felt myself about to slide off the wooden table and onto the dirt floor as the woman moved one foot, then another, over my body while she held on to an overhead pole. It's hard to know what effect these massages might have had on me in the long term, for I wasn't aware of having any particular condition that needed treatment, nor was I in a position to experience a consistent series. But maybe I should consider a return trip, for while I've not lost my hair, it's steadily going gray, and my skin isn't as smooth and supple as it once was.

nervous system and equilibrium throughout the body, when this dosha is out of balance, nervous conditions may appear in the form of anxiety, insomnia from restless thinking, depression from exhaustion, even clinical mental disorders.

The three doshas influence the flow of prana in the body through a network of some seven hundred channels called *nadi*. The goal of Ayurvedic methods is to promote this flow in order to maintain physical, mental, and spiritual health, prevent illness, and cure it should it occur. To do so, Ayurvedic physicians analyze your prakruti and current state by reading twelve pulse positions at the wrists, observing your face, skin, tongue, fingernails, eyes, urine, and feces, listening to your voice, and smelling your breath. To advise you on how best to meet your constitutional needs or regain balance, they make recommendations for using diet, herbal remedies, Yoga, detoxification or purification routines (including oil enemas, vomiting therapy), breathing exercises, meditation, and massage. In Ayurvedic clinics and hospitals in India, massage with great quantities of medicated oils—*abhyanga*—is common in treating a wide variety of physical and psychological ailments. While there is no acupuncture, as in traditional Chinese medicine, there is a massage to stimulate 107 sensitive places on the skin known as *marma* points.

Formerly confined to India and Sri Lanka, Ayurvedic treatments are now available in the United States as well. Since the Indian system is not recognized as a medicine (allopathy) in North America, practitioners are generally otherwise licensed. For example, Deepak Chopra, who has been instrumental in popularizing Ayurveda in the West, is a medical doctor; others may be homeopaths, naturopaths, or chiropractors. The cost of treatments ranges accordingly, from quite expensive at certain centers across the country to average-priced sessions with a local practitioner.

## CHAKRAS AND KUNDALINI

Another aspect of Hindu theory and practice is the *chakras* (Sanskrit for "wheels"), which are centers, vortices, or reservoirs of energy. A chain of seven sits in alignment down the middle of the body. Although the chakras are connected with physical systems, they operate on a subtle sensory level related to states of consciousness. Some Western energetic healing systems focus on these centers, too, seeing a link between Reich's seven body segments and the seven chakras.

The Seven Chakras

sahasrara
ajna
visuddha
anahata
manipura
svadisthana
muladhara

The lowermost or root chakra, *muladhara,* is located at the base of the spine, between the genitals and the anus, and represents the earth, our groundedness, and basic survival. Next follows *svadisthana,* at the sex organs, representing water. The third is *manipura,* at the solar plexus, related to fire, emotions, and power in the world. At the heart level is the fourth center, *anahata,* connected to air and the lungs, the breath linking inner and outer worlds. *Visuddha,* the fifth or throat chakra, has to do with communication. The "third eye" (between the eyebrows) is the sixth center, *ajna,* for intuition. And the uppermost or crown chakra, *sahasrara,* which sits at the top of the head, is the gateway to higher consciousness.

At the base of the spine lies an especially powerful form of prana called *kundalini,* represented as a coiled serpent. When this energy is awakened and moves up the spine, several things may occur—tingling, spasms, shaking, twisting, visions, and so on. Certain meditation and yogic practices are designed to activate this "serpent power" to pass through all the energy centers. But because "kundalini rising" can be a dramatic crisis, it also may be dangerous unless the person is trained to receive it. The intense physical release—including flashes of heat and cold, streaming pulsations, arms and legs flailing, nausea—may cause fear, exhaustion, and a feeling of going crazy. Traditionally in India, a student works with a *guru,* an experienced teacher who can be a guide during this spiritual awakening.

In the West, such occurrences often have been misunderstood as psychotic episodes—break*downs* rather than break*throughs.* Without inner resources or external support to integrate the spiritual experiences, individuals may find their mental health disintegrating. But a growing vanguard of transpersonal psychotherapists now identify these crises as "spiritual emergencies," part of the process of personal transformation.[22]

A variety of catalysts can trigger such phenomena: extraordinary sexual experiences, childbirth, athletics, illness and injury (especially near-death experiences), spiritual practices, certain times of life (for example, adolescence or midlife), drug use, the loss of someone close and other emotional traumas. Individuals having such an emergency may undergo acute distress, including physical symptoms, anxiety, loss of appetite, insomnia, depression, hypersensitivity, disorientation, and an inability to deal with the responsibilities of daily life. When they do not understand what's happening, they may feel terrified, even suicidal.

Since Western society does not have guru-guides as they exist in Asian traditions, most people turn to transpersonal counselors or companions who have had similar mystical experiences. Unfortunately, conventional psychiatrists and other allopathic health-care professionals may dismiss such spiritual responses as biochemical reactions or hallucinations. But as the West continues to become more exposed to Eastern perspectives on body, mind, emotions, energy, and consciousness, we'll keep seeing rein-

Love is a feeling, and we cannot feel it as long as we devalue the body's most subtle messages.

—Robert K. Hall

terpretations of what constitutes health on every level of being. We'll also see a growing number of people able to facilitate the kundalini rite of passage.

RESOURCES:

**For information and health services:** Ayurvedic and Naturopathic Medical Clinic, 10025 NE 4th St., Bellevue, WA 98004, (206) 453-8022, fax (206) 451-2670; Ayurvedic Institute, 11311 Menaul NE, Suite A, Albuquerque, NM 87112, (505) 291-9698; Chopra Center for Well-Being, 7590 Fay Avenue, Suite 403, La Jolla, CA 92037, (619) 551-7788; College of Maharishi, Ayur-Veda Health Center, P.O. Box 282, Fairfield, IA 52556, (800) 248-9050; Rocky Mountain Institute of Yoga and Ayurveda, P.O. Box 1091, Boulder, CO 80306, (303) 443-6923.

**Books:** *Ayurveda:* Bhagwan Dash, *Hand Book of Ayurveda: The Indian System of Medicine* (Asia Book Corp., 1983), and *Massage Therapy in Ayurveda* (South Asia, 1992); David Frawley, *Ayurvedic Healing: A Comprehensive Guide* (Passage, 1989); Vasant Lad, *Ayurveda, the Science of Self-Healing: A Practical Guide* (Lotus Light, 1990); Robert E. Svoboda, *Ayurveda: Life, Health and Longevity* (Viking Penguin, 1993); Subhash Ranade, *Natural Healing Through Ayurveda* (Passage, 1993); Deepak Chopra, *Perfect Health: The Complete Mind/Body Guide* (Harmony, 1990).

*Chakras:* Shafica Karagulla and Dora Kunz, *The Chakras and the Human Energy Field* (Theosophical, 1990); Werner Bohm, *Chakras: Roots of Power* (Samuel Weiser, 1991); Rosalyn Bruyere, *Wheels of Light: A Study of the Chakras,* vols. 1 and 2 (Bon, 1989 and 1992); Harish Johari, *Chakras: Energy Centers of Transformation* (Inner Traditions, 1987); Barbara Brennan, *Hands of Light: A Guide to Healing Through the Human Energy Field* (Bantam, 1988), and *Light Emerging* (Bantam, 1994).

*Kundalini:* Ajit Mookerjee, *Kundalini: The Arousal of the Inner Energy* (Inner Traditions, 1983); Lee Sannella, *Kundalini—Psychosis or Transcendence?* (Integral, 1987); Emma Bragdon, *The Call of Spiritual Emergency: From Personal Crisis to Personal Transformation* (Harper & Row, 1990).

**Audiovisual:** "Ayurvedic Medicine," Dr. Vasant Lad, audiocassette or videotapes, World Research Foundation, 15300 Ventura Blvd., Suite 405, Sherman Oaks, CA 91403, (818) 907-5483, fax (818) 907-6044; "Ayurveda: The Science of Life," Dr. Vasant Lad, 6 audiocassettes, Sounds True, (800) 333-9185; "Ayurveda Healing Massage," L.T., Inc., 1760 Rue des Erables, Charlesbourg, Québec, Canada G2L 1R4, (418) 659-8696; Dileepji Pathak, "Kundalini: Energy of Awakening," audiocassette, Sounds True, (800) 333-9185.

# CHAPTER 13

# Other Energetic Systems

We're fields of energy
in an infinite energy
field.

—e. e. cummings

While the Chinese, Japanese, and now Indian energetic traditions have become the best-known of Asian systems introduced to the West, others, such as Traditional Thai Massage and Kurdish Breema, are also gaining popularity. Some Westerners who have trained in Asia have brought the techniques back to America. Others have evolved their own methods by blending various Asian methods or synthesizing Eastern and Western ways—for example, Polarity Therapy and Zero Balancing. A few innovators, such as Dolores Krieger, have created a modern version (Therapeutic Touch) of an ancient method (laying-on of hands).

## FROM ASIA TO AMERICA

This chapter focuses on energetic bodyways that were developed both in Asia and in America. Although Polynesian rather than Asian, Hawaiian massage also figures here because of its underlying philosophy about energy. These bodyways are not necessarily direct derivatives of either Chinese Acupressure or Japanese Shiatsu, but similarities do exist. Because the exact transmission of health-care practices from one culture to another hundreds or thousands of years ago is difficult to verify, ultimately we don't know precisely who started what. All the bodyways described in this chapter subscribe to the idea that energy exists in and around the body, but they don't all work with it in the same manner: The number of pulses, channels, and points varies, as do procedures and direction of energy flow.

Some are customary practices from indigenous cultures, while others are based on a study of several longtime traditions. Some apply direct pressure to the body to affect the movement of energy, while others don't touch the body at all. Those few that combine pressure-point therapy with psychological theory and practice—Jin Shin Do and Process Acupressure—appear in the last chapter, "Convergence Systems."

# Traditional Thai Massage

Chongkol Setthakorn, a native teacher of Thai massage, describes this latest Asian import to the West as a combination of "the best of Yoga and Acupressure." In *Nuad bo-Rarn* (Thai for "ancient massage"), practitioners apply compression and pressure with their thumbs, palms, feet, forearms, elbows, and knees to stimulate the movement of energy through conduits called *sen*. According to traditional Thai medical theory, there are seventy-two thousand sen, of which ten hold top priority. Emphasis is on following these lines rather than specific acu-points.

Thai massage in no way resembles massage you may have experienced in the West, for there are no long strokes smoothed on with oil. Neither do you take your clothes off or lie on a padded table. It looks like a cross between Acupressure, Yoga, and Zen Shiatsu. In addition to compression and pressure, practitioners include manipulation. They position and stretch you in Yoga-like poses and then gently

Thai Massage

# Massage in Southern Thailand

As soon as I arrived in Bangkok, I went in search of Wat Po, the famous Temple of the Reclining Buddha. On the grounds I found a separate small, one-story building called the College of Traditional Medicine. There I got my first Thai massage. And there I could still see in the walls the stone tablets engraved with diagrams that King Rama III had ordered made at least two hundred years earlier, illustrating the energy lines and points on the human body.

The atmosphere was nothing like what I had been used to in California. Everyone got massaged in the same room filled with cots, one next to another, and open on one side, making us visible to anyone walking by. There were no partitions or drapes. But like all the Thai women and men on the cots around me, I was given a pajama-like outfit to put on for my own modesty and so that the massage practitioner could move my body easily every which way. Instead of a soft, quiet lull in the middle of this busy, noisy city, there was constant chatter among the practitioners as they worked methodically, pushing and pulling muscle tissue, "twanging" nerves, and applying pressure on blood vessels.

All the practitioners started with the feet because, as one woman explained, "They're like the roots of a tree." From there, the massage moved around the body in a specific routine. Practitioners pressed along the sen, and they pummeled, bent, twisted, raised, and stretched body parts, as though trying to turn us into pretzels. They repeat the procedure six times in an hourlong session, three times for a half-hour. Later I saw eighteenth-century versions of what I had just undergone: Among the trees and plants in the temple garden sat statues of individuals in contorted positions, submitting to the hand and foot work of a massage practitioner.

Massage was ubiquitous as I traveled farther south. When I stepped off a ferry in the harbor of an island off the east coast, I noticed men being massaged as they lay in an outdoor wooden pavilion. In a tiny open-air restaurant on the beach near where I stayed, I got an intense sit-down massage from an old man. When I stopped to visit a forest monastery on the return trip to Bangkok, I learned from some Western monks that the head monk frequently received massage to improve his health. And in some monasteries, monks themselves are adept in healing with massage, specializing in one condition or another, including respiratory ailments, drug abuse, or sprains and fractures.

I also learned when I returned to Bangkok the following year that differences in Thai massage exist not only between the Northern and Southern styles but also within a style. A blind Thai man with his own practice told me he studied for many years with one teacher, whereas a certificate can be earned from a formal course at Wat Po after only a month. Another man, then fifty-five years old, had studied massage from the time he was fifteen. He explained that usually a student lives with his teacher for ten years as an apprentice. He distinguished between the popular massage given at Wat Po and the kind he performed, known as "court massage" and used for the Thai king and his family. His was not for the pleasure of relaxation, he pointed out, but for relieving pain. He dealt with cervical disorders, insomnia, strokes, paralysis, headaches, polio, backaches, arthritis, sports injuries, indigestion, constipation, and so on, but not diseases such as diabetes.

In this Thai medical massage, practitioners read three pulses at each wrist and understand what is going on in your body in terms of certain elements rather than Western anatomy and physiology. For example, too much of the element wind could cause digestive disturbances, while wind blowing upward in the body could trigger headaches and wind blowing downward could produce pain in the legs. The objective of traditional massage is to redirect the wind along nerves and veins to restore balance and normal bodily functions.

rock you to more deeply open your joints and have a limbering effect. You wear loose-fitting clothing for maximum comfort and lie on a floor mat or cot to afford the practitioner maximum leverage, balance, and weight. A session can range from one to three hours, depending on how many times the practitioner repeats pressing up and down the sen in four successive positions—lying faceup, facedown, on the side, and seated—and stretching your body parts along the way.

These passive movements relieve you of having to make any effort, and thus eliminate resistance. You may find yourself with feet and legs up in the air or your arms stretched back and the practitioner's feet braced against your back. Both the pressure and the manipulation are intended not only to clear the energy pathways, but also to calm your nervous system, improve blood circulation, relax tense muscles, and stimulate internal organs. Practitioners stretch and move the legs around a lot, and they report that this frees up the pelvis and relieves lower back pain. In Thailand, typically people seek traditional massage to relieve fatigue, swollen limbs, painful joints, and headaches. As with most energetic practices, knowledge of therapeutic benefits comes from anecdotal evidence rather than research in the Western scientific mode.

There are two styles of practice: Northern (Chiang-Mai) and Southern (Bangkok). The Southern style, which some American teachers consider faster and more invasive, even painful, is more widespread in Thailand. The gentler Northern style is what has gained a foothold in the United States. After experiencing Thai massage in the city of Chiang Mai, some Americans decided to go back to study at a traditional massage school there. Now they teach it in the United States in a series of weekend workshops or intensive programs. At least one Thai instructor comes regularly to offer classes in American massage schools. Certification is available, but the requirements vary according to the school.

RESOURCES:

**For instruction and practitioners:** Arthur Lambert, Institute of Thai Massage, 189 Harvard Dr., Lake Worth, FL 33460, (407) 588-8198; Lana David, IPSB, 1366 Hornblend, San Diego, CA 92109, (619) 272-4142; Michael Eisenberg, 1539 Peace Rd., Bow, WA 98232, (360) 724-4673; Maxine Shapiro, 53 Marshall St., Newton, MA 02159, (617) 965-5251.

**Books:** *Northern style:* Arthur Lambert with Chongkol Setthakorn, *Nuad Bo-Rarn: The Traditional Massage of Thailand* (Toucan, 1992); Harold Brust, *The Art of Traditional Thai Massage* (Editions Duang Kamol, 1992); Anthony James, *Traditional Thai Medical Massage, The Northern Style* (Anthony James, 1994).
   *Southern style:* Sombat Tapanya, *Traditional Thai Massage* (Editions Duang Kamol, 1990); Anthony James, *Nuat Thai* (Anthony James, 1991).

**Videos:** *Northern style:* "Traditional Medical Massage of Thailand," Chongkol Setthakorn, 80 mins., IPSB, (619) 272-4142; "Nuad Bo-Rarn: Traditional Thai Massage," Michael Eisenberg, 120 mins., see above; "Thai Massage with Chongkol Setthakorn," 130 mins., and others, through Arthur Lambert, see page 307.
   *Southern style:* "Traditional Southern Style Thai Massage," Pian Sukpakkit, (800) 695-2042.

# Breema Bodywork

The root of all health is in the brain. The trunk of it is in emotion. The branches and leaves are in the body. The flower of health blooms when all parts work together.

—Kurdish saying

For centuries farmers and shepherds of Breemava, a Kurdish village in the mountains between Iran and Afghanistan, have practiced body therapy and traditional exercises as a natural part of daily life. But it wasn't until a village native left his home and eventually settled in northern California that people in the United States were exposed to what now is called *Breema*.

Breema is similar in theory and practice to other Eastern energetic traditions. The concept of a vital center of energy in the body—the Chinese *tantien* or Japanese *hara*—is the Kurdish *del-aka*. Breema views the body as an energy system with three centers—mind, feelings, and physical body. Illness is the result of an imbalance or a weak relationship among them. The objective is to activate the body's self-corrective reflexes to create a bal-

# Self-Breema Experience: The Kidney Charge

Doing the Kidney Charge daily can help energize your kidneys and adrenal glands (located on top of the kidneys) in a nurturing way. This is a key exercise because, according to Asian medical philosophy, this organ-gland combination is the storehouse of your body's energy reserves. High levels of stress and tension, especially predominant in modern living, deplete the adrenals and result in weakness, exhaustion, nervousness, fearfulness, irritability, backache, and higher susceptibility to colds and infections. In addition to governing resistance to mental, emotional, and physical stress, the kidneys and adrenals also affect reproductive energy, preserve water volume and balance the salt-to-water ratio, detoxify and purify the blood, conserve essential elements, and eliminate metabolic wastes.

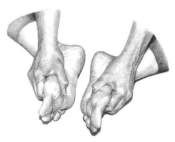

Figure A

To do the Kidney Charge, start by sitting comfortably cross-legged. Now bring the soles of your feet together in front of you on the floor. Alternating your hands, cluster your fingertips and tap around the inner ankle bones of both feet for three full breaths. Then wrap your fingers over the tops of your feet while placing your thumbs on the balls of your feet (figure A). While still holding your feet, on an inhalation straighten your arms as you stretch up and back, straightening your spine, arching your lower back, and opening the soles toward the ceiling yet keeping the edges of your feet connected. On an exhalation release the stretch and bend your arms as you allow your body to collapse forward in total relaxation. Repeat this stretch and release two more times.

Brush your hands up the inside of your legs to the kidneys. Lean forward and vigorously slap the kidneys with alternating open palms for three full breaths (figure B). Then brush from the kidneys down the outside of your legs to the toes three times. Holding your toes, bring one leg and then the other back to the cross-legged position. Brush your knees and sit comfortably and quietly for a moment.

Figure B

—Adapted with permission from Jon Schreiber, *Touching the Mountain: The Self-Breema Handbook: Ancient Exercises for the Modern World* (California Health, 1989).

anced state of energy—clarity in the mind, aliveness in the feelings, and flexibility and readiness in the body.

In its external form, Breema somewhat resembles Thai massage in how the practitioner moves your body. As in Shiatsu and Thai massage, practitioners use their palms, feet, forearms, and knees, but otherwise the practices are not the same. Breema work does not necessarily follow the Chinese or Japanese meridian and acu-point system. Using neither muscular force nor painful pressure, they give your body firm yet gentle and rhythmic leans, brushes, bends, stretches, and holds. There are hundreds of sequences, from delicate to vigorous, for the back, head, neck, internal organs, and so on, and each is an individual dance rather than a strategic pattern of treatment. Wearing loose clothing, you lie or sit on a padded mat on the floor.

*Self-Breema* is a group of exercises for the same purpose as the hands-on work: to support and balance the flow of life energy through your body, release tension, and increase vitality and dexterity. Since Breema is not a medical specialty but common village knowledge, the series of movements parallels those performed in everyday agrarian life: Hulling the Walnut, Dancing on the Grapes, Forming the Dough, Closing the Gate, Cleaning the Trench.

The Institute for Health Improvement offers a 165-hour practitioner certificate in Breema Bodywork.

R E S O U R C E S :

**For Breema instruction and practitioners:** Institute for Health Improvement, 6076 Claremont Ave., Oakland, CA 94618, (510) 428-0937.

**Books:** Jon Schreiber, D.C., *Touching the Mountain: The Self-Breema Handbook: Ancient Exercises for the Modern World* (California Health, 1989).

# Lomilomi

When Captain Cook and other European explorers disembarked on the islands of Polynesia, including what's now the state of Hawaii, the indigenous people healed their aches and pains with therapeutic massage. They revived them after long voyages at sea and strenuous hikes on land. This practice became known as *lomilomi,* "to break up into small pieces with the fingers."[1]

In ancient times, there were several orders of medical priests called *kahunas,* one of which specialized in massage—the *kahuna lomilomi.* Lay members of the community also practiced this healing art. Experts knew how to use it in childbirth, in preparation for bloodletting, and in cases of congestion and inflammation. They restored normal circulation and relieved pain in rheumatism and other musculoskeletal conditions, asthma, and bronchitis. They also applied it to children to strengthen them if weak and to mold their features for physical beauty.

Hawaiian massage contained several elements: both gentle and vigorous rubbing (friction), stroking and kneading with the hands, elbows, and forearms (*lomi*), as well as treading with the feet on the back (*'a'e*), brief pressing at special points (*kaomi*), gentle pressure or light stroking with an open hand (*kahi*), and self-massage with a curved Lomilomi stick usually carved from guava wood. Such sticks are available even today. You hold the long straight handle with both hands in front, at your chest; the other end, which is crooked at an angle of about 45 degrees and flattened, curves over one shoulder. You then can press it up and down the upper muscles of your back. To reach your lower back muscles, you curve the stick around one side or the other of your body.

Lomilomi practitioners used indigenous oils made from coconut and kukui nut trees, working them into the skin in a rhythmic 1-2-3, 1-2-3, 1-2-3 movement. The manipulations were not only physical but also energetic, that is, to stimulate the flow of *mana,* or life force. In its physical aspects, Lomilomi has some resemblance to Swedish massage. However, it is different in its frequent use of the forearm in stroking, its rhythm, and its figure-eight massage pattern. But what specifically distinguishes it from the Western version is its origins in the philosophy or spiritual orientation of the ancient Hawaiians. Aunty Margaret Machado, Lomilomi's chief proponent in the Islands today, teaches it not strictly as a physical practice but as a prayerful work: "the loving touch—a connection of heart, hand and soul with the Source of all life."

It's hard to know how close modern Lomilomi is to what the kahunas traditionally practiced because there was a period in Hawaiian history when the disapproval of Western missionaries and government officials caused native healers to go underground with their knowledge and skills. Hawaiians were even forbidden to speak their native language. Although we'll never know what was lost, Lomilomi today is still a relaxing and therapeutic bodyway.

Students in some massage schools learn the Hawaiian version as part of the certification curriculum. Workshops are also available for those who are already massage therapists and want to add these techniques to their repertoire.

**For instruction and referrals:** Aunty Margaret School of Hawaiian Lomilomi, P.O. Box 221, Captain Cook, HI 96704, (808) 323-2416; Hawaiian Islands School of Body Therapies, P.O. Box 390188, Kailua-Kona, HI 96739, (808) 322-0048.

# Jin Shin Jyutsu®

> There are no incurable diseases, only incurable people.
>
> —Philomena Dooley

Jin Shin Jyutsu (JSJ) is a "physio-philosophy" of life, according to its major exponent in the West, Mary Burmeister. She considers it neither a diagnostic skill nor a curing technique, but the art of reawakening awareness and self-understanding.

Burmeister learned JSJ from Jiro Murai in Japan in the late 1940s, who "rediscovered" this system of healing when he lay in a feverish state alone in the mountains for seven days. As he passed in and out of consciousness, he envisioned sages demonstrating hand gestures, which he then applied to himself. By the seventh day he had completely recovered, and he vowed to spend his life studying the connection between those hand gestures and his miraculous revival. He studied the Bible, ancient Chinese, Greek, and Indian texts, and finally the *Kojiki,* a Japanese text whose name means "Record of Ancient Things." The result was Jin Shin Jyutsu, which, literally translated, means "art of the Creator through man of knowing and compassion." Over a period of five decades, Murai went from calling it the "Art of Happiness" to calling it the "Art of Longevity" and finally gave it the name "Art of Benevolence."

In a JSJ session, as you lay clothed on a padded table, practitioners first "listen" to twelve energy pulses in your wrists and their seven different textures. Then, based on what disharmony they hear, they use their hands as "jumper cables" to revitalize your energy by placing them on your body in a sequence of combinations at twenty-six "safety energy locks." These twenty-six points on each side are where energy may become congested because of abuses to the body and negative thinking. This series of hand placements is called a "flow" and serves to gently balance the course of life energy by redirecting or unblocking it along its pathway. The flow circulates up the back and down the front of the body in twelve major channels. Practitioners never press hard, rub, or knead. They use only light pressure and hold for a couple of minutes with their palms, tips of the thumbs or fingers, or back of the hand until they feel a gentle pulsation.

Practitioners do not talk in terms of treating any condition even though

# Jin Shin Jyutsu Experience:
## Self-Help in Harmonizing Energy

After my first Jin Shin Jyutsu session, the practitioner suggested a self-help project that would strengthen my "main central vertical harmonizing energy." In JSJ thinking, this is our chief source of life, and depending on whether it is harmonious or out of rhythm, so are we. To be in balance with this source, try doing the following sequence of hand placements. I especially appreciate its relaxing effect as I lie in bed to go to sleep.

Begin by resting your right palm or fingers on the very top of your head while simultaneously placing one or a couple of your left fingers between your eyebrows. This is supposed to revitalize the circulation of deep body energy and aid memory. While holding here, breathe fully several times until you're ready to proceed.

Now, keeping your right hand in the same place, move your left finger to the tip of your nose. This position is said to recharge the circulation of superficial body energy and enhance reproductive functions. Remember to take nice slow, deep breaths.

Continue in this way, bringing your left fingers to your sternum (the bony area between your breasts) to reenergize your lungs and pelvic girdle. Don't forget to breathe nice and easy. Next, place your left fingers on the lower tip of the sternum. Hold there before going to the top of your pubic bone, a move that is intended to fortify the spine.

The last position calls for a shift: Leave your left hand on top of your pubic bone and bring your right finger(s) to your coccyx (the tail bone at the base of your spine), for improved circulation of your legs and feet.

—Adapted from Mary Burmeister, *Jin Shin Jyutsu Is Getting to Know (Help) Myself*, book 1 (Jin Shin Jyutsu, Inc., 1980).

---

people come with all manner of physical and emotional complaints, including arthritis, skin ailments, fatigue, digestive disturbances, and other aches and pains. Rather, "taking away the dams"—releasing energy blockages or tensions—allows the body to heal itself. A session usually results in a state of profound relaxation (or realignment of energy), which often leads to the elimination of disease symptoms and the unhealthy mental attitudes underlying them. One of the principal JSJ teachers, Philomena Dooley, was a nurse for twenty-two years and married to a physician, yet she was unable to rid herself of blood clotting difficulties that led to phlebitis and hospitalizations. After ten days of sessions with Burmeister, all of Dooley's symptoms and disharmonies, which had plagued her for almost two decades, disappeared.

There is no certification process. Only associate instructors authorized by Burmeister may lead five-day seminars in parts one and two of JSJ. Practitioners are then able to work with people and teach them self-help "quickie" positions for releasing tension, recharging energy, and serving as a kind of first aid for sprained ankles, nosebleeds, bruises, and headaches. Students who have completed the seminar three times may go on to an advanced class.

RESOURCES:

**For seminars, practitioners, and books:** Jin Shin Jyutsu, Inc., 8719 E. San Alberto, Scottsdale, AZ 85258, (602) 998-9331.

**Books:** Mary Burmeister, *Jin Shin Jyutsu,* self-help books 1, 2, and 3 (Jin Shin Jyutsu, Inc., 1980, 1981, 1985).

# Reflexology (Zone Therapy)

Like other pressure-point therapies, Reflexology works with a reflex response. According to Reflexologists, stimulation to specific points activates the movement of energy to corresponding parts of the body to clear out congestion and restore normal functioning. Various organs, nerves, and glands are connected with certain "reflex buttons" on the feet and hands and even the ears (as in the Chinese practice of auricular acupuncture).

Reflexology probably dates back to ancient Egypt. Two reliefs from Ankh-ma-Hor's tomb (Sixth Dynasty, 2587–2453 B.C.E.) depict two seated men receiving massage of their hands and feet. But it was not until 1913 that Americans heard about it from William Fitzgerald, who had rediscovered it in his work. A medical doctor who specialized in otolaryngology, he was once chief of the Nose and Throat Department at St. Francis Hospital in Hartford, Connecticut. Fitzgerald divided the body into ten vertical zones, five on each side, extending from the head to the fingertips and toes, front to back. Every aspect of the body shows up in one of these ten zones, and each zone has a reflex area on the hands and feet (thus the name *Zone Therapy*). He and a colleague, Dr. Edwin Bowers, demonstrated that by applying pressure in one area of the body, they could anesthetize or reduce pain in another.

Eunice Ingham, a physiotherapist, carried on and expanded Zone Therapy while working in association with practicing physicians. Observing her patients over time, she realized that pressing on various points on the feet had certain effects on other parts of the body. Eventually she was able to map out the entire body onto the feet. A year before her death in 1974, the International Institute of Reflexology was founded to carry on her work.

Reflexologists contend that, as in Shiatsu or acupuncture, energy flows through the ten zones identified by Fitzgerald. When it circulates freely, the body enjoys balance and good health. Massaging specific points, which exist for every organ, stimulates the organ in that zone. If your organ is in a weak condition, it is likely that the reflex point will be extremely tender when pressed. For this reason, a Reflexology massage is not always comfortable or soothing. Reflexologists say that the painful sensations may be due to the breaking up of crystal deposits (an excess of uric acid) that have settled in the feet or to the stimulation of sensory receptors. Sometimes it takes several sessions for acute tenderness to subside.

Practitioners use their thumbs, slightly bent (or simple implements, even a pencil eraser), to press deeply into the reflex points, releasing tension and encouraging better circulation of blood, lymph, and energy. Although diagnosis and curing are not their province, Reflexologists say that by promoting relaxation and stimulating circulation they may have a preventative effect: They help clear up minor blockages before they become major conditions. Also, by following the sore points like a road map, Reflexologists can assess which areas are not functioning at their best and try to correct the imbalance or alert the person to seek medical attention. Although she never

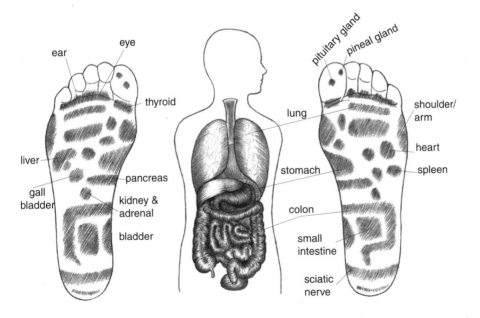

Reflexology: Each organ or other part of the body is represented by a specific point on the foot. Massaging the point is said to stimulate the organ or gland.

volunteered the information on her own, I asked one practitioner what she had detected about my body from working on my feet. Uncannily, her comments were right in line with what an acupuncturist had told me after reading my pulses and with what discomforts I was experiencing. And, as the acupuncturist noticed improvements in my pulses, the reflexologist noticed them in the corresponding areas of my feet.

Most practitioners report a wide range of healings—from inducing a kidney stone to pass (and thus avoiding surgery) to relieving PMS. For example, massaging points on the hands and feet that correspond to the uterus, ovaries, and glands resulted in a 46 percent reduction in total PMS symptoms, according to a study organized by William Flacco, director of the American Academy of Reflexology in Burbank, California.[2] Reflexology appears most suitable for chronic conditions and functional disorders, such as headaches, asthma, difficulty in digestion and elimination, high blood pressure, fatigue, and stress.

For a Reflexology session, all you have to do is remove your shoes and socks; you don't even have to lie down. And if you can't handle pressure in a part of your body because of soreness or inflammation, a viable alternative is massage on the corresponding area in your foot, hands, or ears. You can also learn how to massage yourself or friends and family, but it takes experience to develop enough sensitivity in your fingers to recognize which reflexes are sore in someone else and how to handle them. Generally, it's also more relaxing to have someone work on you.

Some people specialize in Reflexology; others incorporate it into their massage therapy practice. Training varies from weekend workshops to inclusion in massage school programs to one-hundred-hour certification programs recognized by the American Reflexology Certification Board.

## RESOURCES:

**For information, charts, practitioners, instruction, and publications on the Original Ingham Method of Reflexology:** International Institute of Reflexology, P.O. Box 12642, St. Petersburg, FL 33733-2642, (813) 343-4811. For certification programs: American Reflexology Certification Board, P.O. Box 620607, Littleton, CO 80162, (303) 933-6921.

**Books:** Dwight C. Byers, *Better Health With Foot Reflexology* (Ingham, 1983); Mildred Carter and Tammy Weber, *Body Reflexology: Healing at Your Fingertips* (Parker Publishing, 1994); Laura Norman, *Feet First: A Guide to Reflexology* (Fireside/Simon & Schuster, 1988); Nicola M. Hall, *Thorsons's Introductory Guide to Reflexology: A Patient's Guide* (Thorsons, 1992); Kevin Kunz and Barbara Kunz, *The Complete Guide to Foot Reflexology,* rev. ed. (Prentice-Hall, 1991).

**Audiovisual:** "A Complete Guide to Practical Reflexology," 60-min. video-tape by Melva Martin, N.D., Sounds True, (800) 333-9185.

## Polarity Therapy

Polarity Therapy is the creation of Randolph Stone (1888–1981), an Austrian-American who spent decades investigating healing methods all over the world. He became a doctor of osteopathy, naturopathy, and chiropractic, and also studied Reflexology, Chinese medicine, and Ayurvedic medi-

> Energy is the real substance behind the appearance of matter and forms.
>
> —Randolph Stone

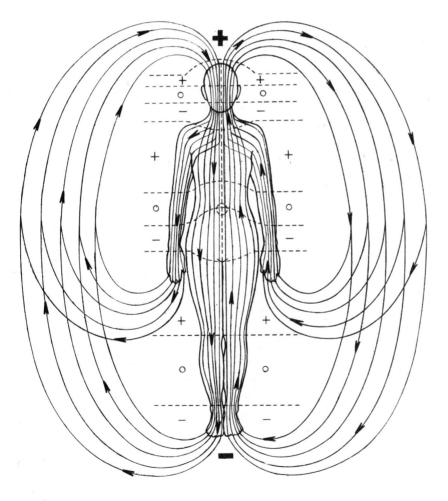

Polarity Energy Lines

# Polarity Therapy Experience

The "tummy rock" is a simple way of doing Polarity Therapy within a few minutes. Try it on a child before bedtime as an easy way to induce sleep; it's a good way to relax a friend at any time; or get someone to do it for you.

Have the person lie down in loose clothes so that there is no restriction. Stand by his or her right side. Rub your hands briskly together so that you feel warmth and energy in them. Rest your left hand on the friend's forehead, your right hand just below the navel. Using your right hand, rock the torso from side to side with an even and gentle rhythm for a couple of minutes. To get the body to move an inch or two, press deeply enough so your hand doesn't slide. Don't impose your own pace, but follow the momentum of your friend's body.

After a couple of minutes stop the rocking but leave your hands in place. Notice sensations in your hands and body while your friend observes energy tingling or rushing in his or her body. Slowly remove your hands. Give the person a chance to get up gradually or take a nap.

The Polarity "Tummy Rock"

—Adapted from Richard Gordon, *Your Healing Hands: The Polarity Experience* (Unity, 1978).

cine. Stone developed a four-part system that integrates both Eastern and Western techniques. It combines pressure-point therapy with diet, exercises (Yoga stretches, breath, and sound), and self-awareness.

Long before the word energy became popular, Stone wrote *Energy: The Vital Principle in the Healing Art* (1948) and believed that a universal energy is what gives rise to the physical world. He theorized that this energy flows between two electrical poles (negative and positive, yin and yang), circulating inside and outside our bodies in specific patterns. Five vertical currents flow up the back and down the front on the right side; another five flow up the front and down the back on the left side. Each current corresponds to a particular chakra, element, body system, and life function. For example, the fire element is related to the chakra just above the navel, to the stomach and intestines (digestion and assimilation), and to will and power. The head holds a positive charge, the feet a negative one; the right palm is positive, the left negative. The body is also divided horizontally into positive, neutral, and negatively charged zones. When life energy is balanced and flows freely between the positive and negative poles, the neutral charge increases. The result is what Stone called the "triune function," a continuous flow of positive-neutral-negative energy.

To unblock and recharge the flow of life energy between the poles, Polarity Therapists first make an energetic assessment, looking for tense or tender areas in your body. Then they place their hands in specific positions to connect negative and positive. The pressure they apply can be deep, moderate, or light. Occasionally they make no contact at all except with the aura or electromagnetic field surrounding your body. Once the energy flows freely again, you experience deep relaxation.

To maintain the sense of well-being achieved through hands-on sessions, practitioners encourage you to adopt cleansing and health-building diets, exercise daily with Polarity Yoga, and resolve negative mental activity. For Stone, thoughts and emotions are vibrations of energy that influence the flow of energy in the body. As in other energetic therapies, musculoskeletal and functional disorders may disappear once your life force is in balance. And a total lifestyle approach is ultimately what will keep you healthy.

There are two levels of national certification to meet the standards for practice set up by the American Polarity Therapy Association (APTA). Level one consists of 165 hours of training for eligibility to register with APTA and become an Associate Polarity Practitioner. Level two is an additional 450 hours to become a Registered Polarity Practitioner. Some people practice Polarity exclusively; others incorporate its principles and techniques into their particular health-care modality. For example, a chiropractor I used to see in California's Monterey Bay area always included some Polarity Therapy along with the spinal adjustments he made.

RESOURCES:

**For information on instruction, practitioners, centers, publications, charts, videos, and tapes:** American Polarity Therapy Association, 2888 Bluff St., #149, Boulder, CO 80301, (303) 545-2080, fax (303) 545-2161.

**Books:** Randolph Stone, *Health Building: The Conscious Art of Living Well* (CRCS, 1985); Franklyn Sills, *The Polarity Process* (Element, 1989); Alan Siegel, *Polarity Therapy: The Power That Heals* (Prism, 1987); John Chitty and Mary Louise Muller, *Energy Exercises* (Polarity, 1990); Philip Young, *The Art of Polarity Therapy* (Prism, 1990); Maruti Seidman, *A Guide to Polarity Therapy: The Gentle Art of Hands-On Healing* (Elan, 1991); Richard Gordon, *Your Healing Hands: The Polarity Experience* (Unity, 1978).

# Watsu

> The body is flexible, a fluid energy field that is in a process of change from the moment of conception until the moment of death.
>
> —Don Johnson

*Watsu,* or water Shiatsu, incorporates elements of Zen Shiatsu, Indian chakra work, meditation, and yoga. Harold Dull, the originator of this unique practice, was a San Francisco Beat poet in the 1950s before he studied with Shizuto Masunaga, the Japanese master who developed Zen Shiatsu; Reuho Yamada, a Zen priest, and Wataru Ohashi, who created OhaShiatsu. Later he became the director of the School of Shiatsu and Massage at Harbin Hot Springs, California.

While practicing Shiatsu, Dull discovered that he could enhance and deepen its effects by working with someone in warm water. The buoyancy and warmth relax the muscles, unlock joints, and support the spine so it can move more fluidly than on land.

Watsu practitioners do not give a traditional Shiatsu session underwater. Although they do press points on your body, they spend a good deal of the time moving you—rocking, arching, cradling, stretching, bending, floating, folding—and just letting your body rise and fall with the breath. In turn, as the spine gets freed up, this stimulates the upward movement of energy.  See "Chakras and Kundalini," page 297. Practitioners report that in the soft, nurturing, relaxing, watery environment, it's not uncommon for someone to have an emotional release—tears, laughter, rage, etc.—as painful or pleasant emotions and memories surface. There is no psychotherapeutic intervention, just quiet, nonjudgmental being with the person. Dull believes that a kind of rebonding to your own center occurs, allowing connectedness to and trust of others as well.

Writer Bill Thompson describes his Watsu session with Howard Dull: "Dull floated me on my back . . . one confident hand balanc[ing] me at my sacrum, the other support[ing] my head and neck. I gradually relaxed and let my muscles loosen, joints unlock, and thoughts drift. . . . Dull swayed me delicately. . . . I became a winding cord of ocean kelp, washing back and forth in rhapsodic slow motion. . . . Coiled around Dull's trunk like a sleepy boa constrictor, I was suspended in clear, soothing waters, worry-free, [weightless], protected from the world. [He] tucked my neck into the crook of his arm . . . [and] drew my head to his chest, holding it to his heart. Then he floated me out and sank his fingers into the muscles along my spine. [After an hour he] steered my semiconscious body to the side of the pool, resting it there on a ledge. I reclined, my limbs oozing like jellyfish, my head bathed in breezy light."[3]

Although some professionals have criticized Watsu for its close contact, which is required for floating someone in water, others have found that this level of nonsexual physical intimacy is what makes Watsu so effective in therapy and recovery. For example, at the Timpany Center in San Jose, California, aquatic specialists and physical therapists report that individuals with severe physical, mental, and emotional disabilities have shown marked improvement in range of motion, ability to relax, and emotional security. Watsu is also now available in some spas.

In addition to Watsu, Dull created *Woga*, or water Yoga, a series of stretches similar to asanas. As in Watsu, the water allows you to stretch beyond what you might be able to do on land and opens you to what Dull calls "the wave." After doing the stretching sequence, Dull sinks into the water to experience a rush of energy through his whole body.

Dull leads a certification program at Harbin Hot Springs. It consists of a series of fifty-hour intensive programs: One hundred hours total are required to become a Watsu practitioner, five hundred to become a Watsu therapist, and more than six hundred hours for an instructor. In 1993 he also founded the Worldwide Aquatic Bodywork Association (WABA).

RESOURCES:

**For instruction and practitioner referrals:** School of Shiatsu and Massage at Harbin Hot Springs and WABA, P.O. Box 570, Middletown, CA 95461, (707) 987-3801.

**Books:** Harold Dull, *Bodywork Tantra on Land and in Water* (Harbin Hot Springs Publishing, 1987), and *Watsu: Freeing the Body in the Water* (Harbin Hot Springs Publishing, 1993).

# Zero Balancing®

> The flesh is not a solid, dense mass; it is filled with life, consciousness, and energy.
>
> —Don Johnson

Zero Balancing (ZB) is the innovation of Fritz Frederick Smith, M.D. He was born in 1929, the son of a chiropractor who later became, in his nineties, the oldest practicing chiropractor in America. Although trained as an osteopathic physician and surgeon, Smith also studied Rolfing with Ida Rolf, Siddha Yoga with Swami Muktananda, acupuncture with J. R. Worsley in England, Jin Shin Do, Shiatsu, T'ai Chi Chuan, and Chi Kung. The result is a model that serves as a bridge or interface between Eastern and Western philosophies.

ZB is a practice that is neither purely an energy system nor purely a structural system. It is a noninvasive hands-on procedure for evaluating and balancing the relationship between your body energy and body structure. Smith considers ZB a skill rather than a therapy or medical tool, one that allows practitioners of any method—psychotherapy, acupuncture, massage, chiropractic—to consciously touch energy and structure simultaneously.

ZB recognizes three domains of energy: 1) the densest energy, or universal life flow, runs vertically through the skeletal system; 2) the internal energy flows move at three different levels; and 3) the background energy field pervades the space inside and around your body.

In a session, you remain clothed and lie on a padded table. Practitioners assess your energy by scanning the field around your body as well as palpating your physical body. They create fulcrums or balance points through pressing, lifting, pulling, twisting, stretching, bending, and sliding movements. To understand how this works, Smith suggests that you take a rubber band and stretch it just far enough to take up the slack. At that point, you will have "contacted" the rubber band. If you go any farther and meet resistance, you will stretch the rubber itself. In essence, this is what practitioners do with the tissues of your body. The fulcrums allow them to take up the physical slack of your tissue in order to "get in touch" with your energy body and provide a stationary point around which your body can organize itself in a balanced way. Practitioners monitor your response to these neutral positions by watching shifts in facial expression, eyelid movement, breathing, and vitality. They also use gentle, pain-free joint balancing, which allows energy to move through and open up a joint.

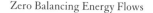

Zero Balancing Energy Flows

According to Smith, your body's tissues hold thought, emotion, attitude, past experience, and memory in a vibratory form. ZB puts a clearer, stronger force field through your body to override or release unclear vibrations. As the unclear vibrations disappear, so do their effects—the charge of the vibration gets discharged. This is where the term *zero balancing* comes in. It refers to your experience of balance after a session, to an expanded state of consciousness. In that regard, ZB is a system of stress reduction and internal reprogramming. In an experience of balance and well-being, you can sense through touch greater possibilities than what you've been living—deeper feelings of harmony, clarity, and connectedness. Although ZB neither diagnoses nor deals with pathology, you may encounter relief of pain, headaches, low back discomfort, and other physical symptoms. And you may find yourself in an easier relationship with gravity: standing more upright, feeling lighter, and moving more fluidly.

ZB is a gentle practice, but Smith advises that people with knee replacements skip it and that those who have had hip replacements be handled delicately.

Students who take the 150-hour Zero Balancing Certification Program are already licensed health-care professionals. Additional advanced intensive programs follow.

RESOURCES:

**For instruction and practitioners:** The Zero Balancing Association, P.O. Box 1727, Capitola, CA 95010, (408) 476-0665.

**Books:** Fritz Frederick Smith, *Inner Bridges: A Guide to Energy Movement and Body Structure* (Humanics New Age, 1986).

**Videos:** "Zero Balancing Video," Fritz Smith, 48 mins., (408) 476-0665 or (800) 233-5880.

# Therapeutic Touch

Some energy-based systems do not rely on applying pressure to specific points to trigger a reflex response elsewhere in your body. In fact, a few, like Therapeutic Touch (TT), don't even directly touch your physical body. Instead, they make contact with and modulate the bioenergetic field surrounding it. This is particularly useful in cases where touching the skin would be painful or otherwise ill-advised, or if you're touch-phobic.

TT is a contemporary modification of the ancient religious practice of laying-on of hands and was popularized by Dolores Krieger, a professor of nursing, and her teacher, Dora Kunz. The basic premise is that your energy extends beyond the skin; in other words, you don't end at your skin. This bioenergetic field surrounding your body is called your aura. Some people are able to see changes in its color and character and interpret them as reflections of internal physical and emotional states. TT practitioners touch this field rather than your physical body to induce relaxation, reduce pain, and accelerate self-healing capacities, which in turn alleviate a variety of symptoms. Krieger says that certain functions seem to be more sensitive to TT than others: the autonomic nervous system, circulatory and lymphatic disorders, musculoskeletal problems, some endocrine glands, and a few psychological disturbances.

Practitioners work in a standard five-step process that follows no network of points or meridians. First, they center themselves to become clear, focused channels for universal healing energy and to affirm their intentions and compassion to help others. For a period of up to twenty-five minutes, they will act as a human energy support system until your own immunological system is strong enough to take over. Then they follow with an assessment of your energy field, generally while you're seated. Holding one palm toward your back, the other at the front, two to three inches away, TT therapists move their hands down your energy field from head to toe. As they pass their

The Aura

hands through your field, they look for cues as to how your energy is distributed—sensations of heat or cold, thickness or emptiness, pressure, heaviness, pulling, or no movement at all. Step three consists of clearing any blockage, imbalance, or congestion of energy they find through a series of sweeping hand movements downward in the person's field.

In step four, they establish harmony by strengthening, quickening, or vitalizing energy where it is either lacking or low, and by toning down or sedating energy where it is extreme or excessive. Instead of using physical pressure to bring about the change, practitioners use their mind. For example, says Krieger, if she senses a lot of heat in the person's field, she can remember what it feels like to be cold and replicate that throughout her own field. Then she consciously focuses that sense of cold through the energy centers in the palms of her hands to the area in the person's field where she first detected heat. Another way the practitioner can redistribute energies is to visualize certain colors—each having a particular quality—while projecting energy to the person.

Finally, step five involves "unruffling" any turbulence in your field and smoothing out "wrinkles" in its surface. Practitioners do this by moving their hands outward, toward the periphery of the field, progressing generally in a head-to-foot direction.

"Although human energies are nonmaterial," says Krieger, "the physical body does register the effects of these invisible forces in its material structures."[4] Her initial investigation of TT, for example, demonstrated that it produces an increase in hemoglobin, the oxygen-carrying component of blood. She and other nurses have observed edema go down, blood pressure lower, headaches melt away, sleep return, digestive conditions disappear, and bone fractures form callus in a third of the average time. Practitioners have used it widely: in pregnancy, labor, and delivery as well as postnatal treatment; for pain management; for treatment of PMS, irritability and anxiety, fever, fatigue and depression, HIV infection, nausea and vomiting associated with chemotherapy and radiation sickness, certain endocrine dysfunctions, manic-depression, catatonia and hyperkinesis, restlessness related to Parkinson's and Alzheimer's; and after surgery.[5] On the other hand, Krieger notes that she has not seen decisive results in cases of pituitary disorders, lupus, and schizophrenia.

Critics of TT have suggested that positive clinical experience is a result of the placebo response. A study conducted among sixty heart patients at St. Vincent's Medical Center in New York by Janet Quinn, associate professor at the University of Colorado School of Nursing in Denver, proved otherwise. TT reduced anxiety levels by 17 percent within five minutes even though the patients had no knowledge of what the technique was supposed to achieve. The control group, whose "healers" merely imitated TT motions while counting backward from one hundred by sevens, showed no change.[6]

# Therapeutic Touch Experience: Assessing the Energy Field

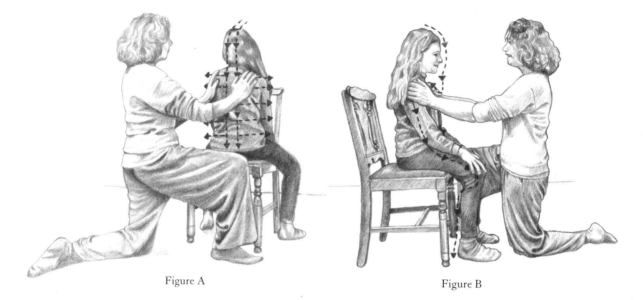

Figure A                                                    Figure B

If you're not familiar with feeling energy in your hands, try the Feeling Energy Experience on ☞ page 281 first. Then if you want to test how much you feel in a person's energy field, do the following.

Have a friend, partner, or your child sit down on a stool so you have easy access to the front and back. Stand in back of the person. Starting near the top of the head, hold your palms facing him or her about two to three inches from his or her body. Slowly bring your hands down through the energy field, moving first along the spinal column, then outward to the sides, back to the spine, and out again, repeating until you've covered the whole back (figure A). Don't stay long in any one place, just proceed level by level until you reach the person's feet. Pay attention to any clues your hands pick up in the field, but don't stop. You may get sensory impression, insights, or vague hunches. If you like, go back again to check the details you noticed in certain areas. Also observe any differences you might feel between your right and left hands.

Next, go to the front of the body (or the back if you started in the front) and do the same thing (figure B). Then test your perceptions with the person for how accurately you are picking up energy cues.

—Adapted from Dolores Krieger, *Accepting Your Power to Heal: The Personal Practice of Therapeutic Touch* (Bear & Co. 1993).

Robert O. Becker, M.D., pioneering researcher in bioelectricity, theorizes that the kind of healing that occurs in a method such as TT is an interaction of electromagnetic energy fields.

Since we know that the body uses electrical control systems to regulate many basic functions and that the flow of these electrical currents produces externally measurable magnetic fields, it does not require a great leap of faith to postulate that a healer's gift is an ability to use his or her own electrical control systems to produce external electromagnetic energy fields that interact with those of the patient. The interaction could be one that "restores" balance in the internal forces or that reinforces the electrical systems so that the body returns toward a normal condition.[7]

Had it not been for Krieger, this esoteric healing art of energy transfer would have remained in the shadows of unacceptability instead of infiltrating mainstream medicine. As a faculty member of New York University, she has taught it to tens of thousands of health-care professionals, particularly other nurses, who use it in hospitals. During the last twenty years, TT has been offered in classes and workshops in more than eighty colleges and universities in the United States and about seventy foreign countries. Practitioners of various methods—massage, Shiatsu, Acupressure, Yoga, physical therapy—use it as an adjunct to their work. Lay people also can learn TT, for Krieger believes we all have the power to heal.

Krieger cautions that in some situations it is better not to receive TT: For example, in the case of cranial injuries, avoid any work directly over your head; also, avoid work when you're near the end of a pregnancy.

RESOURCES:

**For practitioners or classes:** Nurse Healers and Professional Associates Cooperative, Inc., 175 Fifth Ave., Suite 3399, New York, NY 10010.

**Books:** Dolores Krieger, *Accepting Your Power to Heal: The Personal Practice of Therapeutic Touch* (Bear, 1993); Janet Macrae, *Therapeutic Touch: A Practical Guide* (Alfred A. Knopf, 1988).

**Audiovisual:** "The Therapeutic Touch, with Dolores Krieger," 35-min. videotape, Institute of Noetic Sciences, (800) 383-1586.

# Reiki

In Japanese, *Reiki* (pronounced "ray-kee") means "universal life energy." It is a simple hands-on or no-touch technique for channeling this omnipresent energy to promote healing. Also known as the Usui System of Natural Healing, it was named for Dr. Mikao Usui, a Christian minister in Japan who developed Reiki in the middle of the nineteenth century. He passed it on to Dr. Chujiro Hayashi, who in turn transmitted it to Hawayo Takata, a Japanese woman from Hawaii who fully regained her health and avoided surgery after receiving Reiki treatments while visiting her parents in Japan. She introduced Reiki to the United States in the late 1930s.

Before she died, in 1980, Takata prepared her granddaughter, Phyllis Lei Furumoto, to continue the lineage. Along with other Reiki masters authorized by Takata, she formed the Reiki Alliance. A faction, led by Barbara Ray, who claims to have "inherited" leadership from Takata, formed the American-International Reiki Association, now known as the Radiance Technique Association International.

Through a stepped series of weekend intensive sessions in "attunements," practitioners receive direct initiation or training in degrees of mastery (level seven is the highest). Some follow the Usui system, others practice the Radiance Technique. You can give yourself a Reiki treatment or get it from a master. The practitioner places both hands, palms down, side by side or end to end, on or near the person's body in twelve separate locations for a total of five minutes in each site. This laying-on of hands is supposed to relieve pain, even acute ailments and chronic illness, as well as encourage spiritual growth. Practitioners report using it for stress, migraines, cuts, bruises, swelling, tumors, psoriasis, burns, heart disorders, bladder difficulties, high blood pressure, asthma and allergies, rheumatism, whiplash, digestive disorders, insomnia, arthritis, and so on. It is usually gentle and relaxing and is seldom painful, and there are no contraindications.

There is no formal certification process in the Usui system; a Reiki master approves a student when satisfied with his or her competency. In the last few years, there has been concern expressed that what started out as a Japanese tradition has become "a non-specific, generic term referring to all kinds of energy work."[8] In fact, while in 1980 there were only twenty-two Reiki masters personally trained and initiated by Takata, today there are more than 2,000 self-proclaimed masters teaching around the world, making it difficult to know who is doing the work according to the standards of the lineage and who is practicing a homegrown technique. In the mid-1980s Reiki master Ethel Lombardi developed *MariEl* as yet another energetic approach for releasing blockages and attaining health and well-being.

RESOURCES:

**For instruction and practitioners:** Usui System of Natural Healing, Reiki Alliance, P.O. Box 41, Cataldo, ID 83810, (208) 682-3535; Radiance Technique Association International, Inc. (formerly the American-International Reiki Association, Inc.), P.O. Box 40570, St. Petersburg, FL 33743-0570.

**Books:** Hawayo Takata, *Living Reiki: Takata's Teachings* (Life Rhythm, 1992); Barbara Ray, *The "Reiki" Factor* (Radiance, 1989); Marsha Burack, *Reiki: Hands-On Healing for Yourself and Others* (Reiki Healing, 1992); Earlene Gleisner, *Reiki in Everyday Living: How Universal Energy Is a Natural Part of Life, Medicine, and Personal Growth* (WFP, 1992).

**Audiotapes:** "Reiki—Healing Yourself," Marsha Burack, (800) 333-4220 or (800) 634-9057.

# CHAPTER 14

# Eastern Movement Arts

It is only by being
cognizant of our
internal energy and
the natural restorative
powers of the body that
we can take charge of
our own healing and
become active agents of
our own change and
recovery.

—Jerry Mogul

The movement arts of India, China, and Japan—including Chi Kung, martial arts, and Yoga—are like other Eastern healing arts in being both preventative and therapeutic. But they are different in that no one else balances your life force energy by such external treatments as needles, pressure, herbs, or heat. The most important element is your active, involved participation, for it is you who moves and controls chi, making your vital energy flow freely throughout your body. And in learning to do so—that is, becoming sensitive to your own energy—you also learn to interpret or sense the energy in others. That sensitivity is vital in enhancing your health and your personal relationships.

The Indian, Chinese, and Japanese movement arts are useful in attaining or regaining physical health at any age. They loosen and free muscles and joints to improve posture, joint mobility, and flexibility. As weight-bearing exercises, they strengthen bones. They tone internal organs, deepen respiration, and stimulate circulation. They reduce tension in the sympathetic branch of the autonomic nervous system and enhance the parasympathetic aspect. They also develop balance, coordination, and a sense of centeredness.

## MEDITATION IN MOVEMENT

While you can engage in these movement arts strictly for physical conditioning or, in some cases, for defending yourself, they are also methods for quieting the mind. Their highest purpose is unity and harmony, within and without. You can use them to cultivate consciousness and moral character. Some writers contend that these arts originally developed in relation to spiritual practice and that in certain aspects they still reflect such philosophies as Hinduism, Taoism, Buddhism, and Shinto. They are as much a way of being as a prescription for doing. They can foster self-knowledge and strengthen your connection to your own body wisdom.

In learning the movement arts of other countries there is always the danger of misunderstanding what they are and how to use them. Because of language barriers and cultural differences, terms can be easily mistranslated and important philosophical concepts lost or misinterpreted. For example, some Westerners have perceived martial arts as no more than an Eastern version of fighting sports such as boxing or wrestling. They see only external combat and competition without the essential internal development. They are able to imitate the movements without truly knowing the meaning and intention behind them.

As a kind of meditation in movement, these Eastern arts emphasize conscious awareness and effortless action—what the Taoists call *wei wu wei,* "doing nothing" or "not-doing," and the Buddhists call "right effort." In this regard, these bodyways are similar to Western functional approaches. Wei wu wei is not the same as passivity. It is a state of body awareness in which an action happens by itself easefully: The dancer and dance are one; the arrow shoots itself. To perform these arts skillfully, you must rely on proprioceptive cues—sensing yourself from inside—before checking your form on the outside. As a method of sensory-motor training, they are complementary to those body practices that depend on lying down to dispel the effect of gravity.

Although these movement arts may look simple, they demand exquisite body control and balance, which develop from patience, disciplined training, and focused awareness. As Morihei Ueshiba, the founder of Aikido, advised, "In your training, do not be in a hurry, for it takes a minimum of ten years to master the basics and advance to the first rung. Never think of yourself as an all-knowing, perfect master; you must continue to train daily."[1] Those who are adept all cite the importance of having a competent teacher to guide you to good practice.

If you are interested in using the martial arts, for example, as a means of tapping into your body wisdom, beware of macho drillmasters without heart. Look for a good artist rather than a good art. Some schools are concerned with making you a better fighter, while others emphasize making you a better person. Although there are martial arts associations, each with its own standards and rankings, Eastern movement arts are not regulated or licensed by any national agency or board. Anyone can offer classes, so it's up to you to investigate credentials. Even then, if you're inexperienced, you're not qualified to judge an instructor's technical proficiency. They can rattle off the names of teachers they've studied with, but such names might not mean anything to you. However, you *are* qualified to judge whether

Practice not-doing, and everything will fall into place.

—Tao Te Ching

The real value of martial arts study . . . has nothing to do with physical feats such as brick breaking . . . [but] in what the martial arts tell us about ourselves: that we can be much more than we are now; that we have no need of fear; that our capacities for energy, awareness, courage, and compassion are far greater than we have been led to believe. They tell us that all our personal limits can be transcended.

—Don E. Miller

someone is a decent human being who treats you fairly and ethically. The best thing is to try a few classes and see how comfortable you are with the person's instructional style and philosophy. Shop around until you find what you need.

## THE MARTIAL ARTS

The most popular martial arts are from China and Japan, but there are martial arts native to many other countries: for example, *Kalarippayattu* from southern India, *Escrima* from the Philippines, *Taekwondo* from Korea, *Pentjak Silat* from Malaysia and Indonesia, *Capoeira,* a combination of dance, martial art, and sport, from Brazil, and others from Africa.[2] Here I focus on the Chinese systems of chi development *Chi Kung* and *T'ai Chi Chuan,* Japanese *Aikido,* and Okinawan *Karate.* Although they are all involved in the movement of chi, T'ai Chi and Aikido are often described as "internal" or "soft" martial arts, while most Karate is considered an "external" or "hard" art.

Classifying the martial arts, whether as soft or hard, internal or external, or yin or yang, is a troublesome problem about which there is a fair amount of debate.[3] Ultimately, their essence is about the skillful balancing of opposites. As Aikido instructor Paul Linden points out, "The hard arts become soft as hardness is truly understood. They are not brute force but a yang gateway into self-awareness. The soft arts become hard as softness is truly understood. The shadow side of softness is airiness and shallowness. The shadow side of hardness is brutality and murderousness. Without the hard and the soft, people won't have the opportunity to see their shadow parts."[4] Personal growth is the integration of compassion and power, of soft and hard, of internal and external, of light and shadow.

The internal arts focus on yielding and inner strength. They teach you how to respond or defend by giving way. In this attitude, they follow Taoist and Buddhist beliefs, especially as exemplified in the classic Taoist manual on the art of living, Lao-tzu's *Tao Te Ching,* or Book of the Way. The qualities of water are often used for illustrating how best to move. Water is soft and yielding, yet as a river traveling a long way to the ocean, it must surmount innumerable obstructions. It flows around, over, and under them, shifting again and again. "Throw a rock into a pond and the water allows the rock to take its course," explains Michael DeMarco, a martial arts student for more than thirty years. "It yields to the rock while encompassing it. Throw a rock against a tree and see the damage done."[5]

This is not to say that there are no striking, kicking, or punching moves in the internal style. T'ai Chi, for example, is primarily kicking and punching. These martial arts can teach you to become proficient in self-defense, but you also can use them as dynamic meditations. Once employed as fighting systems (and still capable of being used as such), the internal martial arts have evolved into living arts. On the deepest level, they are concerned with life, health, creativity, and self-transformation—physical, mental, and spiritual—rather than with competition and destruction.[6] Training the mind as much as the body, they are methods of mastering yourself rather than conquering others. They depend on your ability to cultivate and apply chi, and to keep your mind still while moving your body. "In the Art of Peace we never attack," said Ueshiba. "An attack is proof that one is out of control."[7]

Philosophically, the soft and hard arts are the same. They are both means for cultivating a quiet, focused, unwavering mind and a peaceful life. However, the hard arts, such as Karate, are also different from the soft arts. They focus on developing muscular power and speed, and the mastery of breaking and throwing techniques delivered with devastating impact. The harsh combative practice functions as a whetstone to polish and sharpen the self.

Depending on the character, attitudes, and behavior of the instructor and student, both the soft and hard arts can be practiced harshly and be abused. Some martial artists are initially attracted to the power, mistaking it for aggression, and never growing beyond their desire to indulge in hostile and destructive action. Others are drawn to these arts out of a concern for increasing self-confidence and self-protection, then transcend the physical strength training and mature into disciplined philosophical and spiritual practitioners.

You're more likely to run into the problem of roughness in a hard form such as Karate than in a soft one such as T'ai Chi. That's because, generally, the external martial arts more obviously seem to be about sheer physical power. Popular movies have portrayed them as a display of brutal force. Nevertheless, they are based on the same principles as the soft styles—centering and respect. You can use them as a vehicle for developing relaxed but alert power. For example, *Goju-Ryu* (*Goju* means "hard/soft"), a style of Karate established on Okinawa, combines external fighting techniques with internal Chinese principles. Although its founder, Master Chojun Miyagi (1888–1953), possessed enormous physical strength, his greatest asset was a gentle manner. He never used Karate to hurt another human being.[8]

Historically, sparring and actual combat have brought about a wide variety of injuries. Many martial artists learned traditional healing practices—herbal preparations, pressure-point therapy, and bone-setting—to treat lesions of muscles, joints, bones, ligaments, and tendons. In Japan *ku-atsu*, a system of emergency care, developed to resuscitate victims of harmful blows. It includes percussive movements with a reflexogenic action,

Mastering others is strength: mastering yourself is true power.

—Tao Te Ching

The more flexible and resilient is your body, the more secure is its relation to gravity and the more enduring its vitality.

—Mary Bond

To lift the spirit up
to the crown,
Sink the chi down to
the tan-tien.

—Wang Tsung-yu

compression for restoring respiration, and external cardiac massage. Traditionally, a martial arts master was likely to demonstrate not only technical proficiency but also competence as a healer.[9]

At the heart of both internal and external martial arts is concentration of the chi at a point two inches or four fingers' width below the navel and deep in the center of the body. This vital place is known as *tantien* ("heavenly field") in Chinese and *tanden* in Japanese. The Japanese term *hara* is the more popularly used word for the belly area.[10] From here, you can then move energy to distant areas in the body. All movements, balance, and power in the martial arts radiate from this core. It is both your physical center of gravity and your psychic center of spirit or essential life force. "The pelvis is the governor of one's whole body," says T'ai Chi Chuan master Alfred Huang.[11]

This foundation can serve you in several ways. When you learn to move from your center, you have a way of facing the world as a whole person—not from your head, not from right or left, but directly from your "home base." By knowing your center, as well as sensing where your body is at all times, where your weight and equilibrium are, you develop strength and confidence for being in the world. Internal martial arts are about meeting constant change with groundedness, fluidity, and a relaxed softness that is resilient and flexible.

### RESOURCES:

For a quarterly review that includes scholarly articles on primary research, informal interviews with master practitioners, reports on particular styles and techniques, and reviews of books and audiovisual materials, see *Journal of Asian Martial Arts,* Via Media Publishing Co., 821 W. 24th St., Erie, PA 16502, (800) 455-9517. See also *Shuhari: A Journal of the Martial Arts,* Atrium Society Publications, P.O. Box 816, Middlebury, VT 05753, (802) 388-0922. There is also the National Women's Martial Arts Federation, P.O. Box 4688, Corpus Christi, TX 78469, (512) 855-6975. For an overview: John Corcoran, Emil Farkas, and Stuart Sobel, *The Original Martial Arts Encyclopedia: Tradition, History, Pioneers* (Pro-Action, 1993); Donn Draeger and Robert W. Smith, *Comprehensive Asian Fighting Arts* (Kodansha, 1981); Paul Crompton, *The Complete Martial Arts* (McGraw-Hill, 1989).

## CHINESE TRADITION

The roots of Chinese movement and martial arts are steeped in legend. Some say that Taoist monks originated these practices as early as the fifth century B.C.E. Out of a need to integrate physical exercise appropriate to their meditation and simple existence, they imitated animal and bird gestures. Other stories focus on the role of Bodhidharma, a monk who came from India around 600 C.E. to the Shao-lin Temple, a Ch'an (*Zen* in Japanese) Buddhist monastery built on Song-shan Mountain in Honan province by Emperor Hsiao-Wen in 496 C.E. Bodhidharma may have taught the monks martial exercises for the purposes of defending against bandits and/or strengthening themselves to withstand the rigors of meditation.[12]

No single individual is responsible for the development of practices for manipulating chi inside and outside the body; more likely it was a collective effort over centuries. Through breathing skills and movement exercises, the monks learned to use their minds to direct energy in the body in order to attain greater physical health, mental clarity, and spiritual depth. Eventually their ways became known in ancient China as a method to promote health and prolong life.

# Chi Kung

If you watched Bill Moyers's trip to China in *Healing and the Mind,* broadcast on PBS in 1993, you probably remember the fantastic demonstrations by masters of *Qi Gong* (the name is a variation of *Chi Kung,* pronounced "chee gung").[13] Translated as "working with life energy" or "breathing skill," it is the art and science of using breath, slow movement, visualization, and meditation to cleanse, gather, and circulate chi. By powerfully concentrating chi in their tantien, elderly men not only resist the attacks of strong young men but actually move their opponents' chi, flinging their bodies away without ever physically touching them. Attaining such levels of mastery can entail at least twenty years of rigorous discipline.

This cultivation of chi can lead to a long and healthy life, martial skill, and spiritual growth. Millions of people in China regularly practice some form of Chi Kung in parks, city plazas, and docks. They use it in health maintenance, sports training, and outpatient medical treatment. For example, extensive research with thousands of hypertension patients at a Shanghai hospital since 1958 indicates that by doing Chi Kung the majority experienced dramatic improvement. Daily practice lowers blood pressure, pulse rate, metabolic rate, and oxygen demand. Chi Kung activates the body's self-regulating systems responsible for balanced functioning of tissues, organs, and glands.[14]

There is also an external Chi Kung, which some masters and traditional Chinese doctors apply to help heal others. They learn how to sense places of excess or deficient chi in a patient and then project chi accordingly, by the lightest touch or, more often, by no touch at all. Standing several feet

If you are centered, you can move freely. The physical center is your belly; if your mind is set there as well, you are assured of victory in any endeavor.

—Morihei Ueshiba

# Ringing the Gong: A Chi Kung Experience

Before you try this, notice how you're feeling. Are you restless, tired, tense, or sleepy? Are you angry, sad, happy, upset?

Stand with your feet hip-width apart, knees and pelvis soft, and shoulders relaxed. You can open your chest by drawing your shoulder blades slightly down and together. Begin turning, starting at your ankles and incorporating your knees, then thighs and hips, before allowing a natural swing of your arms to come into play.

Movement #1: As you twist around to the right and to the left, one arm will fling across the front, the palm of that hand slapping the opposite upper arm. Simultaneously, the upper surface of the other hand will slap the lower back as the arm comes around. It's as though you were wearing a jacket and the sleeves (without your arms in them) were flapping loosely around as you turned your body now this way, now that way. Maintain a soft focus with your eyes as you swing around gently and loosely several times to warm up and get used to the movement.

Movement #2: As you continue turning, let your hands form open fists. Don't close them tight and hard or you will smash your body each time your fists land. Your right fist swings behind and hits your left lower back in the kidney area (just above

Figure A

away from the patient, the Chi Kung master first moves his body and arms in certain classical, formalized ways and then points his outstretched arm at the patient and sends chi.[15] The patient may experience sensations of warmth, weight, vibration, and expansiveness. In traditional Chinese hospitals, this external chi healing is used to treat the same range of illnesses as acupuncture. It has been reported successful in multiple sclerosis, headaches, insomnia, soft tissue injuries, asthma, peptic ulcers and other gastrointestinal illnesses, neurological disorders, arthritis, cancer, internal organ conditions, back pain, joint aches such as arthritis, and even cystic fibrosis.[16]

Through the centuries, there have been some 3,600 schools of Chi Kung, according to David Eisenberg, M.D., the American physician who studied traditional medicine in China and later accompanied Bill Moyers there. Chinese researchers today are investigating a hundred distinct varia-

your waist) as your left fist lands under your right breast (figure A). Then reverse, with your left fist at right lower back and right fist at left lower ribs. Try to do eight repetitions. Stay loose and keep your gaze soft and unfocused at eye level.

Movement #3: Now, repeating this swinging motion, move up your right fist so that it lands on the area between the clavicle (your collar bone) and breast while the left fist continues to hit the kidney area, and vice versa (figure B). Try this eight times.

Now reverse the order of the movements. From #3, move down to repeat #2. Follow that with one last time of doing #1 so that you end by loosely swinging around as you did at the beginning. With some practice, you'll move up and then down smoothly, without having to figure out which hand should go where.

Once you stop, check how you feel. Do you notice any changes? Hitting these areas with your fists means you're making contact with points on different meridians, which can result in a variety of benefits. Gazing softly helps relax your eyes.

Figure B

tions.[17] You can learn to do a Chi Kung massage for yourself and practice the circulation of chi.

## RESOURCES:

For instruction, check with local martial arts supplies stores, practitioners of traditional Oriental medicine, and Taoist centers. You can also find listings of workshops and seminars, books and videos in the magazine *T'ai Chi,* Wayfarer Publications, P.O. Box 26156, Los Angeles, CA 90026 (800) 888-9119 or (213) 665-7773, fax (213) 665-1627.

**Books:** Danny Connor and Michael Tse, *Qigong: Chinese Movement and Meditation for Health* (Weiser, 1992); Tsu Kuo Shih, *Qi Gong Therapy: The*

# Healing with Chi Kung

When Craig Reid moved to the Republic of China in 1979, he was slowly dying from cystic fibrosis. An incurable hereditary disease that causes obstruction in the digestive and respiratory systems, it affects principally infants and children, often killing them before they reach the age of twenty-one. Reid had already been undergoing heavy medication and painful therapies for more than seventeen years when he decided to find a Chi Kung teacher. About five months after learning this healing movement art, he completely dropped his former regimen and has maintained his health ever since.

While in China, Reid witnessed other striking recoveries. Heather Singlewitch, an American gymnast who once ranked sixteenth in the nation, underwent total reconstructive knee surgery after tearing her anterior cruciate ligament. Physicians thought she would never compete again, nor even walk normally. But a Chi Kung doctor "read" her leg, determined exactly where she had pain, and then moved it down her leg and out through her foot. He never touched her, except with chi. For six months she received three treatments weekly. She fully regained her strength and flexibility, returned to gymnastics, and competed without pain, a limp, or a knee brace. Reid also reports the case of an elderly man whose right forearm had been paralyzed for thirteen years. After only a two-hour treatment, he finally reached out his arm, opened his formerly clenched fist, and shook the hand of the Chi Kung doctor who had reversed a condition that physical therapy three times a week for twelve years had barely improved.[18]

*Chinese Art of Healing with Energy* (Station Hill, 1994); Lily Siou, *Ch'i-Kung: The Art of Mastering the Unseen Life Force* (Charles E. Tuttle, 1975); Masaru Takahashi and Stephen Brown, *Qigong for Health: Chinese Traditional Exercise for Cure and Prevention* (Japan Publications, 1986); Bruce Kumar Frantzis, *Opening the Energy Gates of Your Body: Gain Lifelong Vitality* (North Atlantic, 1993); Lam Kam Chuen, *The Way of Energy: Mastering the Chinese Art of Internal Strength with Chi Kung Exercise* (Simon & Schuster, 1991); Mantak Chia, *Awaken Healing Energy Through the Tao* (Healing Tao, 1983), *Iron Shirt Chi Kung* (Healing Tao, 1986), and *Bone Marrow Nei Kung* (Healing Tao/Charles E. Tuttle, 1989); Charles T. McGee, M.D., with Effie Poy Yew Chow, *Miracle Healing from China . . .* Qigong (MediPress, 1994).

**Audiovisual:** "Chi Gung: Opening the Energy Gates" and "Chi Gung: Marriage of Heaven and Earth," 68-min. and 82-min. videotapes, Kumar Frantzis, P.O. Box 99, Fairfax, CA 94978-0099, (415) 454-5243; "Qigong," lecture and seminar videotapes of teachers from People's Republic of

China, World Research Foundation, 15300 Ventura Blvd., Suite 405, Sherman Oaks, CA 91403, (818) 907-5483, fax (818) 907-6044; "Chi-kung for Health," 90 mins., Terry Dunn, White Rose, (800) 374-5505; "The Way of Chi Kung," 5 audiocassettes, and "Chi Kung Meditations," 60-min. tape, Ken Cohen, Sounds True, (800) 333-9185.

# T'ai Chi Chuan

*T'ai Chi Chuan,* or T'ai Chi (pronounced "tie-jee") for short, means "supreme ultimate fist." It is based on the Taoist principles that life is a balance between the opposite forces of yin and yang, health is the unimpeded flow of chi, and the ideal is harmony with nature and our fellow human beings. The T'ai Chi symbol is the same as that for yin and yang, for the practice is a dynamic interaction of both in pursuing a middle state between soft and hard forces. According to Jay Dunbar, an American T'ai Chi instructor, forms of this art go back only to the mid-seventeenth century and the name itself probably originated with Wu Yux-iang (1812–1880). Traditionally, the system had three distinct components: postures done solo, push hands with a partner, and weapons training. However, today the latter is rare, especially in the West. For generations T'ai Chi was handed down only through particular families, which gave rise to four basic styles: Chen and Yang, the two oldest; Wu, which evolved from Yang; and Sun. The Chen Family preserved the early forms and invented "push hands"; the Yang family popularized T'ai Chi starting in the 1800s.

> The soft overcomes the hard; the gentle overcomes the rigid.
>
> —Tao Te Ching

In the twentieth century the family restriction ended and now T'ai Chi is available to the general public, most of whom practice it more for its health-giving aspects than for its combative purposes. For example, a study conducted in eight cities in the United States indicates that exercise such as T'ai Chi for a period of ten to thirty-six weeks helps to improve balance and reduce the risk of falls and injury in people age sixty to seventy-five for up to two to four years.[19] American T'ai Chi instructors report that among their students the practice helps especially in relief of back and spinal conditions, high blood pressure and hypertension, stress-related disorders, arthritis and rheumatism, and knee disorders.[20]

As with Chi Kung, you can see Chinese performing the graceful motions starting at the break of dawn in the parks and plazas of Beijing and other cities, including the Chinatowns and parks of New York City and San Francisco. In fact, T'ai Chi was first taught in North America by Chinese teachers to Chinese students in Chinese communities. The first American to teach was Sophia Delza, beginning in New York in 1960. But the teacher who exerted the greatest influence on T'ai Chi here is Chang Man-Ch'ing, for his Yang short form is more widely practiced than any other.[21]

At the core of T'ai Chi practice is the "long form," a series of 108 linked contrasting movements, each with its own evocative name, such as White Crane Spreads Its Wings, Parting Wild Horse's Mane, and Waving Hands in Clouds. The Yang style short form consists of thirty-seven postures, but others may have as few as eighteen movements.

You do not hold T'ai Chi postures statically or rigidly. Rather, you let yourself flow uninterruptedly from one into another. If you perform them with calmness, clarity, equilibrium, and awareness, they are said to be like a "never-ending river."[22] You constantly shift or "empty" your body's weight from one leg to the other, alternately contract and relax leg muscles, raise and lower arms, rotate from side to side, change directions in space, and so on. All these opposites represent the active interplay of yin and yang. Moving in perfect balance means there is no strain on any part of your body. You are able to embody grounding, alignment, and mindfulness in motion, as well as awareness of the space around you.

Because you move in a slow, circular, and relaxed manner, traditionally practice began at forty, the age at which the Chinese believe you have dissipated the energetic vigor of youth and achieved greater tranquillity and patience. T'ai Chi is about rest and quiet in movement.

Once you learn how to do the form precisely alone, you can study "push hands" with a partner. You face each other on a diagonal, with the back of one wrist and lower forearm resting against those of the partner. Without moving feet, one of you moves your whole body by shifting your weight, gently pushing the other one, who yields, shifting back, rather than resists and then uses circular movement to push you back. You continue in a circle of advance/retreat and yield/initiate. You also learn how to keep your equilibrium. These lessons in weight, balance, and psychological reactions to others afford the opportunity to transform old patterns of being pushed around into new patterns of relaxed alertness and flexible stability.

Awareness of your body from both internal and external perspectives has many advantages. Once you feel where your weight rests and sense your balance from the inside out, you can move entirely from your center. This means you're always facing the world from that core place—the middle of your being—and seeing things directly in front of you rather than looking away. In that regard, it seems to be good training for literally confronting life. And by moving fluidly, connecting to all parts of yourself, you can move efficiently and avoid injuries. You can breathe, relax, and respond more easily. All of this can bring confidence and inner strength. Eventually T'ai Chi becomes more than a brief daily practice; it becomes a new way of life. And you can do it anywhere, wearing no special uniform, only loose, comfortable clothing.

When you stand with your two feet on the ground, you will always keep your balance.

—Tao Te Ching

Nothing in the world is as soft and yielding as water. Yet for dissolving the hard and inflexible, nothing can surpass it.

—Tao Te Ching

# Experience: The Basic T'ai Chi Stance

The basic stance is crucial for doing any T'ai Chi movement. You need to be aware of your center—*tantien*—and your position in space. If it's possible, try to have this experience barefoot outdoors on level ground. To come to the fundamental posture, work from the bottom up. Begin by standing with your feet apart, placed directly under your hips. Feel the contact your soles make with the ground. Check to see that your weight is evenly distributed: Are you leaning more on your heels, toes, balls of your feet, inside or outside edges? Adjust accordingly.

To find that place of balance throughout your body, explore to discover the point between holding yourself rigid and collapsing. For example, first lock your knees, then let them go limp. How does each extreme feel? Do you notice your weight shift forward or backward of center? Do you feel stable and ready for movement in those positions? Play with them until you find an intermediate place from which you could move confidently.

Now focus on your pelvis. Move between the opposites by tilting your pelvis forward and back. Notice what happens to your chest and center of gravity when you do this. Again, do you feel stable and ready for action from these positions, or are you off balance? As before, play between these two extremes until you find the midway point where you can stand relaxed yet alert. Last, involve your head. Notice how you feel when you push your chin forward or pull it in toward your throat. Experiment until you come to the middle, where your head sits comfortably in alignment with your spine. Allow the top of your head to reach lightly upward.

Keep your balance here, simultaneously sinking into the ground and reaching toward heaven, as though you had a sky hook pulling you up and roots in your feet holding you down. Breathe in a relaxed manner from the center of your body. If you can stand with ease, turn your attention to what that feels like inside. What are your checkpoints for knowing you're standing from your center? Use these benchmarks as reminders for finding your way back to this position.

If you want to experiment with this basic posture, let your weight "empty" from one leg into the other as you move from side to side. Notice that you don't have to make your legs rigid to keep your balance. You can move more effortlessly when you let your legs feel soft but not limp.

But don't be surprised if your initial experience is frustrating, especially if you've never engaged in the slow, smooth process typical of such an art. It's nothing like aerobics, Western sports, or calisthenics—you can't go on automatic. Years of exercise and Yoga didn't prepare me for my first T'ai Chi class. It was like starting in kindergarten all over again. I just didn't get it—the fluidity, the stance, the positioning of arms and legs. But I reminded myself that this awkwardness is what most people feel when studying something new. Once learned, it requires only twenty to twenty-five minutes of practice daily for its health benefits to be conferred.

The traditional Asian teaching style emphasized a one-on-one, master-disciple relationship; a teacher individualized instructions and curriculum for each student and judged his or her proficiency. However, in North America, you can learn to do T'ai Chi in a room full of other students without having such a close relationship. Because there are different forms, derived from different lineages, and learned from different instructors, there is no national standard regulating T'ai Chi. Neither does this movement art lend itself to competitions; it is not a sport.

> The soft overcomes the hard.
> The slow overcomes the fast.
>
> —Tao Te Ching

RESOURCES:

To find a T'ai Chi instructor, ask at your local martial arts supplies store and among practitioners of traditional Chinese medicine, and check the "Martial Arts" listing in the Yellow Pages. Seminars and workshops are also listed in *T'ai Chi,* an international magazine published by Wayfarer Publications, P.O. Box 26156, Los Angeles, CA 90026, (213) 665-7773 or (800) 888-9119. See also *Wu Style T'ai Chi Practitioners of North America* (On-Line, 1993). A more scholarly publication is *Journal of Asian Martial Arts,* Via Media Publishing Co., 821 W. 24th St., Erie, PA 16502, (800) 455-9517, fax (814) 838-7811. There are organizations and publications representing the different styles. One such group is T'ai Chi Chuan/Shaolin Chuan Association, P.O. Box 430, Geneva, IL 60134, (708) 232-0029.

**Books:** *The Essence of T'ai Chi Ch'uan: The Literary Tradition,* translated and edited by Benjamin Pang Jeng Lo, Martin Inn, Robert Amacker, and Susan Foe (North Atlantic, 1979); *Cheng Man-ch'ing, Cheng Tzu's Thirteen Treatises on T'ai Chi Ch'uan* (North Atlantic, 1985), and *T'ai Chi Ch'uan: A Simplified Method of Calisthenics for Health and Self-Defense* (North Atlantic, 1981); Chen Wei-ming, *T'ai Chi Ch'uan Ta We: Questions and Answers on T'ai Chi Ch'uan,* translated by Benjamin Pang Jeng Lo and Robert W. Smith (North Atlantic, 1985); Wolfe Lowenthal, *There Are No Secrets: Professor Chen Man-ch'ing and His T'ai Chi Ch'uan* (North Atlantic, 1991), and *Gateway to the Miraculous* (North Atlantic, 1994); Stuart Alve Olson, compiler and translator, *Cultivating the Ch'i: The Secrets of Energy and Vitality* (Dragon Door, 1993).

**Audiovisual:** "T'ai Chi," Waysun Liao, T'ai Chi Center, 433 South Boulevard, Oak Park, IL 60302; "T'ai Chi for Health Series" [short and long forms], Terry Dunn, 120 mins. each, VHS, (800) 333-9185; "T'ai Chi Chuan: Total Exercise for Mind and Body," Nancy Kwan and Bernie Pock, 60 mins., VHS.

## JAPANESE TRADITION

# Aikido

*Aikido* (pronounced "eye-kee-doh") is a relatively new martial art, founded by Morihei Ueshiba (1883–1969) in Japan in the first decades of the twentieth century. *Ai* means "harmony" or "love," *ki* is "vital energy" or "spirit," and *do* is "the way": "the way of harmony with universal energy" or "the way of a loving spirit."

Ueshiba developed Aikido primarily out of *Daito Ryu Aiki-jitsu,* a battlefield combat art. For many centuries, martial arts were used by the *bushi,* the warrior class, for attack and defense (*samurai* were the highest-ranking warriors). However, in the latter 1800s, when Japan emerged from its long feudal period, many military arts shifted and became more concerned with physical, mental, and spiritual training—body-mind unification—than with fighting. Aikido is a modern form that arose out of this change from *Bujutsu* ("techniques of combat") to *Budo* ("way of combat").

As a young man, Ueshiba mastered several Japanese martial arts, including techniques with weapons. But, influenced by Japanese religious beliefs, he became dissatisfied with the warrior philosophy. One day, while drawing water at a well, he had an enlightenment experience, which made him realize that "the heart of *budo* was not contention but rather love, a love that fosters and protects all things."[23] Thereafter, he defined Aikido as "the manifestation of Love," and called budo "a Path of Peace."[24]

Ueshiba preserved the swift and precise movement of the old fighting arts but wanted Aikido to become a nonviolent school of self-mastery, not a way of warring. Thus it is designed to free you of psychological and muscular barriers and enable you to feel alive and in complete harmony with yourself, others, and nature. For example, instructor Wendy Palmer uses Aikido exercises for cultivating awareness and attention, releasing fear, and developing trust in the body's wisdom.[25] In a state of mental and physical balance, you can anticipate the attacking movements of opponents, block or deflect them by harmonizing your ki and movement with theirs, and then immobilize attackers by placing them in a lock or pin where their joints and muscles cannot function.

The true martial art is the one that defeats an enemy without sacrificing a single man; attain victory by placing yourself always in a safe and unassailable position. . . . True budo is for the sake of peace and harmony; train daily to manifest this spirit throughout the world.

—Morihei Ueshiba

# The Unbendable Arm: An Aikido Experience

Aikido emphasizes physical softness and mental energy rather than effort and strength. Focused awareness and full commitment, not physical resistance, are what provide the power behind Aikido defense techniques. To get a sense of this, try doing the Unbendable Arm with a partner.

Stand in front of your partner and put your right arm over his or her left shoulder. Keep your elbow slightly bent and pointed at the floor. Have your partner put both hands on top of your elbow and push down to bend it. She or he can build up to as hard a push as desired, but it has to be gradual so that there is no risk of injury. Your task is to keep your arm strong so it doesn't bend.

After you've tried this, stop to reflect on what you did. Most people get as stiff and hard as they can, and then resist with all their might. If that's what you did, was it successful as a way of not having your arm bent? Was it comfortable? Did it take great effort and energy?

Here's another way to try it. Put your hand back on your partner's shoulder. This time, unclench your hand, gently open your fingers, and point all of them at an imaginary flower growing on a hillside in front of you. Without straining, reach your fingertips toward the flower, moving them a little closer in order to touch it. Let your breathing and whole body stay relaxed. Keep your focus on r-e-e-eaching toward the flower. Now have your partner push down on your elbow to bend it. Be sure not to resist. But don't go limp, either. Just continue your steady concentration on reaching gently toward the flower. Be aware of your partner, but don't get involved in struggling. If you are truly concentrating on the flower and not fighting against your partner, he or she will not be able to bend your arm. It is because you're not resisting that you will not lose. This is the power of gentle focus. Without getting tense and hard, you can remain unaffected by your partner's force.

—Courtesy of Paul Linden, Aikido instructor.

"If one's mind is steady and pure," said Ueshiba, "one can immediately perceive aggression and counter it—that . . . is the essence of *aiki*."[26] Achieving this calls for constant practice in the development of ki, which is the basis of powerful technique. *Kokyu,* deep breathing from the hara, sets the ki in motion and involves perfect synchronization of breathing and movement.

There are hundreds of Aikido movements, including holds, locks, throws, blows, breakfalls, rolls, and escapes. Fundamental are fluid three-dimensional, circular, spiral motions and rapidly changing positions and footwork you use to meet an attack of any force from any direction.

Like the Chinese internal martial arts, Aikido is not a contest of strength. Size and physical power are not factors in whether you can master the art. When you perform the movements precisely, with great skill, they require no undue effort or extraordinary physical force, but call for concentration and groundedness ("sinking down" the hara). Correctly done, Aikido allows the gentle to control the strong.

As physical exercise, Aikido can increase flexibility, strength, and co-ordination. It also fosters control, calmness, focused awareness, and self-confidence so that you can deal with stressful situations and resolve conflicts in a harmonious way. It is instinctive to become tense and make certain self-protective gestures when confronted with aggression, but this response can put you in an unstable stance in which you are less able to defend yourself. Aikido reconditions you so that you learn to stand from a solid base and to move freely and in a relaxed manner with your whole body.

Aikido requires a special training uniform, *aikidogi* (pants, jacket, and belt), and includes a grading system, *kyu/dan,* to indicate level of technical ability. An instructor, *sensei,* teaches students in a training hall, *dojo* ("place for studying the way"), where you observe formal discipline and etiquette. After the basics, training can include a wooden sword or short staff, and you may practice with multiple attackers. As a beginning student, you do not have to take hard falls. You do only as much as is safe and appropriate. In more advanced training, you take hard falls.

In general, most mainstream Aikido styles forbid competitions. The basic techniques are considered too dangerous to do in an unrestrained, aggressive fashion. Also, winning a fight rather than resolving conflict peacefully is antithetical to Aikido's true spirit.

Initially, Ueshiba taught his secret art only to selected pupils, but after World War II Aikido became open to many others, with both women and men practicing under the same conditions on the same level. Since his death, Ueshiba's disciples have established different styles and schools, but the purpose of all of them is "to better people's lives, to make their spirits blossom and become strong, and by making better people to make a better world," according to Mitsugi Saotome, one of his principal students.[27] Some Aikido instructors apply its principles in contemporary life to education, health, conflict resolution, parenting, sports, and spiritual development.[28]

> The hard and stiff will be broken.
> The soft and supple will prevail.
> —Tao Te Ching

RESOURCES:

To find a dojo, look under "Martial Arts" in the Yellow Pages, inquire at martial arts supplies shops, or contact the U.S. Aikido Federation, 142 W. 18th St., New York, NY 10011, (212) 242-6246, or 98 State St., Northampton, MA 01060, (413) 586-7122. Dojo directories, classes, and book and video reviews appear in the two major periodicals: *Aikido Today Magazine,* Areté Press, P.O. Box 1060, Claremont, CA 91711-1060, (909) 624-7770, fax (909) 398-1840, and *Aikido Journal,* c/o Aiki News Business Office, Tamagawa Gakuen 5-11-25-204, Machida-shi, Tokyo 194, Japan, phone/fax 81-427-24-9119, Compuserve 70272,1542, or in the United States (800) 877-2693.

**Books:** Gozo Shioda, *Dynamic Aikido,* translated by Geoffrey Hamilton (Kodansha, 1985); John Stevens, *Aikido: The Way of Harmony* (Shambhala, 1985), and *Abundant Peace: The Biography of Morihei Ueshiba, Founder of Aikido* (Shambhala, 1987); Mitsugi Saotome, *Aikido and the Harmony of Nature* (Shambhala, 1993), and *The Principles of Aikido* (Shambhala, 1989); Morihei Ueshiba, *Budo: The Teachings of Morihei Ueshiba, the Founder of Aikido* (Kodansha, 1991), *The Art of Peace,* translated by John Stevens (Shambhala, 1992), *The Essence of Aikido: The Spiritual Teachings of Morihei Ueshiba,* translated by John Stevens, edited by Eric Chaline (Kodansha, 1994); A. M. Westbrook and O. Ratti, *Aikido and the Dynamic Sphere* (Charles E. Tuttle, 1970); Yoshimitsu Yamada and Steven Pimsler, *The New Aikido Complete: The Arts of Power and Movement* (Carol, 1981); Kisshomaru Ueshiba, *The Spirit of Aikido,* translated by Taitetsu Unno (Kodansha, 1988).

**Audiovisual:** Check the two Aikido periodicals for listings.

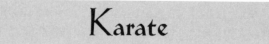

# Karate

*Karate* ("empty hand" or "bare fist") is a native Okinawan fighting style. Like most martial arts of that island, it traces its origin to Chinese schools. It developed when, starting in the late 1400s, the Okinawans were forbidden by Chinese and Japanese invaders to possess any arms. Gichin Funakoshi (1869–1957) brought this weaponless self-defense system to Japan in the early 1900s.

When most people think of Karate, they conjure an image of people breaking boards, or bricks. But that is not the objective of this martial art. You train in Karate to develop coordination of mind and body and to be calm and aware in any situation, whether fighting for your life or embracing a loved one. In Japanese this is called *fudoshin,* imperturbable mind. Contrary to its movie image, Karate is not merely aggression and brutality. It is a system of personal development by means of hard, physical training that generates power. By forcing yourself to produce maximum physical power in both attacking and defending, you can break through the limitations and restrictions that obscure your true self.

It's true that, originally, the striking techniques were intended for genuine combat. But in the twentieth century Funakoshi's son, Yoshitaka,

## An Experience in Karate: Breaking the Pencil

Get a new wooden pencil. Hold one end of it firmly in your left hand (if you're right-handed; otherwise, switch), with your palm down and the length of the pencil sticking out to the right; put the exposed end on the edge of a table. Hold your right hand in front of you with your palm facing left (thumb on top). In that position, your hand is positioned the way a knife blade would be. Raise your hand, bring it down on the pencil, and chop through it.

What do you think of before you do this? Are you hesitant? Are you afraid of getting hurt? Do you feel your muscles drawing away from the pencil even as you chop down on it? That self-doubt is the focus of much learning in Karate. Imagine the feelings you might have as you prepare to break a brick with your hand. Or imagine having to break a thousand pencils, one after another. The point of employing physical force and repetition is to encourage your self-doubts to surface—and then to master them.

—Courtesy of Zachary Smith and Paul Linden, black belts in Karate.

transformed Karate from a lethal sporting method into the gentler, modern Karate-do (*do* is Japanese for the Chinese *tao*) whose main motto, *Karate ni sente nashi,* means "Never strike the first blow," or "There is no first attack in Karate." A student must always aim to be "inwardly humble and outwardly gentle. True karate . . . strives internally to train the mind to develop a clear conscience enabling one to face the world truthfully, while externally developing strength until one may overcome even ferocious wild animals. Mind and technique are to become one."[29]

Karate practice is composed of *kihon* (basic movements of blocking, punching, and kicking), *kata* (linked movements, a shadow dance of fighting an opponent), sparring (unprogrammed combat practice), and self-defense applications. The power behind these actions is derived not from body size but from mastery of balance, timing, speed, and degree of movement. Proficiency results from precisely combining these factors with muscular strength, concentration, rhythm, proper breathing, and centeredness.

Practice takes place in a *dojo,* or training hall, where you wear a two-piece white outfit (*gi* or *keikogi*) and a colored belt to indicate your grade or degree of mastery according to a *kyu/dan* scale. In that setting you follow formal rules of etiquette and ethics. You learn basic stances and moves alone before working with a partner. A common expression in Karate is: "Learn the form. Keep the form. Break the form." Only after mastering the form can you give it up and do whatever movements emerge spontaneously, not unlike a classically trained musician who later becomes an improvisational jazz pianist. Just as in the soft form of T'ai Chi, freedom comes only after many years of discipline.

Today, you can get involved in Karate as self-defense art, meditation form, or sport (for which there are competitions and tournaments).

> The highest form of martial arts is love, with an awareness of yourself and everything around.
>
> —Anonymous

## RESOURCES:

For instruction in your area, check the "Martial Arts" listing in the Yellow Pages or contact Pan-American Union of Karate-do Organizations (PUKO) and USA Karate Federation, 1300 Kenmore Blvd., Akron, OH 44314, (216) 753-3114.

**Books:** Gichin Funakoshi, *Karate-do Kyohan,* translated by Tsutomu Ohshima (Kodansha, 1973); Shoshin Nagamine, *The Essence of Okinawan Karate-do* (Charles E. Tuttle, 1976); Masatoshi Nakayama, *Dynamic Karate: Instruction by the Master* (Kodansha, 1974).

## INDIAN TRADITION

# Yoga

As with Chinese movement arts, the origins of Yoga are lost in the mists of time. Indian stone sculptures from as early as 3,000 B.C.E. demonstrate Yoga postures; five hundred years later, Hindu scriptures called the *Vedas* mention Yoga. While some people mistake it for an Indian religion, it is a universal art or discipline of conscious living. In fact, it may be the world's most ancient system for personal development—physical, mental, emotional, and spiritual.

Although it seems that Yoga is a newcomer on the American scene, it actually made its debut in the mid-1800s among groups of intellectual writers interested in the esoteric philosophies of the East. Then, when Swami Vivekananda appeared before thousands at the World's Fair in Chicago in 1893, he sparked even more interest, which led eventually to Yoga's current widespread popularity.

For a long time, Yoga was thought to be nothing more than bizarre cult practices: fakirs, snake charmers, and turban-wearing swamis bending themselves into human pretzels, walking on hot coals, or levitating. Gradually people realized they could enjoy and benefit from Yoga without subscribing to the traditional lifestyle of a foreign culture. They didn't have to give up their jobs, don white robes, and join an ashram. They could engage in Yoga for physical exercise and stress reduction.

Today Yoga is as much a part of Western daily life as jogging. You're more likely to meet a Yoga teacher wearing a colorful leotard than a white turban. You can get instruction on TV, in health spas and community centers, or at your local Y. Yoga has become mainstream enough to attract everyone from housewives to Fortune 500 executives and to appear in publications from *Good Housekeeping* to *The New York Times*. It even has become part of stress management programs at medical centers, such as those established by Dean Ornish, M.D., and Jon Kabat-Zinn, Ph.D. And for those individuals who want to explore the path of Yoga beyond its physical aspects and mental calming, its basic philosophy is still accessible.

*Yoga,* from the Sanskrit *yug,* means "yoke." This does not refer to an onerous yoking, but rather a union or joining of the individual self with the Divine, Universal Spirit, or Cosmic Consciousness, for that is the ultimate goal of Yoga. The Indian epic poem *Bhagavad Gita* (ca. 500 B.C.E.) calls it the "path on the Eternal and freedom from bondage."[30] The first systemized treatise on Yoga was the *Yoga Sutras* (ca. 200 B.C.E.), attributed to the physician-scholar Patanjali.

There are several paths of Yoga, including selfless service, devotion, and knowledge—all of which can help you reach the same final destination. In the West, *Raja* ("science of physical and mental control") is the most well known and most widely practiced. It consists of eight limbs, three of which comprise *Hatha* ("powerful" or "forceful") *Yoga asanas* (postures or poses), *pranayama* (breath regulation), and progressive relaxation. The other subdivisions of Raja are concerned with ethical and moral discipline, concentration, meditation, and unification.

Yoga is based on a fundamental principle in Indian philosophy that there are five layers or dimensions to human existence: the physical frame; the vital body, which is made up of *prana* (life energy); mind, which consists

Yoga is not a religion, it is crystallized truth.

—Selvarajan Yesudian and Elisabeth Haich

One always finds a form of yoga whenever there is a question of experiencing the sacred or arriving at complete mastery of oneself.

—Mircea Eliade

of emotions and thoughts; higher intellect; and the "abode of bliss," where inner peace and union with the Divine occur. Various elements of Yoga practice address all these levels as well as serve both preventive and therapeutic functions.

For example, asanas can release muscle tension, stretch and tone muscles, lubricate joints, massage internal organs, increase circulation, and, when used aerobically, even help in weight control. Pranayama slows the breath, expands lung capacity and respiration, builds up prana, and regulates its flow through invisible body channels called *nadis*. Other reputed benefits of Yoga are greater resistance to stress, a stronger immune system, a balanced nervous system, decreased cholesterol and blood sugar levels, and lower blood pressure. Practitioners report that it has alleviated such conditions as arthritis, scoliosis, back pain, insomnia, chronic fatigue, asthma, heart conditions, difficult menses, and more.

Because of Yoga's therapeutic results, the Preventive and Rehabilitative Cardiac Center at Cedars-Sinai Medical Center in Los Angeles combines gentle postures and breathing techniques for heart disease patients. At the University of Massachusetts Medical Center, the Stress Reduction and Relaxation Program includes Yoga poses along with its Mindfulness Meditation classes for patients with a wide range of medical problems, from headaches, blood pressure, and AIDS to chronic pain, cancer, and heart disease.

The physical practices were designed to develop a strong and healthy body and mind in preparation for self-transcendence. By intentionally awakening the body's psychospiritual energy, known as *kundalini shakti,* the yogi (practitioner of Yoga) can experience this "serpent power" rise through the seven centers or *chakras* of the body, ending in ecstasy at the crown. ☞ See page 297.

Asanas are comprised of movement sequences performed while standing, sitting, lying down, or balancing on your head, shoulders, or hands—bending forward, backward, and sideways, and twisting the spine. Generally you perform them slowly and meditatively, combining them with deep breathing. In a structured routine, each pose counterbalances the preceding one, stretching and strengthening. The asanas have names that reflect the animals and other forms they imitate—Fish, Cobra, Locust, Bow, Lotus, Crow, Triangle, Plough, Bridge, etc.

You can use these physical poses to explore your own limits in pain, fear, resistance, or separation, and investigate your attitude toward yourself, your body, and others. Do you rush into a posture, or do you carefully and consciously move into it? Do you release into a pose, or do you force your body to the point of pain and injury? Do you judge yourself and compete with others, or do you patiently and sensitively train your body so that you develop greater precision, flexibility, strength, balance, and groundedness?

Hatha Yoga is based on the principle that changes in consciousness can be brought about by setting in motion currents of certain kinds of subtler forces in the physical body.

—I. K. Taimni

In each pose there should be repose.

—B.K.S. Iyengar

# Experience: A Yoga Asana

The basic stance in Yoga is called Tadasana, or Mountain Pose. Like a mountain, you stand still, steady, and upright. Begin by placing your feet two to three inches apart. Establish your grounding by evenly distributing your weight between both legs, between both sides of the feet, and neither fully on your toes or heels. Keep your legs awake and alive but not rigid. Let your spine and neck stretch up. Let your arms hang straight by your sides, palms facing but not touching your thighs.

From Tadasana you can move into other standing postures, such as Vrksasana, or Tree Pose, which can increase muscle tone in your legs and give you a sense of poise and balance. Standing in Tadasana, bend either your right or left leg at the knee, placing the heel at the top of the inside of the opposite thigh, right where it meets your groin. Let your foot rest there (or if that's difficult, leave it just above the knee), with your toes pointing down. If you can maintain your equilibrium on the extended leg, join your palms at the center of your chest and slowly raise them together overhead as you straighten your arms. Breathe deeply several times before lowering your arms, separating your palms, and releasing your bent leg to return to Tadasana. Then repeat all of the above steps standing on the other leg.

Return to Tadasana and relax. Take a moment to notice how you feel.

Vrksasana: Yoga Tree Pose

Do you endlessly repeat the same postures you're comfortable with and proficient at, or do you challenge yourself to perform others?

In 1964 the renowned violinist Yehudi Menuhin expressed what he had already learned from doing Yoga:

The brain is the hardest
part of the body to ad-
just in asanas.
—B.K.S. Iyengar

Strength that has effort
in it is not what you
need; you need the
strength that is the
result of ease.
—Ida Rolf

The practice of Yoga over the past fifteen years has convinced me that most of our fundamental attitudes to life have their physical counterparts in the body. Thus comparison and criticism must begin with the alignment of our own left and right sides. . . . Impetus and ambition might begin with the sense of weight and speed that comes with free-swinging limbs. . . . Tenacity is gained by stretching in various Yoga postures for minutes at a time, while calmness comes with quiet, consistent breathing and the expansion of the lungs. Continuity and a sense of the universal come with the knowledge of the inevitable alternation of tension and relaxation in eternal rhythms.

What is the alternative? Thwarted, warped people condemning the order of things . . . the tragic spectacle of people working out their own imbalance and frustration on others.[31]

A wide variety of Yoga styles have arisen, either influenced by particular teachers and their lineage or as innovations in the West. Although the basic asanas and breathing exercises remain the same, how you do them, the order in which you do them, and what you focus on while doing them constitute the differences among the many schools. However, no matter which style you try, you don't need a special outfit, just comfortable, loose clothes and a mat.

If you don't know which style of Yoga you want to learn—for example, slow and inward-oriented, athletic, or philosophical—try several different classes. Once you decide what you prefer, be careful in choosing someone to work with. Traditionally, a Yoga disciple trained for years, even decades, until the guru felt he or she was ready to teach. Today, teacher training programs range from a few intensive days to a few years, and all of them may grant certification. Unlike the British Wheel of Yoga and the European Yoga Union, there is no North American official organization that regulates standards for Yoga teachers.

If you're a beginner, you'll have difficulty judging a teacher's level of expertise. Instead, look for other qualities, such as respect and carefulness. Beware of instructors who try to push you into poses you're not ready for. Trust your own judgment, for overly forceful adjustments can result in torn muscles, busted knees, and vertebral damage. Beware also of your own aggressiveness and competitiveness, for they'll just as easily lead to injuries. Check on how you feel after you've tried a class: Are you relaxed yet vitalized by the challenge? Do you look forward to more? Or are you depressed and upset, and does your body hurt?

# Yoga Styles

Although the Yoga teachers in India who are most well known in the West—Iyengar, Desikachar, and Jois—all studied with the great Yoga master Krishnamacharya, each one took the practice in a different direction. In turn, their students have also developed their own versions.

• Iyengar Yoga was founded by B.K.S. Iyengar, who is renowned for his rigorous and scientific approach to Yoga. His approach emphasizes great precision in the poses. You achieve this by paying strict attention to alignment and anatomy and, when necessary, by using such props as straps, blocks, blankets, and sandbags. This dramatically changed the nature of teaching Yoga, for the props allow anyone—even the rigid, weak, or elderly—to get into a pose. Classes tend to focus in great detail on only a few asanas so you can refine the movements. Because of Iyengar's kinesiological emphasis, teachers have been able to apply his style in a therapeutic or rehabilitative way. Iyengar Yoga is taught at hundreds of centers around the world, including in the British school system. Iyengar taught Yoga to Queen Elizabeth.

• Kripalu Yoga, developed by Amrit Desai, is less interested in structural detail and more concerned with your mental and emotional states as you hold a pose. It encourages a gentle, compassionate, and introspective approach toward yourself. By staying in a posture for a longer time than in most other styles, the Kripalu approach gives you the opportunity to explore and let go of emotional and spiritual blocks. This led practitioner Michael Lee to develop Phoenix Rising Yoga Therapy, in which Yoga therapists hold you at your physical limits until emotional tensions surface and release.

• Ashtanga Yoga, made popular by K. Patabhi Jois, seeks to generate heat through each fast-paced series of vinyasa (flowing asanas linked by the breath) and thus to purify and strengthen the body while also generating prana and channeling it up the spine. Each of the six progressively more difficult series has a different focus and intention. For example, the initial series is supposed to realign and purify the physical body, especially the spine. This style of Yoga provides such a vigorous workout that some people call it "power Yoga." It has become the latest fave rave as an aerobic fitness system that's calorie-burning, fat-melting, and body-sculpting, yet still meditative. Sweating is essential here because when your body heats up, your muscles will loosen, enabling you to prevent injuries and get into postures more easily. Working up a good sweat also eliminates waste products through your skin.

• White Lotus Yoga is Ganga White's modified version of the flowing energetic Ashtanga style.

• Tri Yoga, developed by California teacher Kali Ray, combines an Ashtanga-like nonstop, dancelike flow of postures with pranayama and meditation, there is music in the background.

• <u>Viniyoga,</u> as taught by T.K.V. Desikachar, is a highly individualized, gentle approach that adapts the poses to each student's unique body type, emotional needs, cultural heritage, and interests. Desikachar's school in Madras, India, has led the way in research on Yoga's positive effect in cases of schizophrenia, depression, mental retardation, asthma, and diabetes.

• <u>Integral Yoga,</u> from Swami Satchidananda, combines all the paths of Yoga—asanas, pranayama, selfless service, prayer, chanting, meditation, and self-inquiry—into one approach. The emphasis is more meditative than anatomical.

• <u>Sivananda Yoga,</u> originated by Swami Vishnudeva-nanda, is similar to Integral Yoga in integrating the same elements of Yoga, along with dietary restrictions and scriptural study. Lilias Folan, the TV Yoga teacher, studied this system first.

• <u>Istha Yoga,</u> established by Mani Finger and his son Alan, from South Africa, concentrates on opening subtle energy channels through postures, visualizations, and guided meditations.

• <u>Kundalini Yoga</u> focuses on arousing the kundalini energy, using asanas, pranayama, and meditation.

• <u>Hidden Language Yoga,</u> from Swami Sivananda Radha, a Western woman influenced by Jungian psychology, combines physical practice, journal-writing, and group discussion to investigate the symbolic meaning of each asana and the posture's effect on a student's mind and spirit.

• <u>Bikram Yoga,</u> developed by Bikram Choudhury at the University of Tokyo, focuses on repeating twenty-six specific postures and two breathing techniques in each class to stretch and tone the whole body. Based in Los Angeles, he is known as "Yoga teacher to the stars."[32]

### RESOURCES:

**For instruction:** look for classes at local YMCAs or YWCAs, community centers, schools, and health centers in your area. Leaf through the *Yoga Journal,* P.O. Box 3755, Escondido, CA 92033, especially the July/August issue, when the annual directory of Yoga teachers comes out; or try *Yoga International,* Himalayan Institute, RD 1, Box 88, Honesdale, PA 18431. You can also contact the International Association of Yoga Therapists (IAYT), 4150 Tivoli Ave., Los Angeles, CA 90066.

**Books:** There are several hundred books on Yoga presently in print, dealing with different aspects, not just Hatha. Some authors specifically address the practice to runners, pregnant women, children, older people, people in recovery, people with back problems, and so on. Here is only a sampling.

A. G. Mohan, *Yoga for Body, Breath, and Mind* (Rudra, 1995); Eleanor Criswell, *How Yoga Works: An Introduction to Somatic Yoga* (Freeperson, 1989); B.K.S. Iyengar, *Light on Yoga* (Schocken, 1975), and *The Tree of Yoga* (Shambhala, 1989); Georg Feuerstein and Stephan Bodian, eds., *Living Yoga: A Comprehensive Guide for Daily Life* (Jeremy P. Tarcher, 1993); Judith Lasater, *Relax and Renew: Restful Yoga for Stressful Times* (Rodwell Press, 1995); Lucy Liddell et al., *The Sivananda Companion to Yoga* (Simon & Schuster, 1983); Swami Vishnudevananda, *The Complete Illustrated Book of Yoga* (Crown, 1988); Beryl Birch, *Power Yoga: The Total Wellness Workout for Mind and Body* (Macmillan, 1995); Richard Hittelman, *Yoga for Health* (Ballantine, 1985).

**Audiovisual:** "*Yoga Journal*'s Yoga Practice Series," Patricia Walden, 4 videos, 60–80 mins. each, (800) 2-LIVING; "Yoga: A Complete Video Guide," Sivananda Yoga Retreat, 1 hr.; "Lilias! Alive with Yoga," 3 videos, 60 mins. each, (800) 280-0403 or (800) 876-7798; "Aerobic Yoga" (64 mins., video) and "Total Yoga" with Ganga White and Tracey Rich, (800) 544-FLOW; "Tri-Yoga, Level 1," Kali Ray, 70 mins., video, (800) 359-YOGA; "Iyengar on Video," many tapes, Mystic River Video, P.O. Box 716, Cambridge, MA 02140, (617) 483-YOGA; "Astanga Yoga: An Aerobic Yoga System," K. Patabhi Jois and Ray Rosenthal, video and book, Hart Productions; "Yoga in Motion" (Vinyasa), Theresa Elliott, (800) 781-4990; "Yoga with Richard Freeman" (Ashtanga), 120-min. video and booklet, (800) 334-8152; "Yoga Alignment and Form" (Iyengar), John Friend, (800) 334-8152.

# Convergence Systems

In a moment of empty
time, one can begin to
listen to the story of
one's flesh, and begin to
reformulate the meaning
of one's life. In the
hearing of the story,
past and future can
begin to be reconciled.

—Robert Kugelmann

In convergence systems, working with the body converges with working with the emotions, like two branches of the same creek flowing together.[1] The originators of these approaches found that, in touching or moving the body, they inevitably contacted the emotions as well. Through their hands, convergence practitioners help provide the context for an experience of healing. There is no decision ahead of time whether that healing is physical or emotional. These approaches are concerned not only with the convergence of body and psyche, but also with that of body and spirit, energy and structure, psyche and energy, psyche and spirit, and so on.

## WHERE BODY AND PSYCHE MEET

The convergence systems may be particularly helpful when you are confused, frustrated, or disappointed after many unsuccessful efforts to resolve stubborn physical difficulties. By dealing with your body and psyche simultaneously, they can penetrate to the core of persistent aches and pains. Their basic premise is that the body stores unresolved emotional experiences, those you could not handle and had to suppress. You may have had a healthy impulse to express yourself—for instance, to cry or yell—but if it was considered unacceptable behavior or you were in a life-threatening situation, you restrained yourself by tensing your muscles. Now, each time an event triggers a similar impulse to sadness or anger, you may find yourself automatically responding in that old way, even though it's no longer necessary. ☞ See Chapter 6: "Psychological Dimensions of Bodyways."

You may not be aware of the emotions you felt in the past and how you coped with them, but they still affect you. Those incidents shaped your body the way water and wind sculpt a canyon. You can see the old emotions in a collapsed or puffed-up chest, a head that hangs forward, or hunched-over shoulders. And they may be the source of troubling symptoms.

To facilitate lasting change, convergence practitioners believe intellectual understanding of your condition is inadequate; it is essential to address—indirectly or directly—the emotional holding behind the physical tension. While you cannot change the initial impact of long-ago incidents, you can release emotions, memories, and feelings held in the body and modify the postures into which they have formed you.

Convergence practitioners see themselves as facilitators or catalysts of change, not creators of it. They endeavor to follow your lead in which direction to take—that is, they align themselves with your inner efficiency expert. A truly skillful practitioner does not impose a particular therapeutic outcome, but provides a supportive and caring environment so that issues can emerge and be attended to.

To help you become consciously aware of your holdings, these bodyways add verbal dialogue to physical handling and/or movement. The originators of these approaches often discovered the value of talk during hands-on work with the body. For example, as a physical therapist, Marion Rosen, who created the Rosen Method®, noticed that those patients who spoke with her about the circumstances in their lives at the time of an accident or injury recovered most quickly. The combination of hands-on work and verbal techniques fosters a letting go of both physical and emotional tension.

Convergence practitioners acknowledge a client's emotions and help her or him to recognize, experience, and understand those emotions. But they are not psychologists, psychotherapists, or psychiatrists, and they don't claim to be. In striving for body-mind integration, their point of entry is the body, not the psyche. Their approaches are not talk therapy.

While the intention of these bodyways is not necessarily to instigate catharsis, repressed feelings often come out. However, such feelings do not have to be overpowering or overwhelming; they can produce useful information and insight. In turn, that new awareness can enable personal transformation; you see other ways you can express yourself and behave.

In the convergence systems, there is no massage with oils or lotions, nor is it necessary to remove clothing. You may find that resolution of a physical-emotional difficulty occurs in only one session, or you might explore certain issues over time. You make up your mind how long to engage in one of these therapies as you go along.

Unexpressed emotions tend to "stay" in the body like small ticking time bombs—they are illnesses in incubation.

—Christiane Northrup

Emotional release and muscular release are interdependent—one does not occur without the other.

—Elaine Mayland

# Rosen Method®

What is in your body is in your unconscious. If you think you know what it is, that isn't what it is. The holding is an unconscious holding. You cannot tell that story. The story you can tell is made up of what you have already handled.

—Marion Rosen

Marion Rosen was born in Germany in 1914 and started taking movement classes seven years later. In the 1930s she studied with Lucy Heyer, one of a group of therapists who used massage and breathwork with patients of Swiss psychoanalyst C. G. Jung. ☞ See Chapter 6: "Psychological Dimensions of Bodyways." Heyer's influences included, among others, Elsa Gindler and Rudolf Laban. ☞ See "Sensory Awareness," page 226, and "Laban-Bartenieff," page 248. When the Nazis forced Rosen to flee, she learned physical therapy in Sweden while awaiting a visa to the United States; she also graduated from the physical therapy program at the Mayo Clinic in Minnesota.

Rosen believes that people are born open—not holding back, down, or in. But as situations arise requiring you not to move or express emotions (for example, if your parents expected you to be a picture-perfect princess—quiet, well behaved, and never sad or needy), you lose your spontaneity and your muscles remain frozen in those holding positions. The Rosen Method aims at helping you gain or regain your natural state, in which the widest range of possibilities for expression and authentic spontaneous behavior exists. When chronic muscle tension no longer prevents it, you can move out of the contracted body and restricted worldview you've gotten cornered in and find your true space and size. A quote from *The Gnostic Gospel of Thomas* is often cited as the philosophy behind Rosen's approach: "If you bring forth what is within you, what you bring forth will save you. If you do not bring forth what is within you, what you do not bring forth will destroy you."

Rosen practitioners observe where you hold tension in your body and thus where your breath cannot move freely. Both your musculature and your breath are their guides to your emotions. They touch your body to determine which muscles remain tense even when you are lying down. With your awareness, you follow the practitioner's hands as they "meet" the tight muscles, also called "barriers." She or he uses a firmer or lighter touch depending on the amount of tension encountered. This touching reminds your muscles that they are holding and can let go. Emotional release and muscular release are interdependent—one does not occur without the other.

During the session, practitioners also ask you what is happening in your body. You may feel long-forgotten emotions and have insights about past events. Discussing them may give rise to using your body in new ways and gradually discarding habitual patterns.

People choose to engage in Rosen work because of physical discomfort

# A Rosen Experience: Opening the Chest

The following sequence of movements, done with a partner, is designed to open the upper chest and stimulate the diaphragm. As the partner in the sitting position, it will help you become aware of the difference between the depressed or slumped position and a nondepressed or uplifted one. When your chest is up, then your arm movements and gestures can also be free and inviting.

Have your partner sit on the floor while you stand behind her with your knees gently bent against her back to help support it. If you can, try to provide a bit of massage by slowly pressing your knees into her back. As you deepen your bend, your knees can move down to touch the lower back; as you straighten, you can reach the upper back.

Take your partner's hands and move each arm, elbows bent, out to the side. As you hold the arms apart, turn her torso from side to side so that the chest stretches. In the same position, slowly move the arms backward to stretch her chest wider (figure A).

Now let go of your partner's hands and place your hands on her shoulders. Gradually move your hands down her back as you gently push forward so she bends in the lower back and hip joint (figure B).

Figure A

Figure B

To finish, stand in front of your partner (her knees are bent), take both of her hands, and pull her to standing. Reach up high, extending all hands and arms, and stretch. Ask your partner if she noticed any difference between having her chest open as you stretched her out and back and having her chest fold up as you pushed her forward. Switch places and repeat the entire series of movement.

—Adapted from Marion Rosen and Sue Brenner, *The Rosen Method of Movement*
(North Atlantic, 1991).

---

> This work is about transformation—from the person we think we are to the person we really are. In the end, we can't be anyone else.
>
> —Marion Rosen

or the desire for personal growth. In working with emotions held in muscles, practitioners use no chart, blueprint, or map of the body, but deal with your unique situation. However, if you need medical or psychological treatment, they refer you to the appropriate specialist. They do not work with clients who appear psychotic, who have a poor sense of boundaries, or who need their defenses or barriers to get through such circumstances as grief.

Along with the table work, there is the Rosen Method of Movement. Rosen developed it because a friend wanted to know how to prevent aches and pains before she needed physical therapy. In 1956 Rosen began teaching movement classes using exercise sequences set to music. After thirty years of "dancing" with her, some students are now in their seventies and eighties, yet still limber and active. The movements enable you to attain full range of motion in every joint and to release the diaphragm so that there is more space in the chest for breathing. Swings, stretches, bounces, and twists loosen and lengthen the muscles around the joints. The movements also help increase balance and rhythm, prepare your body for more strenuous activity, and facilitate moving with ease and pleasure rather than strain and effort.

Rosen workers come from diverse backgrounds—including physical therapy, nursing, psychotherapy, art, and teaching. They are certified by the Rosen Institute after a two-year training program plus an extensive internship.

RESOURCES:

**For workshops, training programs, and practitioners:** Rosen Method, The Berkeley Center, 825 Bancroft Way, Berkeley, CA 94710, (510) 845-6606.

**Books:** Elaine L. Mayland, *Rosen Method: An Approach to Wholeness and Well-Being Through the Body* (Inksmiths, 1992); Marion Rosen and Sue Brenner, *The Rosen Method of Movement* (North Atlantic, 1991).

# Rubenfeld Synergy® Method

Ilana Rubenfeld developed the Rubenfeld Synergy Method for the integration of body, mind, and emotions out of her own frustration with the split that existed among different therapies. She never intended to become either a body therapist or a psychotherapist, let alone both rolled into one as a synergist. Her heart and hands belonged to music. A graduate of the Juilliard School of Music, where she studied with Pablo Casals, Rubenfeld played the viola, oboe, and piano. She also became an orchestral and choral conductor and served as assistant to Leopold Stokowski. But a rigorous program of honing her musical skills left a painful tune in her body, first as a student, then as a professional. Medical help relieved her back and shoulder spasms only temporarily.

It was the late 1950s. No one had ever instructed Rubenfeld in how to use her body efficiently. Then someone referred her to Judith Leibowitz, an Alexander teacher. Although she found the experience "inscrutable intellectually," she continued because the lessons made her feel better. Also, to her amazement, the light touch spontaneously evoked sadness, anger, and other emotions as memories surfaced. Because they weren't dealt with in the Alexander work, Rubenfeld had to go elsewhere to process her feelings. She felt divided, seeing one person for her body and another for her mind.

Rubenfeld herself became an Alexander teacher and trainer, but the psychotherapeutic component was still lacking. Starting in 1965, she studied Gestalt Therapy with Fritz and Laura Perls, who encouraged her to incorporate their work with her body practice. Then, six years later, she began training with Moshe Feldenkrais and became part of his first core group of teachers in America. And last, Rubenfeld incorporated Ericksonian hypnotherapy. Her synthesis of all these elements became the Rubenfeld Synergy Method after Buckminster Fuller suggested the word *synergy* to her in 1975.

As a result of Rubenfeld's journey, the practitioners she has trained employ a variety of approaches in their work. Generally, they work with you on a massage table, but if you feel a desire to sit or move around, the table is set aside. They use gentle touch with "open and listening hands." They also incorporate verbal expression, movement, breathing patterns, body posture, kinesthetic awareness, imagination and visualization, sound, intuition, and humor. All of these components help practitioners gain access to emotions and memories stored in your body as energy blocks, tensions, and imbalances—what Rubenfeld calls "holding patterns." "As many times as you help clients get rid of their physical symptoms," she says, "unless their emotions are also dealt with simultaneously, these symptoms may return."[2]

Bodies can tell a tale that ideas cannot master and words cannot convey.

—Hugh and Gayle Prather

Every muscular rigidity contains the history and the meaning of its origin. Its dissolution not only liberates energy . . . but also brings back into memory the very infantile situation in which the repression had taken place.

—Wilhelm Reich

# Jack's Back

"Appropriate humor seems to lighten the dark and painful places in people's lives," says Ilana Rubenfeld. "It makes those places bearable and assists clients to go deeper into their feelings."[3] Here's how she handled a man she calls Jack, a thirtysomething therapist, during a Rubenfeld Synergy session.

Sitting on the edge of the padded table, Jack tells Rubenfeld that he's had an agonizing pain in his back behind his right shoulder blade for twenty years despite having tried massage, Rolfing, chiropractic, etc. He voices great expectations.

"If nobody else has helped you, what makes you think I can?" she says, and laughs. "Let's forget about my curing you and instead we'll see what emerges. No agenda, okay?"

Jack lies down, and Rubenfeld slips her hand under his back and discovers an "iron ball" on the spot that has bothered him for years. She senses no energy pulsating through this area. Its texture tells her it's a very old hurt.

"Can you remember a time when you did not have this pain?" she asks.

"I was around twelve years old," he replies.

"Close your eyes and go down to that spot. What unusual or outstanding event happened to you in your early teens?"

After a long pause, he says flatly, "My mother died. She abandoned me, left me alone."

Rubenfeld feels the ball of tight muscle remain hard and unyielding. That signals to her that abandonment may not be the issue. In fact, his voice sounds as though he's told this story many times before. She moves her hands away from Jack's back and gently touches his head.

"I'm sad that she died and abandoned me and now she's in my back," he says, then suddenly realizes the connection. "That's what it is: She's in my back." He starts to sob and gasp for air. Rubenfeld begins to feel energy pulsating through the area. To her, this is a sign that his body, emotions, and mind agree as to what's going on, for "the body tells the truth." She suggests Jack direct his attention to that spot in his back. She asks him, "What would you like to say to your mother?"

"Leave my back! Get out!" Jack screams.

Rubenfeld's hands are under his back again; the iron ball is not releasing its hold. "How many years has she been in your back?"

"I guess about twenty years."

"Hmmm . . . twenty years. . . . How much rent does she pay?"

"What?"

Rubenfeld realizes she has caught Jack off guard. He is startled and confused.

"You heard me, rent. Is your back rent-controlled, rent-stabilized, a condo, or a co-op?"

"She doesn't pay any rent!"

"That's the problem. We need to create an eviction notice." Rubenfeld asks him to visualize himself writing an eviction notice and presenting it to his mother. His back softens slightly. She senses they are getting closer to the issue. She moves to his legs and supports them gently, preparing him for the next juncture. "Imagine that you could talk to your mom now and say whatever you want."

"Mom, you've been in there causing me pain for twenty years." Then he screams, "Get out, get out," and his back softens a little more.

"You've been carrying your mother around for all these years. Don't you think it would be worthwhile to find out how she feels? Speak with her."

"Mom, why are you in my back? Why don't you go?"

"If she could answer, Jack, what would she say?" Rubenfeld feels a dramatic shift in her hands. The iron ball is beginning to soften and spread out.

Jack's voice goes up, and an ethereal sound emerges from his throat. "Jack, I'm very tired of being in your back. I died many years ago. I need to go on my journey, and you're holding me back. Please let me go! What do you want from me?"

Jack starts to sob again, and the iron ball melts even more. He is surprised that she doesn't want to stay in his back at all and that he is the one who's been holding on to her by means of all the pain and rigidity. He stops crying and says, "I never thought of it that way . . . that I'm holding on to her." As he integrates this insight, Rubenfeld feels pulsating energy stream through his now soft back.

Jack slowly sits up, looks around the room, and smiles. He moves his back without pain. "I never felt my shoulder and back like this before," he says.

Rubenfeld explains that her hands gave her important feedback all during the session. Her intention was to help support the emergence of Jack's story and allow him to release this deep, tight spot himself. But it was his journey that melted the spasm and allowed him to let go of a very sensitive life issue.

—Courtesy of Ilana Rubenfeld.

To assist you in expressing and resolving those emotions, the Synergist supports you in gradually reexperiencing your memory and feelings of the incident that originally led to the physical holding patterns and tightness. This then allows you to assess your present situation based on a new awareness. You also have the opportunity to respond differently to similar circumstances in the future. Making these connections occurs in a nonjudgmental and natural (rather than forced) atmosphere.

Training for certification in the Rubenfeld Synergy Method takes place in intensive segments three times a year for four years. It also includes regional training between the week-long intensive segments and regular sessions with certified Synergists.

RESOURCES:

**For trainings and practitioners:** The Rubenfeld Synergy Center, 115 Waverly Place, New York, NY 10011, (212) 254-5100, fax (212) 254-1174.

# Phoenix Rising Yoga Therapy

*The mind can forget what the body, defined by each breath, subject to the heart beating, does not.*

—Susan Griffin

Michael Lee was an Australian college educator when he first learned Yoga at an ashram in Adelaide in 1978. He later directed programs at the Kripalu Center for Yoga and Health in Lenox, Massachusetts, while studying humanistic psychology. One day, he was holding a particular Yoga pose when suddenly he found himself crying as he remembered a fearful incident from his childhood. He felt a shift inside and, for days afterward, noticed a new ease of movement in his hips as well as a change in consciousness—from fear to fearlessness. From that experience, Lee developed Phoenix Rising Yoga Therapy, after the legendary bird that burned itself on a pyre, then rose from the ashes to live again.

Lee devised ways for a Yoga therapist to assist a client in maintaining sixteen well-known forward- or backward-bending, inverted, and spinal-twisting poses. The therapist gently holds you in the asana longer than you might be able to on your own, playing at your physical limit until emotional tensions begin to surface and release. Then she will engage you in verbal dialogue about your experience to stimulate awareness of, insight into, and integration of the emerging emotions. In this way, the Yoga therapist does not impose a particular direction on you, but follows where your internal process leads. To complete the session, you will be guided through a kind of meditation, and you will generate your own affirmations to reinforce self-awareness.

The introductory session has a twofold purpose: It helps you get in touch with your body, and it enables the therapist to locate major areas of holding as an indicator for future sessions. This general session can include nine assisted postures as well as transition stretches. It's not necessary to have a background in Yoga practice in order to do them.

Yoga therapists report that people come to sessions with emotional difficulties and/or physical discomforts—such as scoliosis, skin conditions, asthma, and back pains. In exploring their body through the poses, clients often find the emotional component underlying the physical symptoms. For one Yoga therapist, Barbara Kaplan, the greatest benefit she has derived is gaining the wisdom of her body. "I can really trust and listen to it—it guides me," she says.[4]

My session in Phoenix Rising Yoga Therapy began with a body scan while I remained standing. "Feel your feet on the ground," the therapist said. "Is there more weight on your heels or toes, outer edges or inner arches?"

As we continued up my body—ankles, shins, calves, knees, thighs, buttocks—I was to be aware of softness or tightness in any area. When we got to the pelvis, she suggested, "Imagine your pelvis as a bowl of water. Would the water spill forward or backward or to one side?" Once we went through my entire body in this fashion, she said, "Now take a deep breath to come back to a sense of your whole body, connecting all the parts."

Then we focused on the right and left sides of my body. She asked me to be receptive to any colors, memories, or feelings that might arise and to come up with an "I am" statement about how I felt, first on one side, then on the other. After another full breath to sense my body as a whole, I opened my eyes, sat down, and shared what I'd noticed during the body scan. My right side felt heavy and dark; "I am dragged down" was its communication to me. My left side said, "I am open, straight, strong, comfortable, light."

After taking some nice deep breaths, with my eyes closed, I looked inside myself for whatever intention I had in this session, that is, any issues I wanted to examine. I shared that with the Yoga therapist.

The Yoga part came when I lay down on my back and she began to work with my legs. She bent my left knee and warmed up the hip area before bringing my leg straight back into a hamstring stretch. She moved it gradually until I got to my limit—seven on a scale of one to ten—and then she backed off. When a tightness appeared in my right leg during this delicious stretch of the left, she asked, "Does it have a color? What would the sensation say if it could talk? Does that voice have an age or gender?" She eased me out of that stretch and into a different one for the inner thigh, moving my leg out to the side. I kept feeling a holding in my right hip—a pulling forward and tightness—that wouldn't release.

"What is an 'I am' statement about it?" she asked.

"I am a fist," I spontaneously responded.

"Can you relate to that in some area of your life? Where do you feel like a fist?"

"The only thing I can come up with is being a fist around P., that I tighten up around him."

"Can you tell me more about tightening?"

"There's a protection."

Because of her assistance, I was able to stay in this posture much longer than I could have on my own and to sink deeply into relaxation. I had lots of time to observe the physical sensations I was experiencing as well as the feelings that they conveyed. I noticed that my left leg, which was enjoying the stretch immensely, said, "I am wide open."

"Where does that show up in your life?" she asked.

"With somebody else," I told her.

Then she asked my two sides to talk to each other: "What does 'I am wide open' have to say to 'I am a fist'?"

"You're missing out, you're losing."

"What does 'I am a fist' say to that?"

"I don't really want to be tight there. It's not fun to be that way. I'd like to come out."

"What's in the way?"

"Hurt. I feel pushed away by P."

My body gave me an accurate reading of what was going on in my life at that time. I took a few more deep breaths. The therapist stretched my leg across my body before bringing it back down and switching to my right side. During the right stretches, again she checked in with me and conducted a similar dialogue. At the end, we worked on lifting my pelvis, exaggerating the position to turn the bowl so that the imagined water would not spill forward. My task was to remember this wide-open feeling and find ways to recapture it on my own.

To become a certified Phoenix Rising Yoga Therapy Practitioner involves training in a three-part, 310-hour program, consisting of two four-day intensive sessions and a six-month internship-practicum.

RESOURCES:

**For training and practitioners:** Phoenix Rising, P.O. Box 819, Housatonic, MA 01236, (800) 288-9642.

# Integrative Yoga Therapy

Joseph LePage was a certified Kripalu Yoga teacher and experienced practitioner of various bodyways before he created Integrative Yoga Therapy (IYT) in 1991. IYT uses the technology of Yoga to facilitate health and wellness in the physical body, balance and integration of the mind and emotions, and an awakening to the spiritual dimension of life. According to Yoga philosophy, the ultimate human quest and potential is a sense of unity and our innate connection with all of life. Suffering and illness result from searching for it in the wrong place.

"Physical and emotional problems are often symptoms of that separation," says LePage. "Yoga is a set of techniques for pointing us back to that unity consciousness. As we discover it within ourselves, we release the stress-producing patterns that block the flow of *prana* (vital life energy) in the physical body. As the flow of prana is restored, our body has the opportunity to balance and heal itself."[5]

IYT works on various levels. From the perspective of Yoga, we are a multidimensional creation with coexisting "bodies" or *koshas*. Our physical body is composed of matter; our subtle body is energy, thought, and emotion; and our causal body is a spiritual source of energy. Health is the integration of all aspects of our being.

IYT practitioners combine traditional elements of Yoga with the latest insights in mind-body health research to work with your different koshas, using breath as the bridge between them. A session generally begins with the therapist guiding you on a journey of awareness through your entire body. He or she may also have you draw a body map. Out of a series of twenty asanas, the IYT practitioner selects and modifies only those that are appropriate to your specific condition. For example, with your knees bent and feet flat on the floor, as you inhale you may slowly roll up your spine toward the shoulders, one vertebra at a time. As you exhale, you gradually roll back down. The practitioner will ask you to explore what you're feeling inside, without directing you to have any particular experience. Then he or she will instruct you in a counterpose as well as adjust pranayama (Yogic breathing) to your individual needs.

Imagery, meditation, and deep relaxation are part of a session, too. For example, you may see colors and shapes in the area you're focusing on; words may accompany them. During a session, I "saw" in my pelvis a soft rose-colored circle tinged with a purple edge emerge from a rectangular foundation. The phrase "sensual spirituality" came up right after it. The practitioner does not impose such images or phrases on you, but waits for them to be generated from within you, and may suggest that you expand the healing imagery to encompass your whole body.

Although IYT practitioners do not solicit catharsis as part of the process, you may find yourself crying or otherwise discharging emotionally. If you have not had success with doing Yoga poses alone, this emotional component could be what's behind whatever difficulty brought you for the deeper but gentle work of Yoga therapy. Therapists will dialogue with you as needed. Don't be surprised if looking to heal your physical symptoms— whatever they are—turns into a greater interest in your spiritual life.

Training to be a certified Integrative Yoga Therapy practitioner consists of a thirteen-week program and a three-month internship with a medical center, clinic, senior center, or similar health agency. An extended version of the training is also available at a northern California college as a master's degree with a focus in Yoga and mind-body health.

Our bodies tell our stories: Where we have been; what we have been encouraged to do and prevented from doing; what we have attended to or ignored in our daily lives; what we have learned directly through felt experience; and what we have acquired by way of education.

—Leonard Pitt

RESOURCES:

For training programs and practitioners: Integrative Yoga Therapy for Body, Mind, and Spirit, 305 Vista de Valle, Mill Valley, CA 94941, (800) 750-YOGA or (415) 388-6569.

# Somatosynthesis

*We are not merely freefloating minds but minds embodied. A genuinely holistic viewpoint cannot but see the body as the visibility of the mind and the mind as the expression of the particular individual self's way of embodiment.*

*—Edward Whitemont*

As a chiropractor, Clyde W. Ford found that when he did even the simplest and gentlest manipulation, it would evoke unexpected spontaneous responses in some patients. They would experience vivid mental imagery, a feeling of leaving the body, changes in perception of time, and insights into spiritual or psychological issues underlying their pain or illness. To be able to deal with the emotions that his touch elicited—chiropractic school hadn't prepared him for this—Ford trained in Psychosynthesis, a therapy developed by Italian psychiatrist Roberto Assagioli. It enabled Ford to interact more effectively with patients, but since his work is based in the body (soma) rather than in the mind (psyche), he originated the term *somatosynthesis* to indicate the difference.

Somatosynthesis practitioners are "guides" and the people they work with are "travelers"—rather than patients or clients—on a journey toward healing. Typically, a guide begins by assessing where to work with you based on one of two things: physical manifestations of emotional issues or emotional expressions of physical issues. Once an area of restriction is found, the guide asks you to bring your awareness to that area. Both of you dialogue with your body to determine what type of touch is needed. The guide then uses a variety of hands-on techniques to release the limitation. Together, you also come up with counterimages for that area, such as moving from "churned-up" intestines to a "calm sea."

By anchoring the work in your body, Somatosynthesis helps you gain important insights about bodily and psychological states that otherwise—for example, by merely talking—might not be as readily accessible. The ultimate goal is to assist you in realizing how essential it is to listen to your body and to discover new ways to keep listening. In turn, its messages will inform you how to face the conflicts in your life and free yourself from their physical, emotional, or mental binds. Somatosynthesis is concerned not only with the effect of your personal difficulties on your well-being, but also with the impact of social issues, such as racism.

# Talking Hands: An Experience in Somatosynthesis

To make this experience easier, memorize the following instructions or have someone else read them to you.

Lie down or sit in a comfortable place and loosen your clothing so you can breathe without restrictions. Close your eyes and focus your awareness on how you're breathing. Take deep, full breaths. As you inhale, silently repeat to yourself, "I am." As you exhale, say, "Relaxed." Spend a few minutes getting relaxed.

Now bring your awareness to whatever area of your body needs your attention because it is in pain or under some other stress. Don't try to analyze why it's so, nor try to change or control it. Just notice it as it is. As you become aware of this area, are you also aware of any emotions? Again, don't analyze, change, or control them. Just notice what they are.

With your eyes open or closed, make your right hand into a shape that expresses how the area you're focusing on feels. You might want to stretch your fingers long or curl them into a hard fist. Let your hand do whatever it needs to do to reflect how your body feels. Hold your right hand in that position for several minutes and observe it. Then let your left hand take on the shape of how you'd like your body to feel if it were not in pain. If your right hand is closed and tight, maybe your left hand is open and loose. Do what feels right to you.

Slowly move your attention between your two hands, between the shape that represents how you're experiencing your body now and how you'd like to experience it. Gradually let your right hand change into the shape of your left hand. Notice how your body feels after you do that and how you experience the related emotions.

When you've finished, if you've had your eyes open, close them and bring your awareness back to your breathing. Breathe deeply several times before you open them.

—Courtesy of Clyde Ford, D.C.

---

Ford trains only licensed health-care and social-service professionals—including medical doctors, massage and other body therapists, chiropractors, psychotherapists, and social workers—in intensive workshops and certification programs of varying length.

RESOURCES:

**For workshops and practitioners:** Clyde Ford, D.C., ISTAR, P.O. Box 3056, Bellingham, WA 98227, (360) 398-WELL, fax (360) 398-7631, e-mail: 71426.72@Compuserve.com.

**Books:** Clyde Ford, *Where Healing Waters Meet: Touching Mind and Emotion Through the Body* (Station Hill, 1989), and *Compassionate Touch: The Role of Human Touch in Healing and Recovery* (Simon & Schuster, 1993).

# SHEN® Physio-Emotional Release Therapy

*Healing can occur in the present only when we allow ourselves to feel, express, and release emotions from the past that we have suppressed or tried to forget.*

*—Christiane Northrup*

SHEN is an acronym for "Specific Human Energy Nexus." According to its founder, Richard Pavek, the energy field that permeates and surrounds the physical body is involved in producing sensations that we call "emotions." In turn, they trigger so-called psychosomatic conditions, such as eating disorders, premenstrual and menstrual distress, sexual dysfunctions, irritable bowel syndrome, and migraine and cluster headaches.

According to Pavek, the body contracts around pain, whether it is physical or emotional, coming from the inside or the outside. He identified the Auto-Contractile Pain Response (ACPR) as the physiological mechanism through which the body traps painful emotions and disrupts normal physical functioning. The main purpose of SHEN is to clear trapped emotions from your body.

To do this, SHEN practitioners hold their hands at various places on your body without applying pressure. They wait at each spot a few seconds or minutes, until they sense a release as energy passes from one of their hands to the other. "Doing a flow" through the body relaxes it, dissolving tensions, unlocking contractions, and encouraging you to let go of debilitating emotions, traumas, or memories. Provided there is no ongoing biological cause, Pavek says you may experience relief of pain and faster recovery from illness.

Although there are no specific meridians or acu-points, as in the Chinese and Japanese systems, practitioners follow a pattern of hand placement in a series of flows—peripheral, spinal, shoulder-head, roots, arm-hand. In SHEN theory, the natural flow in your body is up the right side and down the left. Therapists also work with four emotion centers, which are located at or near the sites of four of the seven chakras. ☞ See "Chakras," page 297. For example, they call the second chakra "the *Kath*"; it is located from the top of the pubic bone almost to the navel and relates to issues of self-esteem, self-worth, and sexuality.

SHEN protocols have been developed for chronic-pain units and psychiatric treatment programs as well as for drug and alcohol treatment programs. According to Pavek, SHEN can be used in such stress-linked and emotion-related disorders as depression, anxiety, shock, and phobias, and in such crises as kundalini episodes. ☞ See "Kundalini," page 297. It has only a small, indirect effect on viral or bacterial diseases. But, says Pavek, SHEN can reduce local swelling by releasing tensions in the surrounding tissues so that drainage occurs, and it also can cause the passage of gallstones.

To become certified in SHEN Physio-Emotional Release Therapy, practitioners enter a three-phase program: an eight-day fundamental-techniques training session; a six-month mentored internship; and master-class

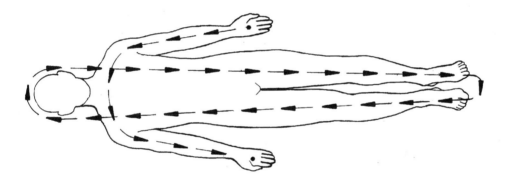

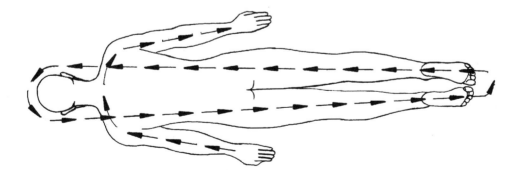

SHEN Energy Flows

intensive sessions. Various professionals, including nurses, psychotherapists, counselors, physical and occupational therapists, massage and other body therapists, and physicians, also incorporate SHEN into their practice after learning only the fundamental techniques.

## Resources:

**For publications, instruction, and practitioners:** International SHEN Therapy Association (ISTA), 3213 W. Wheeler St., #202, Seattle, WA 98199, (206) 298-9468, fax (206) 283-1256.

**Books:** Richard Pavek, *Handbook of SHEN* (SHEN Therapy Institute, 1987).

# Somatic Experiencing®

Every disturbance of the ability to fully experience one's own body damages self-confidence as well as the unity of the bodily feeling.

—Wilhelm Reich

Peter Levine, who holds doctorates in medical biophysics and psychology, developed Somatic Experiencing (SE) as a short-term, biological, body-oriented approach to shock or highly traumatic experience. He believes that trauma is the result of physiology, not psychology. Thus, healing it is possible without long hours of therapy, the painful reliving of memories, or continued reliance on medication. Instead of emphasizing psychological meaning, as in verbal psychotherapy, SE activates intense responses that are both physiological and emotional. But, unlike certain techniques that seem to favor catharsis purely for the sake of catharsis, SE renegotiates these responses without retraumatizing the person.

SE evolved from a study of animal behaviors in the wild. It draws on the body's innate, instinctual wisdom that has developed over millions of years—in particular, the powerful fight/flight drives. Levine explains that at the level of physiology, we remain animals—we still have primitive, nonconscious structures within our nervous systems, bodies, and psyches that perceive certain events as potentially damaging or dangerous to survival. Our ability to react effectively to danger—to flee or fight—and then to discharge the energy our body and mind have mobilized is crucial to avoiding traumatization.

If your orienting and defensive resources (your neuromuscular system, autonomic nervous system, and senses) for confronting potentially life-threatening situations were missing or inadequate at the time of the incident, your ability to respond appropriately probably got frozen and resulted in panic and post-traumatic anxiety reactions. According to Levine, when the appropriate response process happens naturally, then trauma doesn't occur. The nervous system doesn't get stuck and is able to return to its accustomed level of functioning. "Traumatic symptoms are not due to the triggering event, per se," says Levine, "but occur when we fail to resource and move completely out of immobility after the event."[6]

If, however, you are stuck, SE tracks survival resources and helps you rework and restore active-adaptive responses. It does this not by eliciting emotional catharsis and a story line about what happened, but by working with bodily sensation or the "felt sense." ☞ See the "Felt Sense" Experience, page 371. Levine uses a variety of strategies, ranging from directed touching and gentle manipulation to the use of imagery, movement patterns, and hypnoidal state. In SE you focus on the many different kinds of sensation going on in your body as well as images, sounds, smells, taste, and touch. The practitioner will notice subtle shifts in posture or a part of the body trembling, vibrating, pulsing, or moving in other ways. You share your observations from the inside and the practitioner shares them from the outside, proceeding gradually rather than going into the trauma too quickly.

Levine believes that abreactive approaches, which get you to discharge repressed emotions, do not address underlying developmental or psychophysiological stress patterns. They may also drive the trauma deeper and cause further dissociation and fragmentation. "People feel relieved because they've released this energy," he says. "They're high on endorphins and catecholamines, but an hour or two later, they go back into the trauma vortex. Then they need to release something again, so a pattern becomes set."[7]

Levine likens SE's noninvasive way of working to the chemical procedure of titration. If you mix together a powerful acid, such as hydrochloric acid, and a powerful base, such as caustic soda, all at once, you get a huge explosion and damage, he explains. You also get, as a final product, salt and water—basic ingredients of life. However, if you add the base drop by drop into the acid, you get an Alka-Seltzer fizzle and, about thirty drops later, you still get the same net effect—salt and water—but without the explosion. The same is true when dealing with traumatized clients, he says. Instead of going for a big discharge of emotion, you let the person move right up to the edge of the traumatic experience, then stay with the feeling, with no pushing, until there's an automatic somatic integration of the old experience but through a different present consciousness. It's as though the body's pH changes by gradually retuning the nervous system from long-term sympathetic arousal to parasympathetic homeostasis.

Levine conducts workshops to train health-care professionals in Somatic Experiencing as an adjunct in their practices. To become certified in SE, over a three-year period practitioners undergo a 100-hour training program as well as supervised practicum.

The body always leads us home . . . if we can simply learn to trust sensation and stay with it long enough for it to reveal appropriate action, movement, insight, or feeling.

—Pat Ogden

# Nancy's Story

A woman named Nancy had her first attack of panic and agoraphobia while taking the Graduate Record Examination. Although she suddenly was terrified in the crowded room, she forced herself to finish and then ran out. Afraid to get on a bus or into a taxi, she frantically paced the streets for hours until she met a friend, who took her home. For two years, her symptoms grew worse and more frequent. She was afraid to leave her house alone and could not attend graduate school, though she had done well on the test and been accepted by a major university. After a lack of success with psychotherapy and only minimal relief from tranquilizers and antidepressant drugs, she went to see Peter Levine on her psychiatrist's recommendation.

As Nancy recalled the experience of her first panic attack, Levine tracked such physiological signs as her neck pulse, posture, and breathing. After recounting certain details, suddenly her heartbeat accelerated and her eyes glazed over. To focus her attention, Levine asked if she had written the exam with a pen or pencil. "With a pencil, I think . . . yes, it's a pencil," she said.

"Can you feel it?"

"Yes, I can. . . ."

Nancy's face paled and her hands began to tremble. "I'm real scared . . . stiff all over . . . I feel like I am dying . . . I can't move . . . help me," she exclaimed. Her throat became so constricted that she could hardly breathe or speak. "Why can't I understand this? . . . I feel so inferior, like I'm being punished . . . I feel like I'm going to be killed but there's nothing . . . it's just blank." Levine exhorted her to feel the pencil. "I remember now, I remember what I thought: 'My life depends on this exam.' " Then her heart rate went up again.

Suddenly, Levine announced loudly: "You are being attacked by a large tiger; see the tiger as it comes at you; run toward that tree, climb it, and escape!" In reaction, Nancy let out a bloodcurdling scream and her legs started trembling in running movements. After sobbing and shaking for almost an hour, she recollected a terrifying memory of being three years old and strapped to an operating table for a tonsillectomy with ether anesthesia. The physical discharge she experienced in moving out of her passive, frozen response into an active, successful escape allowed her nervous system to return to a normal level of functioning. Body sensation, rather than intense emotional catharsis, was the key to healing her trauma.

Levine worked with Nancy for a few more sessions, and she stopped taking medication to control her attacks. Two decades after her trauma, Nancy mastered the threatening situation she had experienced as a helpless little girl. She also finally entered graduate school, completed a doctorate, and never had a relapse.

—Courtesy of Peter Levine.

# An Experience of Felt Sense

The felt sense is the foundation or ground of everything that forms your internal experience. It is the means through which you can learn to hear what your body and mind are saying. It can heighten your sensual enjoyment and provide the entryway to certain spiritual states. It can enhance your sense of balance and coordination and improve your memory. And it can make physical and psychological therapies more effective.

To experience what the felt sense is, sit comfortably in a chair, on your bed, or on the floor. Feel the way your body makes contact with the surface that is supporting you. Notice how your clothes feel on your skin. What do you sense underneath your skin?

Gently remembering these various sensations, what makes you sure that you are comfortable? Is it a mental knowing? What sensations contribute to your overall feeling of comfort? As you become more aware of these sensations, do they make you feel more or less comfortable? Does that change?

Sit quietly and fully enjoy the felt sense of your comfortableness. Recognize that it comes from you—your felt sense of comfort—not from the chair, mattress, carpet, or pillow that you're sitting on. You can never know whether a piece of furniture is comfortable until your bodily felt sense of the sitting experience tells you so.

—Courtesy of Peter Levine.

RESOURCES:

**For training programs and practitioners:** Ergos Institute, P.O. Box 1730, Lyons, CO 80540, (303) 823-9524.

# Hakomi Integrative Somatics

Our movement and action in the world are disconnected from a depth of body knowing. We literally do not feel the effects of our actions, because we are not connected to the sensation in the body where feeling resides. . . . If we were somatically sensitive and present in the sensation of the body . . . we would change our actions.

—Pat Ogden

Hakomi Integrative Somatics (formerly known as Hakomi Bodywork) regards the body as a living source of information, intelligence, and change. "It is centered around developing the resource of the body to establish and maintain the deepest felt sense of who we are," says Pat Ogden, a founding member and trainer of the Hakomi Institute and originator of Hakomi Integrative Somatics.[8]

Practitioners combine movement, body awareness, and hands-on work to help you establish a new awareness of and sensitivity to the sensations you experience in your body. Together you explore your psychological and physiological habits and translate the language of your body. When the meaning of a physical condition becomes clear, you discover greater choice and freedom in your body and behavior, according to Ogden. Pain that stubbornly resists other therapeutic attempts may finally release. She illustrates this with the story of her client Tom.

In the two-week period after his father died, Tom suffered shooting pain in one shoulder, but he could find no relief after working with massage therapists, doctors, and chiropractors. By the time he went to see Ogden, he couldn't even sleep. First she helped him become sensitive to the tensions and impulses in his shoulder and listen to any messages coming from that area. When Tom exaggerated the tension in his shoulder, he discovered an impulse to hit the physicians who had uncaringly attended his father. By tightening his shoulder, he had been able to hold back his anger and frustration. As soon as he translated the message of his body and expressed his rage, his shoulder immediately let go.[9]

Hakomi Integrative Somatics also addresses traumas and developmental beliefs registered in the body. While resolving developmental issues may call for a reinterpretation on your part—an exercise in cognition—resolving trauma demands an actual physical release. Because trauma arouses our primitive physiological instinct to fight or flee, merely rethinking and talking about the traumatic incident that got "frozen" in the body are inadequate for transforming its negative impact. Instead, the practitioner helps you become aware of and stay with bodily sensations that get rearoused. This affords your body a chance to "defrost" and complete the fight-or-flight response that got stuck during the trauma.

Hakomi Integrative Somatics training begins with a long weekend, and then sessions meet every four or five weeks over a period of seventeen to twenty months to allow for ongoing practice. They are open to practicing body therapists, social workers, psychotherapists, movement or dance therapists, Yoga teachers, and other health-care professionals who want to integrate the skills and strategies into their work. To become a Certified Hakomi Therapist involves an additional two to three years of study and practice.

# An Experience in Hakomi Integrative Somatics

To help you become more sensitive to your body—its impulses, tensions, movement patterns, sensations—and find words to describe your physical experience, a practitioner of Hakomi Integrative Somatics might ask you a series of questions even before you lie down on the table. These inquiries are useful in discovering how your body is reflecting your psychospiritual state and in making you aware—giving you a felt sense—of the connection among body, mind, emotions, and spirit during the hands-on work. ☞ See the "Felt Sense" Experience, page 371.

You'll find this experience easier if you record and play back the questions or have someone read them to you. Pause at each ellipsis (. . .) for a response.

As you're standing, become mindful of your body by sensing what's going on in it. Are some places tight and others relaxed? . . . If you feel tension, which way is it pulling—up, down, forward, backward, on a diagonal? . . . What are the qualities of the tension: dull, sharp, heavy, thick, narrow? . . . Turn your ears inward to listen to sounds that might be coming from the body. . . . Do you hear weeping, laughing, screaming, singing? . . . If you hear a song, does it have words? . . . Is the music fast or slow, sad or happy? . . . What instruments are playing? . . . Turn your eyes inward to look inside your body. Do you see colors, shapes, faces, landscapes? . . . If you're feeling relaxed in one part of your body, expand that feeling into other areas. Where in your body does it want to grow? . . . If you're feeling tense, how does exaggerating that tension affect the rest of your body? Do other areas tighten or loosen? . . . If you feel a movement, express it in slow motion and notice all the details of what happens as you do. . . .

—Courtesy of Pat Ogden.

RESOURCES:

**For training and practitioners:** Hakomi Integrative Somatics, P.O. Box 19483, Boulder, CO 80308, (303) 447-3290.

# Jin Shin Do®

Jin Shin Do (JSD), the "way of the compassionate spirit," is Iona Marsaa Teeguarden's synthesis of Eastern and Western theories and practices. It combines classic Chinese acupuncture theory, Taoist Yogic philosophy and breathing methods, and Japanese Acupressure techniques (Teeguarden studied Jin Shin Jyutsu with Mary Burmeister and Haruki Kato in Japan). To this foundation, Teeguarden added Wilhelm Reich's view of the body as a series of segments that hold certain experiences and emotions. ☞ See Chapter 6: "Psychological Dimensions of Bodyways."

JSD differs from other Acupressure systems in working with eight energy channels called the Strange Flows, or four pairs of Extraordinary Meridians. These pathways serve as reservoirs for storing and releasing energy to the twelve organ-related meridians and the entire body. ☞ See "The Chinese Tradition," page 274. JSD practitioners stimulate your body's own system of self-regulation by activating the Strange Flows and allowing your body to balance its energy. You can sense this flow of energy as a pleasant tingling, pulsing, or streaming sensation.

Practitioners generally begin with an assessment, listening to why you've come. As you lie clothed on your back on a padded table, they will palpate your body for tense areas, feel points along the meridians, and read your pulses. Then they use firm but gentle pressure at points for a minute or two until they feel the tissue soften. With one hand they hold a "local point" in a tense area, and with the other hand they hold "distal points," which help that part let go more easily and deeply. They do not try to break down tension with muscular force, but rather contact it. The touch brings your attention to that area so you can release the tension from the inside out. Practitioners ask you to notice what's going on in your body and how the points feel. In response, you may observe sensations, colors, images, words, or sounds.

Incorporating Western psychology, JSD works with the way acu-points in Reich's horizontal rings of "armoring" (body segments of chronic tension) influence one another and certain related emotions. For example, according to Reichian theory, the chest contains joy, grief, and sadness, while the abdomen harbors motivation, anger, and assertion. When you are not allowed to vent such feelings, you tighten the muscles that would ordinarily express them. JSD uses Acupressure to loosen the segments and restore expressiveness. Learning to be aware of your feelings and permitting yourself to air them appropriately can enable you to prevent the emotional and physical distress that often results from either repressing or overreacting.

JSD practitioners also work with the Emotional Kaleidoscope, a detailed map of emotional states that Teeguarden developed based on the

Our body remembers without censoring. Our conscious mind often edits, filters, and selects what we retain.

—Clyde W. Ford

Five Elements theory. ☞ See "The Chinese Tradition," page 274. Each element is related to certain strong or pleasant emotions (shock, fear, anger, joy, etc.). The Kaleidoscope correlates one hundred different feelings and emotions with the twelve organ meridians. Practitioners use this tool to identify which meridians your personal issues are affecting.

At the most basic level, JSD facilitates relaxation. For example, pressure to a series of points can release stubborn tensions in the neck and shoulder area. According to practitioners, JSD is also effective in relieving certain physical difficulties: headaches, menstrual or menopausal imbalances, gastrointestinal problems, sinus pain and allergies, insomnia, back pain, eye strain, and fatigue. Trained therapists who use JSD say they can help free you of the effects of childhood abuse and other traumas. Your experience may range from intense catharsis to quiet imagery and trance.

To attain the title of Registered Jin Shin Do Acupressure Practitioner, the person must be a licensed or certified health-care professional and complete 125 hours of Acupressure classes, 25 hours of training in counseling and process skills, 125 practicum hours, and other requirements.

RESOURCES:

**For information, books and charts, teachers, and practitioners:** Jin Shin Do Foundation for Bodymind Acupressure, Box 1097, Felton, CA 95018, fax (408) 338-3666.

**Books:** Iona Marsaa Teeguarden, *The Acupressure Way of Health: Jin Shin Do* (Japan Publications, 1978); *The Joy of Feeling: Bodymind Acupressure* (Japan Publications, 1987); and *A Complete Guide to Acupressure* (Japan Publications, 1995).

# Process Acupressure

Aminah Raheem, Ph.D., originated Process Acupressure (PA) after studying both Jin Shin Jyutsu and Jin Shin Do (which she also taught) and Western psychology. She designed PA to release tension, promote awareness, and enhance personal development. It blends a hands-on Acupressure approach to the body with a process orientation to the psyche and a transpersonal psychology focus on the soul.

PA works with your body's energy systems through the pathways or meridians of traditional Chinese medicine and the centers or chakras of Indian medicine. ☞ See Chapter 12: "Eastern Energy." It defines energy as a force or wave motion that interpenetrates the matter of the body; it's an

> The only thing permanent about behavior patterns is our belief that they are so.
>
> —Moshe Feldenkrais

Without the body, the wisdom of the larger self cannot be known.

—John Conger

The body must be credited with an immense fund of know-how.

—Deepak Chopra

interface between consciousness and matter. The objective of a PA session is to bring a clearer, stronger energy field through your whole being and through whatever issues or symptoms you're dealing with. You can also use PA simply for relaxation.

In a session, a practitioner first orients and opens your body's energy. She or he uses dialogue and a twelve-step hands-on procedure to release the flow of energy in the meridians and chakras, relax you, and deepen consciousness so that you're aware of those parts of your body that are signaling for attention. You remain clothed to receive the gentle to very deep finger and thumb pressure on acu-points (energy windows). The practitioner doesn't hold these points but applies fulcrums to them, as in Zero Balancing. Once your energy flows freely and in a balanced way, your other body systems—muscular, skeletal, circulatory, nervous, organs, and so on—will tend to come into harmony on their own. Blocked feelings, chronic body tensions, and sometimes old, unhealed traumas of the past may also release, says Raheem.

Into this traditional energetic foundation, PA incorporates the fundamental principles of Process-Oriented Psychology, as developed by physicist and Jungian analyst Arnold Mindell. PA practitioners see you as an ever-fluctuating complex of body, mind, emotions, and soul. Thus, depending on what arises from parts, points, or centers of your body, they will help you process that material and go to the deepest level possible with it, including the spiritual dimension. They don't try to "fix" a particular symptom, condition, attitude, or idea you have. Nor are they intent on imposing some predetermined structure, balance, or alignment on your body. Instead, they follow your organic process to help you reveal yourself to yourself. A core belief of the process orientation is that there is a center of healing wisdom within each of us, and that it is the best guide to transformation. Practitioners honor your own timing and style because the most important emphasis in PA is on soul-centered development. In closing a session, they may balance the chakras to consolidate and smooth out the work.

You can work with a practitioner or learn to do it on yourself, family, and friends. Practitioners of PA have dealt with body symptoms such as headache, back pain, and digestive difficulties, with emotional distress, and with confusion about personal goals.

Professional certification in Process Acupressure requires three four-day courses and some additional training and practice.

RESOURCES:

**For workshops and practitioners:** Upledger Institute, (800) 233-5880, ext. 164, or Process Acupressure Association, 2621 Willowbrook Ln., #104, Aptos, CA 95003, (408) 476-7721.

**Books:** Aminah Raheem, *Soul Return: Integrating Body, Psyche, and Spirit* (Asland, 1991)—theoretical background of Process Acupressure. There are three textbooks that are part of the training program.

---

# Being In Movement®

Being In Movement (BIM) is a practical way of doing philosophy in the body. Paul Linden, who created BIM, believes that how you breathe, how you hold your body, and how you move are shaped by and also shape your beliefs about yourself and the world around you. BIM uses movement experiments to examine and refine your philosophy of being. They involve investigating and improving your responses to the challenges you face. The physical details of your habitual responses to those challenges reveal your habitual ways of thinking. Trying out new ways of using your body in handling various situations breaks you free from old ways of thinking and being.

> Movements are expressions of people's beliefs about and strategies for handling themselves and the world.
>
> —Paul Linden

The roots of BIM go back as far as the philosophical journal Linden kept in high school, in which he wrote about perceived truth as being somehow connected with how we are "constructed." It was only after many years of education and training that he developed a means of understanding how physical structure is the foundation for mental functioning and vice versa. Linden has a B.A. in philosophy and a Ph.D. in physical education. He holds a fourth-degree black belt in Aikido as well as a black belt in Karate, and is an instructor of the Feldenkrais Method.

Students come for BIM lessons or classes because they are not handling some challenge as well as they would like: walking easily after an automobile accident, working at a computer for hours without strain, playing a flute with a richer sound, delivering a better tennis serve, moving gracefully while eight months pregnant, overcoming the fear of public speaking, and recovering from self-loathing generated in childhood sexual abuse.

The challenge is the starting point for movement exploration in a safe, limited setting. BIM uses five key methods of learning. The first is the development of self-awareness through *body-based language*. For example, instead of saying, "I am angry," you would observe the details of physical events in your body that you name "being angry." You might report, "My fists are tight, my breathing is shallow, my eyes are squinting." By noticing what you are physically doing moment by moment, you not only become aware of and feel much more of what is going on inside of you but also are able to communicate that with more richness.

# Intentional Projection:
## An Experience in Being In Movement

When you drive up to a stoplight just as it turns yellow, does your foot waver between the brake and the accelerator because you can't decide whether to stop or to go? By paying attention to the sensations of intention in your body, you can uncover and understand your intentions and actions. This same awareness of intention is helpful in perceiving and understanding others as well. It leads to a sense of how choice and responsibility operate in your life, and by refining your intentions, you can refine your actions and your self.

You can feel what intentional projection means by doing the following. Put a pencil down on the floor, about ten feet in front of you. Standing up, look at the pencil and want to walk over to get it. Feel that in your body. Truly want the pencil. Don't just think about wanting it. If you have found the right internal process, you will feel your body involuntarily tip toward the pencil just a bit. That tipping is the interface between the mind and the body. When you form a clear intention to execute a specific movement, your muscles automatically respond by beginning to do the movement.

—Courtesy of Paul Linden.

A second area of practice has to do with *intentional projection* (see Experience). A third method includes *proper body alignment and movement organization*. This is the development of power, sensitivity, and compassion, which BIM sees as one and the same. The physical processes of stability and strength, delicacy and sensitivity are the concrete manifestations of the emotional and spiritual processes of determination and courage, empathy and lovingness.

A fourth application involves belief testing, that is, testing intentions and strategies. Intentions are particular muscular movement plans for executing specific actions in certain circumstances. Strategies are the stored plans that you have learned throughout your life and use in a broad variety of situations. For example, as a child you may have made your chest rigid and stiffened your breathing to suppress the fear you felt when your mother yelled at you. You learned that being strong means being hard. In a BIM lesson, you can test the validity of this concept physically as it applies to a difficulty you might be experiencing, such as backache when playing the violin. Does hardening your chest actually offer more strength, or does it make your movements slower and more awkward?

Does softening your chest lead you in the direction of relaxation, power, love, and freedom?

The final key element of BIM is *tracing body sensations and movement patterns.* By going deeply into your body experience of the patterns you find yourself stuck in, you can become aware of their meaning and origin. Through dialogue with the body, you can reconnect to the first moment you ever experienced a specific difficult sensation and work with that memory. Generally, such emotional patterns have a component of learned powerlessness and some unfinished action, says Linden. Once you know what that is, by approaching the situation from a balanced state of compassionate power, you can successfully perform the action you were previously unable to and thus resolve the body pattern.

Linden teaches public workshops as well as professional training programs for such groups as physical therapists, mediators, psychotherapists, and bodyways practitioners.

R E S O U R C E S :
_____

**For information, published articles, and instruction:** Columbus Center for Movement Studies, 221 Piedmont Rd., Columbus, OH 43214, (614) 262-3355. Internet: paullinden@aol.com. Compuserve: 71175, 3146.

**Books:** Paul Linden, *Compute in Comfort: Body Awareness Training: A Day-to-Day Guide to Pain-Free Computing* (Prentice-Hall, 1995).

_____

Helping people to experience themselves as living bodies on the living earth . . . is necessary in achieving any solution to the problems we all face . . . Only with the reawakening of body awareness will people fully feel themselves and what they are doing to the world. Only with the bodily experience of power and compassion will people have the courage and the desire and the ability to undertake what must be done to heal the planet.

—Paul Linden

# ACKNOWLEDGMENTS

I was able to put together a book as comprehensive as *Discovering the Body's Wisdom* only because a great number of people were so generous with cooperation, information, and support. I extend much heartfelt gratitude to all of you and apologize to anyone I have inadvertently left out.

Fellow writer and editor Bill Thomson was the first person to sprinkle water on the seed that became this book and express confidence in my being the right person to cultivate it. Later, his critical comments helped improve the manuscript.

Literary attorney Neal Gantcher stepped in at the right moment to turn my book proposal into a contract. I am fortunate to have him as my advocate and friend, and I thank Martin Furman for the pivotal introduction.

Massage therapist and former lawyer Maria Fire encouraged and challenged me from the beginning. Without her, it would have been a harder and lonelier journey. Stimulating discussions with this clearheaded thinker strengthened my resolve to stay my own course.

Artist Judith Selby sent clippings, read an early draft, took photographs, and, as always, cheered me on with her boundless enthusiasm. Her friendship, support of my work, and confidence in me go back to my first days as a massage therapist. I am continually awed by her unwavering courage to fully embrace the creative life.

Chiropractor and writer Clyde Ford listened and played devil's advocate whenever needed. Our ongoing conversations are a treasured source of shared intellect, heart, and humor.

Toni Burbank, my knowledgeable and personable editor at Bantam, skillfully yet gently recommended editorial changes for greater clarity and readability, and she did so without ever compromising my own voice. I appreciate the great trust she complimented me with from the start. It has been a pleasure and a privilege to work with and learn from her. Her assistant Adrienne Chew was especially helpful and friendly. I thank the whole Bantam team for all their efforts in producing my book as beautifully as they did.

Therapist and teacher Aileen Crow graciously offered materials and insights, carefully critiqued an early draft, and gave me a taste of her work, all in her wise and "spritely" manner.

Body and movement awareness educator Paul Linden provided valuable feedback, dialogue, writings, and exercises, especially regarding the martial arts. His camaraderie as we both composed our books was the equivalent of a big hug.

Artist Laura Lanier devoted countless hours to making sure her fine illustrations were both lovely and accurate. I appreciate her professional conscientiousness in getting things right and sharing the journey of this book with me with such dedication.

Many other individuals were kind enough to take the time to do some or all of the following: read portions of the manuscript and sharpen my explanations for accuracy and clarity; discuss issues with me; donate articles, books, tapes, and videos; give me an experience of their particular bodyway through private sessions or workshops; and contribute exercises for readers to experience it as well. I am grateful for everyone's assistance:

Krista Acevedo, Janet Adler, Judith Aston, Ann Marguerite Axtmann, Ellen Barlow, John Barnes, Ben E. Benjamin, Pat Benjamin, Janet Bertinuson, Mariska Bigos, Raymond Blaylock, Stephan Bodian, Karen Bolesky, Joan Breibart, Alexis Brink, Fran Brown, Rodney Buchner, David Burmeister, Victoria Carmona, Daphne Chellos, Linda Chrisman, Bonnie Bainbridge Cohen, Leonard Cohen, Connie Cook, Sandra Bain Cushman, Emilie Conrad Da'oud, Skye Daniels, Gene Dobkin, Philomena Dooley, Irene Dowd, Carl Dubitsky, John Dzubay, Pavana and Harold Dull, Michael Eisenberg, Adeha Feustel, Linda Foster, Cynthia Gaydos, Cat Gilliam, Elliott Greene, Lynn Harris, Jane Hein, Leigh Hollowell, Barry Kapke, Barbara Kaplan, Robert K. King, George Kousaleos, Arthur Lambert, Ronald Lavine, Jane Lawson, Joseph LePage, Peter Levine, Dana Levy, Jeffrey Maitland, Gilles Marin, David Masters, Kamala Masters, Meredith McIntosh, Kathleen McLoughlin, Gene Miller, Adrienne Mohr, Kate Tarlow Morgan, Brent Neely, Laura Norman, Pat Ogden, Liesel Orend, Ronnie Neufeld Oliver, Luann Overmeyer, Richard Pavek, Karen Perlroth, Rich Phaigh, Robin Powell, Bonnie Prudden, Aminah Raheem, Joyce Riveros, Mary Alice Roche, Ilana Rubenfeld, Phyllecia Rommel, Ellen Saltonstall, Lisa Sarasohn, Taum Sayers, Connie Schrader, Jon Schreiber, Don Schwartz, Anne Terrel Senechal, Barbara Shaw, Joan Skinner, Fritz Smith, Zachary Smith, Iona Marsaa Teeguarden, Philip Anthony Trigiani, Lynn Uretsky, Paula Vaden, Thea Van Houten, Pamela Vantress, Lynn Vaughn, Judyth Weaver, Jerry Weinert, Carol Welch, Deborah Wenig, Betsy Wetzig, David Zemach-Bersin, and the staffs of the many organizations, schools, and institutes cited.

I thank Sue Warga for meticulously copyediting the manuscript.

For their willingness to pose for photographs and/or provide them for illustrations, I thank Zach Allen, Ellen Barlow and The Round Company, Erik Bendix, Joan Breibart and Physicalmind Institute, Anthony Byrd, Kathryn and Conner Elliott, Cat Gilliam, Rose Griscom, Kim Hardiman, Beck Horne, Arthur Lambert, Laura and Joseph Lanier, Laurel Mamet, Elizabeth Squire, and Alima Wieselman.

I want to express my appreciation to all the reference librarians at Pack Memorial Library and the University of North Carolina, Asheville, for their assistance no matter how many times I called with requests. The crew at Malaprop's Bookstore also answered my questions. I thank Jane Voorhees and Emoke B'Racz for giving me the opportunity to be in one of my favorite environments and avail myself of its resources.

Thanks to Scott Smith and Alan Moss at In-Line Creative for generously allowing me to use their equipment before I got better equipped.

Some people had no direct involvement in this project but contributed to my life and my work at different times in various ways. They were kindhearted in their support and encouragement as "uncle," mentor, counselor, friend, editor, or fellow writer. I'll always be grateful to them for believing in me: Sam Steckelman, Scott C.S. Smith, Rita Knipe, Bette Jackson, Dana Devereaux and Tony Mekisich, Mark Mayell, Rafael Tuburan, James G. Callan and my Maui writers' group.

Though I was not able to include a separate section on their practices, I appreciate the following professionals for the interviews and/or materials they were considerate enough to give me: Thomas Pope of Lomi Institute, Peter Bernhardt of Bodynamic Institute, Siegmar Gerkin of Institute of CORE Energetics West, Marjorie Rand of Rosenberg-Rand Institute of Integrative Body Psychotherapy, Janet Smith for Pesso System, Daria Halprin Khalighi of Tamalpa Institute, Ann Weiser Cornell and Luke Lukens for Focusing, Richard Overly, and Ellen Goldman.

Meredith Balgley and Erik Bendix provided the cottage in the woods, where the birds, wind in the trees, and water running down the mountain were the only sounds that punctuated the quiet of what proved to be the perfect writer's retreat. I thank them for their magnanimity.

Patrick Newman Dennison built my office, tailor-made for my writing needs. I appreciate the gift of his considerable talents as a designer-builder and the room in which to write. He helped make my retreat in the Blue Ridge Mountains possible.

My sister Rebecca Knaster made it easy to be in New York whenever I needed to take care of business. She's been generous in so many ways.

My dharma sister Kamala Masters, even thousands of miles away, is always there with a pure heart, wise counsel, and girlish laughter to help me through the challenges and to share the joys.

And thanks to Larry for serendipitously reappearing just when I needed his love.

# How to Deal with Sexual Misconduct

An attempt by a body practitioner to engage in sexually intimate behavior with a client is inappropriate and violate of professional ethics. When such boundaries of ethical conduct are crossed, you have the right to refuse further treatment and to report the illegal behavior. In dealing with the unfortunate incident, you may go through a dizzying array of emotions, wonder what recourse you have, and want help in getting over the offense.

## COMMON EXPERIENCES

If sexual behavior occurs with a body practitioner, you may experience:

*Confusion.* You may feel angry, yet also loving and protective of the therapist. Maybe you wonder whether you're being controlled by the other person.

*Fear, isolation, distrust.* You may feel alone in your experience, that you have no one to talk to, that no one will believe what happened.

*Indecision.* You may experience a temporary inability to make decisions, deal with your job, or cope with personal needs.

*Guilt, shame, responsibility.* If you feel that somehow what occurred was all your fault, remember that it is the ethical responsibility of professionals to avoid a sexual relationship with clients.

*Depression.* It's not unusual to get depressed and feel out of control (and in some cases even suicidal) when your trust has been betrayed.

*Recurrent nightmares.* You may experience nightmares, fears, flashbacks about what happened, and difficulty concentrating.

## Options for Recovery

*Do not isolate yourself.* In every state there are people who have experienced sexual misconduct on the part of health, education, or religious professionals. Find someone you trust to talk with—friend, family, therapist, support group.

*Therapy.* To assist you in effectively healing from the incident of sexual misconduct, carefully choose a therapist experienced in dealing with people who have had this happen to them.

*Networking.* Contact other individuals who have been through the same thing. Remaining silent may hurt you and keep others from avoiding such painful experiences.

*Reporting misconduct.* It is important to report abusive practitioners to help prevent the same thing from occurring over and over.

## Possible Actions

If the incident was not dangerous or overt, give the practitioner a chance to admit the mistake and apologize. Let the person know how you're feeling. On the off chance that you may have misinterpreted the practitioner's impropriety or are projecting your own unconscious desires, it is important to thoroughly consider what happened and what you're feeling. It is helpful to be clear in yourself before accusing someone of unethical behavior.

If you can't speak directly or if your first attempt is unsuccessful, try again in the presence of a neutral third party, such as another body practitioner, psychotherapist, or someone from a local advocacy group.

If you're satisfied with the response you've gotten from the practitioner or organization where you had your session—an apology, a refund for the session, as well as disciplinary action, educational measures, and psychotherapy for the practitioner—you may find that's enough.

If you're not happy with how the matter has been handled, you might consider filing a complaint and taking legal action.

## Registering Complaints

State government agencies called Licensing Boards receive and investigate complaints. They have the authority to discipline someone if the law has been broken. Just as we can have our driver's license taken away, so can a practitioner have a professional license revoked. However, such boards cannot award monetary damages or criminally prosecute anyone; and many bodyways are not licensed modalities.

You can also register a complaint with professional organizations about members who have violated their code of ethics (e.g., American Massage Therapy Association, American Oriental Bodywork Therapy Association).

## LEGAL ACTION

*Civil.* Through a civil lawsuit, you may be able to derive some financial compensation for losses incurred and damages suffered. You can locate attorneys specializing in such cases through a victim advocacy group.

*Criminal.* To pursue criminal prosecution, you have to work through the Office of the District Attorney in the county of the violator.

This outline is an adaptation of "Sexual Misconduct: An Informational Brochure for Consumers of Health Care Services," in *Massage Therapy Journal* (winter 1992). I am grateful to Ben E. Benjamin, Ph.D., who generously invited others to make the information freely available to all consumers of health-care services.

# References

## INTRODUCTION

1. On how healers become healers, see, for example, Stanley Krippner and Alberto Villoldo, *The Realms of Healing* (Celestial Arts, 1986).

2. For a review of clinical research, see John Yates, *A Physician's Guide to Therapeutic Massage: Its Physiological Effects and Their Application to Treatment* (Massage Therapists' Association of British Columbia, 1990).

3. I have mixed feelings about using the word *bodywork* for the field I am discussing. It sounds mechanical, as though we were nothing more than automobiles to be taken to a body shop to have our dents smoothed out and structure realigned after an accident. Yet in some ways the metaphor is apt. We too strive for a "smoothing" and "straightening out" of our physical and emotional "dents."

I've thought of using *bodymindwork* but find it too thick a word, too clunky for a process that is essentially about movement—fluids coursing through blood vessels and lymph vessels, electrochemical messages speeding along nerves and jumping across synapses, muscles lifting bones, and so on. And while *bodymindwork* is an attempt at integration, it leaves out yet other aspects of our being that should not be split off: spirit and emotions.

The late Thomas Hanna made a distinction between *body* and *soma* and introduced the term *somatics* in 1970. The difference between perceiving ourselves as body or soma lies in where we're looking from. As a soma, we are observing or experiencing ourselves from our personal point of view, that is, from inside. It's like being a first-person narrator in a novel: I tell the story through my own eyes, through *I* and *me*. As a body, we are examining ourselves from a third-person perspective, from outside, and we are noticed and acted upon as an object—measured, diagnosed, and treated. When we look at ourselves in the mirror, we see a body; when we feel ourselves from within, we are a soma. It's vital that we do both, for culturally we have exaggerated the importance of what's in the mirror to the total neglect of what exists on the inside. Too many of us have beaten ourselves up, literally and figuratively, over our outer appearance, forgetting or denying our inner core. Anorexia nervosa, bulimia, self-hatred, and excessive dieting and exercising to the point of amenorrhea are some of the destructive results. Though the distinction between soma and body is valid, I'm sticking with *body* because it is recognizable and easily understood. We don't have to change the word, only our attitude toward the body.

4. David M. Eisenberg, M.D., et al., "Unconventional Medicine in the United States," *The New England Journal of Medicine* 328 (Jan. 28, 1993), pp. 246–52.

5. Jordan Fisher-Smith, "Field Observations: An Interview with Wendell Berry," *The Sun* (Feb. 1994), p. 13.

6. Robert Frager, ed., *Who Am I?: Personality Types for Self-Discovery* (Jeremy P. Tarcher/Putnam, 1994), p. 14.

7. Ted Kaptchuk and Michael Croucher, *The Healing Arts: Exploring the Medical Ways of the World* (Summit, 1987), p. 37.

## CH. 1: THE BENEFITS OF BODYWAYS

1. Deane Juhan, *Job's Body: A Handbook for Bodywork* (Station Hill, 1987), p. xviii.

2. Jon Kabat-Zinn, *Full Catastrophe Living: Using the Wisdom of Your Body and Mind to Face Stress, Pain, and Illness* (Delta, 1990), pp. 8–9.

3. James Lynch, quoted in Henry Dreher, "Why Did the People of Roseto, PA, Live So Long?" *Natural Health* (Sept./Oct. 1993), pp. 130–31.

4. Anita Greene, "Giving the Body Its Due," *Quadrant* (fall 1984), p. 10. See also Christiane Northrup, M.D., *Women's Bodies, Women's Wisdom: Creating Physical and Emotional Health and Healing* (Bantam, 1994). The introduction includes her story about not paying attention to her body's needs, masking pain with medication, and winding up with an abscess cavity under her right breast, which necessitated surgery (pp. xxi–xxiii).

5. Jean Shinoda Bolen, *Crossing to Avalon: A Woman's Midlife Pilgrimage* (HarperCollins, 1994), pp. 244–45.

6. James Lynch in Dreher, "Why Did the People of Roseto, PA, Live So Long?" p. 131.

7. Clyde Ford, *Compassionate Touch: The Role of Human Touch in Healing and Recovery* (Simon & Schuster, 1993), ch. 3.

8. Richard Strozzi Heckler, *The Anatomy of Change* (Shambhala, 1985), pp. 23–25.

9. Primo Levi, *Survival in Auschwitz and the Reawakening* (Summit, 1986), p. 395.

10. Barry Neil Kaufman, *Son-Rise: The Miracle Continues* (H. J. Kramer, 1994).

11. Ken Wilber, *No Boundary: Eastern and Western Approaches to Personal Growth* (Shambhala, 1979), p. 108.

12. Michael Murphy, quoted in Richard Smoley, "Knowledge of the Body: The *Gnosis* Interview with Michael Murphy," *Gnosis Magazine* (fall 1993), p. 33.

13. Ashley Montagu, *Touching: The Human Significance of the Skin* (Harper & Row, 1978), pp. 76–81.

14. Derived from Joseph Heller and William A. Henkin, *Bodywise* (Wingbow, 1991), p. 179.

15. Robert Ornstein and David Sobel, *Healthy Pleasures* (Addison-Wesley, 1990), pp. 25, 38.

16. Lionel Tiger, *The Pursuit of Pleasure* (Little, Brown, 1992), p. 23. This is a thought-provoking, witty celebration of our ability to experience pleasure and our need to seek it out.

17. Gloria Steinem, *Revolution from Within* (Little, Brown, 1993), pp. 199–200.

18. Derived from Ida Rolf, *Rolfing: Reestablishing the Natural Alignment and Structural Integration of the Human Body for Vitality and Well-Being* (Healing Arts, 1989), pp. 25–26.

19. Information comes from PASS, American Sports Medicine, P.O. Box 1837, Mill Valley, CA 94942; (415) 383-5750.

20. The suggestion for these body movements comes from William "Dub" Leigh, *Bodytherapy: From Rolf to Feldenkrais to Tanouye Roshi* (Water Margin, 1989), p. 73. A master bodyways practitioner, he tried adjusting his posture after feeling overwhelmed by waves of sadness while driving. Thirty miles down the highway, Leigh found himself whistling and tapping his foot to his own music.

21. Information is from *P.R.E.S. Releases,* 1984–1990 (Project P.R.E.S., Office of Education, County of Santa Cruz, 809 Bay Ave., Suite H, Capitola, CA 95010); Eve Hill Pecchenino and Jeanne St. John, "Let Your Fingers Do the Walking," *Academic Therapy* 19:1 (Sept. 1983); Jeanne St. John, "A Hands-On (Literally) Approach to Stress Reduction: What's New in Schools?" *Thrust* 13:7 (June 1984), pp. 12–14; Jeanne St. John, "P.R.E.S.: Physical Response Education Systems; The Oriental Model Goes to School," *The Journal of Traditional Acupuncture* 99:2 (spring/summer 1987), pp. 30–35, "Acupressure Therapy in a School Environment for Handicapped Children," *American Journal of Acupuncture* 15:3 (July–Sept. 1987), pp. 227–32.

22. Tiffany Field, director, Touch Research Institute keynote speech at 50th-anniversary American Massage Therapy Association convention, Chicago, Oct. 13, 1993.

23. Reported in Thomas Armstrong, *Seven Kinds of Smart* (Plume/Penguin, 1993), p. 84.

24. Ashley Montagu, *Touching*, especially ch. 4 and ch. 6; Mirka Knaster, "Premature Infants Grow with Massage: Dr. Tiffany Field's Research," *Massage Therapy Journal* (summer 1991), pp. 50–60; Amelia Auckett, *Baby Massage: Parent-Child Bonding Through Touching* (Newmarket, 1982), esp. pp. 85–88; *News at Duke Med* (July 1995), p. 6; James W. Prescott, "Body Pleasure and the Origins of Violence," *The Futurist* (Apr. 1975), pp. 64–74; Gary Mitchell, "What Monkeys Can Tell Us About Human Violence," *The Futurist* (April 1975), pp. 75–80. See also Catherine Caldwell Brown, ed., *The Many Facets of Touch* (Pediatric Round Table: 10; Johnson & Johnson Baby Products Co., 1984) and Nina Gunzenhauser, *Advances in Touch: New Implications in Human Development* (Pediatric Round Table: 14; Johnson & Johnson, 1990).

25. Ashley Montagu, *Touching,* pp. 321-22.

26. Michelle Locke, "Human Touch Soothes Surgery Patients," *Marin Independent Journal* (June 21, 1992), pp. A1, A7.

27. Deane Juhan, *Job's Body,* p. xxix.

28. Sidney Jourard, "Some Ways of Unembodiment and Re-embodiment," *Somatics* (autumn 1976), p. 4.

29. Adapted from Julie Firman and Dorothy Firman, *Daughters and Mothers: Healing the Relationship* (Crossroads, 1992).

30. Don Johnson, *Body* (Beacon, 1983), pp. 3, 20.

# CH. 2: BODY ALIENATION: WHERE WE LOST THE BODY

1. Alan Watts, *Does It Matter?* (Vintage/Random House, 1971), p. 29.

2. Marija Gimbutas, *The Gods and Goddesses of Old Europe: 7000–3500 B.C.: Myths, Legends, Cult Images* (Thames & Hudson, 1974) and *The Language of the Goddess* (Harper & Row, 1989); Merlin Stone, *When God Was a Woman* (Dial, 1976); Riane Eisler, *The Chalice and the Blade: Our History, Our Future* (Harper & Row, 1987).

3. Judith Duerk, *Circle of Stones* (LuraMedia, 1989), p. 7.

4. Matthew Fox, *Original Blessing* (Bear & Co., 1983), pp. 76–77.

·5. Negative body terms are from an early Christian text and the fifteenth-century German ecclesiastic Thomas à Kempis; the Samuel Johnson quote is in *R. W. Chapman's Edition of Boswell's Life of Johnson* (Oxford University Press, 1969), p. 175.

6. Wendell Berry, *The Unsettling of America: Culture and Agriculture* (Avon Books, 1977), p. 107.

7. The material about original sin is from Matthew Fox, *Original Blessing,* p. 54; the quote beginning "We must keep down . . ." is by Philo, quoted in Matthew Fox, *Whee! We, Wee All the Way Home* (Bear & Co., 1981), p. 4.

8. Andrew Kimbrell, *The Human Body Shop: The Engineering and Marketing of Life* (HarperSanFrancisco, 1993), ch. 13.

9. Frederick Lee of Columbia University, *Public Health Reports,* 1918, quoted in Leonard Pitt, "The Grounding of America," *Somatics* (spring/summer 1987), p. 6.

10. Leonard Pitt, "The Grounding of America," pp. 5-6.

11. Arthur Burton and Robert E. Kantor, "Touching the Body," *Psychoanalytic Review* 51:2 (spring 1964), p. 122.

12. Charles Péguy, quoted in Morris Berman, *Coming to Our Senses: Body and Spirit in the Hidden History of the West* (Simon & Schuster, 1989), p. 136. This excellent book charts the cycles of heresy and orthodoxy in the West.

13. Berman, *Coming to Our Senses,* p. 147.

14. Larry Dossey, *Healing Words: The Power of Prayer and the Practice of Medicine* (HarperSanFrancisco, 1993), pp. 57–58.

15. Dossey, *Healing Words,* pp. 15, 17.

16. Andrew Kimbrell, *The Human Body Shop.*

17. Statistics from U.S. Census Bureau and National Center for Health; ideal model from PBS program *The Famine Within,* produced, directed, and written by Katherine Gilday in association with the National Film Board of Canada and TV Ontario, Kandor Productions, Ltd., aired on North Carolina public television, Mar. 1993.

18. Statistics from *The Famine Within* (see note 17).

19. Judith Rodin, "Body Mania," *Psychology Today* (Jan./Feb. 1992), pp. 58–59.

20. "Vital Signs," *Health* (Oct. 1994), p. 12.

21. Gloria Steinem, *Revolution from Within,* p. 237. For a provocative collection of fiction and nonfiction on the complex and peculiar relationship women have with their bodies, see *Minding the Body: Women Writers on Body and Soul,* edited by Patricia Foster (Doubleday, 1994). See also "Joyous Body: The Wild Flesh," in Clarissa Pinkola Estés, *Women Who Run with the Wolves: Myths and Stories of the Wild Woman Archetype* (Ballantine, 1992), pp. 199–213.

22. Judith Rodin, "Body Mania," p. 57. See also Judith Rodin, *Body Traps: Breaking the Binds That Keep You from Feeling Good About Your Body* (William Morrow, 1992) and Rita Freedman, *BodyLove* and Kimbrell, *The Human Body Shop.*

23. Charlotte Selver, in Gerald Kogan, ed., *Your Body Works* (And/Or Press, 1981), p. 119.

24. Mikal Gilmore, *Shot in the Heart* (Doubleday, 1994), quoted in Kathryn Harrison, "In His Brother's Shadow," *New York Times Book Review* (May 29, 1994), p. 12.

25. Gay Hendricks and Kathlyn Hendricks, *At the Speed of Life: A New Approach to Personal Change Through Body-Centered Therapy* (Bantam, 1993), p. 77.

26. Julius Lester, *Lovesong* (Henry Holt, 1988), pp. 146–47.

27. Clyde Ford, *Compassionate Touch,* ch. 1.

28. Robin Powell, "Body Awareness: The Kinetic Awareness Work of Elaine Summers," unpublished doctoral dissertation, New York University, 1985, p. 172.

29. Christiane Northrup, *Women's Bodies, Women's Wisdom,* p. 21.

30. J. Kevin Thompson, "Larger Than Life," *Psychology Today* (Apr. 1986), p. 42.

31. Joseph Campbell, *The Joseph Campbell Companion: Reflections on the Art of Living* (HarperCollins, 1991), p. 15.

## CH. 3: BODY WISDOM

1. For a discussion of experiments on muscle activity and thinking, see Thomas Hanna, *The Body of Life: Creating New Pathways for Sensory Awareness and Fluid Movement* (Healing Arts, 1993), pp. 146–49.

2. Maxine Sheets-Johnstone organized "Giving the Body Its Due: An Interdisciplinary Conference" (Nov. 1989, Eugene, Oregon), which later led to *Giving the Body Its Due* (SUNY Press, 1992).

3. Gary Snyder, "The Etiquette of Freedom," in *Practice of the Wild* (North Point, 1990), p. 16.

4. David Bodanis, *The Body Book: A Fantastic Voyage to the World Within* (Little, Brown, 1984), pp. 16, 18.

5. Deepak Chopra, "Timeless Mind, Ageless Body," *Noetic Sciences Review* 28 (winter 1993), pp. 17–18.

6. Ibid., p. 18.

7. Janet Burroway, "Changes," in Patricia Foster, ed., *Minding the Body: Women Writers on Body and Soul* (Doubleday, 1994), p. 226.

8. Laura Riding, *Four Unposted Letters to Catherine* (Persea, 1993), pp. 23–24. The body and bodily awareness are central in the very genesis of language. See Mary LeCron Foster, "Body Process in the Evolution of Language," in Maxine Sheets-Johnstone, *Giving the Body Its Due,* pp. 208–30.

9. Jean Shinoda Bolen, *Crossing to Avalon: A Woman's Midlife Pilgrimage* (HarperCollins, 1994), pp. 259–60.

10. Deane Juhan, *Job's Body,* p. 35.

11. Alicia Appleman-Jurman, *Alicia: My Story* (Bantam, 1988), p. 134.

12. Harriet Goldhor Lerner, *The Dance of Deception: Pretending and Truth-Telling in Women's Lives* (HarperCollins, 1993), p. 186.

13. Mary Field Belenky et al., *Women's Ways of Knowing: The Development of Self, Voice, and Mind* (Basic Books/HarperCollins, 1986), p. 53.

14. Jean Houston, *The Possible Human: A Course in Extending Your Physical, Mental, and Creative Abilities* (Jeremy P. Tarcher, 1982), pp. 26–27.

15. Thomas Armstrong, *Seven Kinds of Smart* (Plume/Penguin, 1993), pp. 81–82.

16. Sidney Jourard, "Some Ways of Unembodiment and Re-embodiment," pp. 5–6.

17. Ibid.

18. Terry Tempest Williams, "In the Country of Grasses," *An Unspoken Hunger* (Pantheon, 1994), pp. 3–12.

19. Harriet Witt-Miller, "The Soft, Warm, Wet Technology of Native Oceania," *Whole Earth Review* (fall 1991), p. 67.

20. Jacques Lusseyran, *And There Was Light* (Parabola, 1987), pp. 31–33.

21. Clyde Ford, *Where Healing Waters Meet: Touching Mind and Emotion Through the Body* (Station Hill, 1989), pp. 22–23, 90–92; Lusseyran, *And There Was Light,* p. 33.

22. Naomi Epel, ed., *Writers Dreaming* (Carol Southern, 1993), pp. 96–97.

23. Jon Kabat-Zinn, *Full Catastrophe Living: Using the Wisdom of Your Body and Mind to Face Stress, Pain, and Illness* (Delta, 1990), p. 26.

24. Harriet Goldhor Lerner, *Dance of Deception,* p. 179.

25. Ibid., p. 26.

26. Eugene Gendlin, *Focusing* (Bantam, 1988), pp. 32–33. You can use Focusing to gain access to your body's wisdom. This book explains the technique step by step.

27. Robert Frager, *Who Am I?* p. 25.

28. For a basic course in proprioception—a kind of textbook in self-sensing—see Anna Halprin, *Movement Ritual* (San Francisco Dancer's Workshop, 1979).

29. Lusseyran, *And There Was Light,* pp. 126–28.

30. Oliver Sacks, "The Disembodied Lady," in *The Man Who Mistook His Wife for a Hat and Other Clinical Tales* (Summit, 1985), pp. 42–52.

31. Joanne Wieland-Burston, *Chaos and Order in the World of the Psyche* (Routledge, 1992), p. 123.

## CH. 4: CHOOSING AND WORKING WITH A PRACTITIONER

1. Aileen Crow, "What Is Bodywork?" unpublished manuscript (May 1992), unpaginated.

2. Ibid.

3. Mirka Knaster, "Philosopher Turned Somatic Educator: An Interview with Jeffrey Maitland," *Massage Therapy Journal* (spring 1992), p. 61.

4. See Peter Rutter, M.D., *Sex in the Forbidden Zone: When Men in Power—Therapists, Doctors, Clergy, Teachers, and Others—Betray Women's Trust* (Jeremy P. Tarcher, 1989).

5. Jack Engler and Daniel Goleman, *The Consumer's Guide to Psychotherapy* (Simon & Schuster, 1992), p. 26.

6. Don Johnson, quoted in Michael Murphy, *The Future of the Body* (Jeremy P. Tarcher, 1992), pp. 398–99; originally appeared in Don Johnson, "Somatic Platonism," *Somatics* (autumn 1980), pp. 4–7.

7. Anita Greene, "Giving the Body Its Due," p. 16.

8. Aileen Crow, "What Is Bodywork?" op. cit.

## CH. 5: DECIDING ON A BODYWAY

1. D. Patrick Miller, "The Voice of the Earth: A Conversation with Theodore Roszak," *The Sun* (Apr. 1994), p. 9. See also Don Johnson, *Body,* p. 157: Before the somatic pioneers "became publicly recognized experts with defined methods, they all experienced similar conversion from alienation to authenticity. During those events they learned valuable lessons about how we all might reconnect with our bodily wisdom. . . . Our emphasis on the variety of techniques they developed obscures their unity in a radical commitment to the authority of sensual experience."

2. Richard Grossinger, "Beyond the Ideology of Healing," *Gnosis* (winter 1995), p. 51.

3. Ronald Kotzsch, "Treating an Injured Back," *Natural Health* (Sept./Oct. 1993), pp. 60–62.

4. This three-paradigm view of the scope of practice was originally formulated by Jeffrey Maitland, director of academic affairs, Rolf Institute.

5. Mirka Knaster, "Researching Massage as Real Therapy: An Interview with Dr. Tiffany Field," *Massage Therapy Journal* (summer 1994), pp. 56–65, 112–113.

6. This story appears in Ted Kaptchuk and Michael Croucher, *The Healing Arts,* pp. 25–26.

7. William S. Leigh, *Bodytherapy,* p. 96.

8. Ibid.

9. The idea for making body maps was contributed by Clyde Ford and appears in his book, *Where Healing Waters Meet.*

10. For example, Rosie Spiegel draws on two decades of experience as a Yoga instructor and Rolfer in explaining how Hatha Yoga and Rolfing mirror the values and philosophies of each other while serving as complementary disciplines. See *Bodies, Health, and Consciousness: A Guide to Living Successfully in Your Body Through Rolfing and Yoga* (SRG, 1994).

## CH. 6: PSYCHOLOGICAL DIMENSIONS OF BODYWAYS

1. Richard Grossinger, *Planet Medicine: From Stone Age Shamanism to Post-Industrial Healing* (Anchor Press/Doubleday, 1980), p. 249.

2. Sigmund Freud, *The Interpretation of Dreams* (Avon, 1965), p. 617.

3. Recounted in Jeffrey Moussaieff Masson, *The Assault on Truth: Freud's Suppression of the Seduction Theory* (Penguin, 1985).

4. Susan Griffin, *A Chorus of Stones: The Private Life of War* (Anchor Books/Doubleday, 1992), pp. 97–98.

5. Ibid., p. 98.

6. Reich didn't originate the use of catharsis. Austrian doctor Josef Breuer (1842–1925) introduced the principle of the cathartic method to Freud after he learned it from one of his patients.

7. Wilhelm Reich, quoted in William E. Mann and Edward Hoffman, *The Man Who Dreamed of Tomorrow: A Conceptual Biography of Wilhelm Reich* (Jeremy P. Tarcher, 1980), p. 122.

8. Ron Kurtz and Hector Prestera, *The Body Reveals: An Illustrated Guide to the Psychology of the Body* (Bantam, 1976), pp. 88–89. Stanley Keleman, *Emotional Anatomy: The Structure of Experience* (Center, 1985), pp. 136–45. For a sophisticated and highly readable account of body reading, see Ken Dychtwald, *Bodymind,* rev. ed. (J. P. Tarcher, 1986).

9. On Reich's death, see Mann and Hoffman, *Wilhelm Reich,* and Myron Sharaf, *Fury on Earth: A Biography of Wilhelm Reich* (Da Capo, 1994).

10. David Boadella, "Somatic Psychotherapy: Its Roots and Traditions," *Energy and Character* 1 (1990), pp. 2–26.

11. For a variety of articles, see fall 1984 issue of *Quadrant;* see also John P. Conger, *Jung and Reich: The Body as Shadow* (North Atlantic, 1988).

12. Candace Pert, "The Wisdom of the Receptors: Neuropeptides, the Emotions, and Bodymind," *Advances* 3:3 (summer 1986), p. 11.

13. Saul Schanberg, telephone interview, Sept. 18, 1992.

14. Ilana Rubenfeld, personal interview, New York City, Oct. 14, 1992.

15. Clyde W. Ford, *Where Healing Waters Meet.,* pp. 21–22.

16. Peter Levine, telephone interview, May 26, 1993.

17. Ibid.

18. John E. Upledger, *Your Inner Physician and You: CranioSacral Therapy, Somato Emotional Release* (Upledger Institute/North Atlantic, 1991), pp. 67–68.

19. Paul Linden, "Applications of Being In Movement in Working with Incest Survivors," *Somatics* (autumn/winter 1990–91), p. 46.

20. Peter Levine, "The Body as Healer: Transforming Trauma and Anxiety" (unpublished manuscript).

21. Gerald Edelman, *Brilliant Air, Brilliant Fire: On the Matter of the Mind* (Basic Books/HarperCollins, 1992).

22. Peter Levine, telephone interview, May 26, 1993.

23. Ibid.

24. Jon Kabat-Zinn, *Full Catastrophe Living,* p. 14.

25. For an overview of research on meditation, see Roger Walsh and Frances Vaughn, eds., *Paths Beyond Ego: The Transpersonal Vision* (Jeremy P. Tarcher, 1993); Jon Kabat-Zinn et al., "Four-Year Follow-up of a Meditation-Based Program for the Self-Regulation of Chronic Pain," *The Clinical Journal of Pain* 2:3 (1986), pp. 159–73.

26. Pema Chödron, *The Wisdom of No Escape and the Path of Loving-Kindness* (Shambhala, 1991), p. 4.

## CH. 8: WESTERN STRUCTURE AND FUNCTION

1. See, for example, the works of Herodotus, Hippocrates, Asclepiades of Bithynia, Celsus, Paulus Aeginata, Caelius Aurelianus, Aretaeus of Cappadocia, Soranus of Ephesus, Galen, Flavius Philostratos, Oribasius, and Avicenna.

2. For an explanation of the therapeutic effects of massage, see E. C. Wood and P. D. Becker, "Effects of Massage," in *Beard's Massage* (W. B. Saunders, 1981), pp. 23–36; John Yates, *A Physician's Guide to Therapeutic Massage.*

3. Associated Press, "RX for Tension Headache Sufferers: Relax," *Asheville Citizen-Times,* Feb. 16, 1995, p. 2A; Michael Weintraub, "Shiatsu, Swedish Massage, and Trigger Point Suppression in Spinal Pain Syndrome," *American Journal of Pain Management* 2:2 (Apr. 1992), pp. 74–78.

4. G. Joachim, "The Effects of Two Stress Management Techniques on Feelings of Well-being in Patients with Inflammatory Bowel Disease," *Nursing Papers* 15:4 (1983), pp. 5–18.

5. Tiffany Field, personal communication, Feb. 20, 1994. The Office of Alternative Medicine (National Institutes of Health) is also funding a study of the effect of massage therapy on immune response among forty HIV-1 patients recruited from the Infectious Disease Clinic at the Medical College of Ohio in Toledo. See " 'A Fighting Chance': Massage Therapy and Immune Response," *PT Magazine* (Sept. 1994), pp. 54–55.

6. For a discussion of how pregnancy causes structural distortion and visceral displacement, see Dale G. Alexander, "Freeing the Breath Wave During Pregnancy," *Massage Therapy Journal* (summer 1994), pp. 51–55.

7. Margaret Duncan Jensen, Ralph C. Benson, and Irene Bobak, *Maternity Care* (C. V. Mosby, 1981), pp. 290, 958; Bette Waters, *Massage During Pregnancy* (Research Triangle Publishing, 1995), pp. 26–28.

8. Frédéric Leboyer, *Loving Hands: The Traditional Indian Art of Baby Massage* (Alfred A. Knopf, 1976).

9. See Frank A. Scafidi, Tiffany M. Field, Saul M. Schanberg, et al., "Massage Stimu-

lates Growth in Preterm Infants: A Replication," *Infant Behavior and Development* 13 (1990), pp. 167–88; Tiffany M. Field, Saul M. Schanberg, Frank Scafidi, et al., "Tactile/Kinesthetic Stimulation Effects on Preterm Neonates," *Pediatrics* 77:5 (May 1986), pp. 654–58; Patricia Bodolf Rausch, "Effects of Tactile and Kinesthetic Stimulation on Premature Infants," *JOGN Nursing* (Jan./Feb. 1981), pp. 34–37; Margret Schaefer, Roger P. Hatcher, and Peter D. Barglow, "Prematurity and Infant Stimulation: A Review of Research," *Child Psychiatry and Human Development* 10:4 (summer 1980), pp. 199–212; Jerry L. White and Richard C. Labarba, "The Effects of Tactile and Kinesthetic Stimulation on Neonatal Development in the Premature Infant," *Developmental Psychobiology* 9:6 (1976), pp. 569–77; Norman Solkoff and Diane Matuszak, "Tactile Stimulation and Behavioral Development Among Low-Birthweight Infants," *Child Psychiatry and Human Development* 6:1 (fall 1975), pp. 33–37.

10. Amelia Auckett, "Birth Trauma in the Newborn," in *Baby Massage: Parent-Child Bonding Through Touching* (Newmarket, 1982), pp. 85–88.

11. The Touch Research Institute at the University of Miami School of Medicine has been conducting studies on the effects of massage on cocaine-exposed and HIV preterm infants and babies born to depressed adolescent mothers.

12. John Yates, *A Physician's Guide to Therapeutic Massage,* pp. 15–27; Kimberly D. Jordan and Dwight Jessup, "The Recuperative Effects of Sports Massage as Compared to Passive Rest," *Massage Therapy Journal* (winter 1990), pp. 57–59, 62–64, 66–67.

13. Lee C. Overholser and Ramona A. Moody, "Lymphatic Massage and Recent Scientific Discoveries," *Massage Therapy Journal* (summer 1988), pp. 55–59; Robert Harris, "An Introduction to Manual Lymph Drainage: The Vodder Method," *Massage Therapy Journal* (winter 1992), pp. 55–66; and "Report on the Eighth International Congress on Dr. Vodder's Manual Lymph Drainage," *Massage Therapy Journal* (spring 1993), pp. 48–50.

14. Milton Trager with Cathy Guadagno-Hammond, *Trager Mentastics: Movement as a Way to Agelessness* (Station Hill, 1987), p. 9.

15. *The Trager Journal* (fall 1982 and fall 1987); and Trager with Guadagno-Hammond, *Trager Mentastics.*

16. "Kicking the Legs" is adapted from Trager with Guadagno-Hammond, *Trager Mentastics*, pp. 116–27.

17. John E. Upledger, *Your Inner Physician and You,* pp. 46–47.

18. Ibid., p. 81.

19. Stephanie Golden, "Yamuna Zake's Body Logic," *Yoga Journal* (Sept./Oct. 1991), p. 24.

## CH. 9: STRUCTURAL APPROACHES

1. Ida Rolf was the first to use this sweater image of the body in describing the fascia. See Ida Rolf, *Rolfing.*

2. John Barnes, "Myofascial Release," *Physical Therapy Forum* (Sept. 16, 1987).

3. Ida Rolf used the image of an orange in her book, *Rolfing,* p. 38.

4. John F. Barnes, "Fascia," in *Myofascial Release: The Search for Excellence* (MFR Seminars, 1990), p. 4.

5. This is an adaptation from an exercise in *Sitting: What You Don't Know Can Really Hurt!* (Health Dynamics, 1983), p. 10.

6. Don Johnson, *Body,* p. 126.

7. Ibid., p. 103.

8. Ibid., p. 126.

9. Ibid., pp. 109–10.

10. Ida P. Rolf, "Structural Integration, Gravity: An Unexplored Factor in a More Human Use of Human Beings," in Gerald Kogan, ed., *Your Body Works,* p. 95; also in *The Journal of the Institute for Comparative Study of History, Philosophy and the Sciences* (June 1963), vol. 1, no. 1; and as a separate booklet published by the Rolf Institute of Structural Integration (1962), p. 15.

11. Judith Leibowitz, "For the Victims of Our Culture: The Alexander Technique," *Dance Scope* (fall/winter 1967–68), p. 34.

12. Mary Bond, *Rolfing Movement Integration: A Self-Help Approach to Balancing the Body* (Healing Arts, 1993), p. 18.

13. Rosemary Feitis, ed., *Ida Rolf Talks About Rolfing and Physical Reality* (Rolf Institute, 1978).

14. John T. Cottingham and Stephen Porges, "Effects of Soft Tissue Mobilization (Rolfing Pelvic Lift) on Parasympathetic Tone in Two Age Groups," *Journal of the American Physical Therapy Association* 68:3 (Mar. 1988), pp. 352–56, and "Shifts in Pelvic Inclination Angle and Parasympathetic Tone Produced by Rolfing Soft Tissue Manipulation," *Journal of the American Physical Therapy Association* 68:9 (Sept. 1988), pp. 1364–70; Julian Silverman, "Stress, Stimulus Intensity Control, and the Structural Integration Technique," *Confinia Psychiatrica* 16 (1973), pp. 201–19; Robert S. Weinberg and Valerie V. Hunt, "Effects of Structural Integration on State-Trait Anxiety," *Journal of Clinical Psychology* 35:2 (Apr. 1979), pp. 319–22; V. V. Hunt, *A Study of Structural Integration from Neuromuscular, Energy Field and Emotional Approaches* (Rolf Institute, 1977); David Robbie, "Tensional Forces in the Human Body," *Orthopaedic Review* 6:11 (Nov. 1977), pp. 45–48.

15. "Getting to Know Your Standing and Walking Patterns" is adapted from Mary Bond, *Rolfing Movement Integration*, pp. 19–21.

## CH. 10: FUNCTIONAL APPROACHES

1. Moshe Feldenkrais, *The 1975 Annual Handbook for Group Facilitators* (reformatted by Feldenkrais Resources, 1991), p. 2.

2. Sandra Bain Cushman, personal communication, Sept. 12, 1994.

3. David Zemach-Bersin, personal communication, Oct. 17, 1994.

4. Robin Powell, "Body Therapies: Body Awareness Techniques," *Journal of Holistic Nursing* (spring 1987), p. 40.

5. Moshe Feldenkrais, *Awareness Through Movement: Health Expressions for Personal Growth* (Harper & Row, 1972), p. 31.

6. Ibid., p. 54.

7. Juhan, *Job's Body,* pp. 340–41.

8. There are exceptions: Bonnie Bainbridge Cohen, who originated Body-Mind Centering, also works with sleeping infants and adults in a sleep/trance state.

9. Thomas Hanna, *The Body of Life: Creating New Pathways for Sensory Awareness and Fluid Movement* (Healing Arts, 1993), pp. 197–98.

10. Moshe Feldenkrais, "Bodily Expression," *Somatics* (spring/summer 1988), p. 55.

11. Thomas Hanna, *The Body of Life,* p. 35.

12. See, for example, Jeff Haller, "Sensory-Motor Education and Transpersonal Psychology," Ph.D. dissertation, Institute of Transpersonal Psychology, 1988.

13. Edward Maisel, "Introduction," in *The Resurrection of the Body: The Essential Writings of F. Matthias Alexander* (Shambhala, 1986), pp. vii–xlvi.

14. Gerda Alexander, *Eutony: The Holistic Discovery of the Total Person* (Felix Morrow, 1985), p. 7.

15. Carola Speads, *Ways to Better Breathing* (Felix Morrow, 1986); Ilse Middendorf, *The Perceptible Breath* (book and audio tapes), from Feldenkrais Resources, (800) 765-1907 or (510) 540-7600, or the Middendorf Breath Institute, 198 Mississippi, San Francisco, CA 94107, (415) 255-2174.

16. Moshe Feldenkrais, *Awareness Through Movement,* p. 71.

17. Moshe Feldenkrais, *The 1975 Annual Handbook for Group Facilitators,* p. 2.

18. Moshe Feldenkrais, *Awareness Through Movement,* p. 36.

19. Chava Shelhav-Silberbush, "Feldenkrais Method with Cerebral Palsy," master's thesis, Boston University, 1986; Reuven Ofir, "Heuristic Investigation of the Process of Motor Learning Using the Feldenkrais Method in Physical Rehabilitation of Two Women

with Traumatic Brain Injury," Ph.D. dissertation, Graduate School of the Union Institute, 1993.

20. "Owing to the close proximity to the motor cortex of the brain structures dealing with thought and feeling, and the tendency of processes in brain tissue to diffuse and spread to neighboring tissues, a drastic change in the motor cortex will have parallel effects on thinking and feeling." Moshe Feldenkrais, *Awareness Through Movement,* p. 39.

21. Ibid., p. 57.

22. Moshe Feldenkrais, "Mind and Body," in Gerald Kogan, ed., *Your Body Works,* p. 79.

23. S. Ruth and S. Kegerreis, "Facilitating Cervical Flexion Using a Feldenkrais Method: Awareness Through Movement, *Journal of Orthopaedic and Sports Physical Therapy* 16 (1990), pp. 25–29; Meena Narula, "Effect of the Six-Week Awareness Through Movement Lessons—The Feldenkrais Method on Selected Functional Movement Parameters in Individuals with Rheumatoid Arthritis," M.S. thesis, Oakland University, 1993.

24. Thomas Hanna, *Somatics: Reawakening the Mind's Control of Movement, Flexibility, and Health* (Addison-Wesley, 1988), pp. 67–68, 79–81.

25. Hanna, *Somatics,* pp. 17–19.

26. Thomas Hanna, "Clinical Somatic Education: A New Discipline in the Field of Health Care," *Somatics* (autumn/winter 1990–91), p. 9.

27. Hanna, *Somatics,* p. xiii.

28. Hanna, "Clinical Somatic Education," p. 7.

29. For information on balls and workshops, contact Body-Mind Centering Practitioner Ellen M. Barlow, The Round Company, (202) 686-3635, fax (202) 686-0228, or (212) 978-9426. The photograph for illustration on page 247 is courtesy of The Round Co.

30. Lisa Nelson and Nancy Stark Smith, "Perceiving in Action: Interview with Bonnie Bainbridge Cohen on the Development Process Underlying Perceptual-Motor Integration," *Contact Quarterly* (spring/summer 1984), p. 26.

## CH. 11: WESTERN MOVEMENT ARTS

1. Ted Kaptchuk and Michael Croucher, *The Healing Arts,* p. 150. For a discussion of the developmental process, see Bonnie Bainbridge Cohen, *Sensing, Feeling, and Action: The Experiential Anatomy of Body-Mind Centering* (Contact Editions, 1993), especially "Perceiving in Action: The Developmental Process Underlying Perceptual-Motor Integration," pp. 98–113.

2. See, for example, Sandra Kay Lauffenburger and Nancy Winters, "Merging Massage and Movement Therapy: Getting Back to Normal," *Massage Therapy Journal* (winter 1992), pp. 71-76.

3. Joseph Pilates, *Pilates Forum,* introductory issue (Sept. 1991), unpaginated.

4. See Mabel Elsworth Todd, *The Thinking Body: A Study of the Balancing Forces of Dynamic Man* (Dance Horizons/Princeton Book Co., 1959).

5. Cynthia Novack, *Sharing the Dance: Contact Improvisation and American Culture* (University of Wisconsin Press, 1990), p. 151.

6. Bonnie Bainbridge Cohen explains how these repatternings or healings occur in *Sensing, Feeling, and Action,* pp. 58–59.

7. Emilie Conrad Da'oud, Continuum workshop, Santa Cruz, CA, Oct. 1994.

8. Ibid.

9. Mary Starks Whitehouse, "Physical Movement and Personality," *Contact Quarterly* (winter 1987), pp. 16–19.

10. Janet Adler, "Who Is the Witness? A Description of Authentic Movement," *Contact Quarterly* (winter 1987), p. 20.

11. Ibid.

12. Valerie Hunt and Mary Ellen Weber, "Validation of the Rathbone Manual Tension Test for Muscular Tension," *Archives of Physical Medicine and Rehabilitation* (Oct. 1964), pp. 525–28.

13. For exploring your body and self, you can also try movement exercises alone or with a partner in Sandra Cerny Minton, *Body and Self: Partners in Movement* (Human Kinetics Books, 1989).

## CH. 12: EASTERN ENERGY

1. Quoted in David Eisenberg, *Encounters with Qi* (W. W. Norton, 1985).

2. Richard Chin, *The Energy Within: The Science Behind Every Oriental Therapy from Acupuncture to Yoga* (Paragon, 1992), p. 80.

3. Robert O. Becker, *Cross Currents: The Perils of Electropollution, the Promise of Electromedicine* (Jeremy P. Tarcher, 1990), p. 129.

4. Robert O. Becker and Gary Selden, *Body Electric: Electromagnetism and the Foundation of Life* (William Morrow, 1985), pp. 234–35.

5. The research was reported at the World Research Foundation Congress of Bio-Energetic Medicine, November 7–9, 1986, Los Angeles, CA. For a video of the lecture/demonstration, contact the World Research Foundation, 15300 Ventura Blvd., Suite 405, Sherman Oaks, CA 91403, (818) 907-5483, fax (818) 907-6044.

6. Richard Jackson, *Holistic Massage* (Drake, 1977), p. 40.

7. See Jeanne St. John, *High Tech Touch: Acupressure in the Schools;* for P.R.E.S. Releases and other materials, contact Project P.R.E.S. (Physical Response Educations Systems), Santa Cruz County Office of Education, 809-H Bay Ave., Capitola, CA 95010.

8. James Clavell, *Shogun: A Novel of Japan* (Dell, 1975), p. 64.

9. U. A. Casal, "Acupuncture, Cautery and Massage in Japan," *Journal of Asian Folklore Studies* 21 (1962), pp. 231–35; W. N. Whitney, "Notes on the History of Medical Progress in Japan," *Transactions of the Asiatic Society of Japan* 12:4 (July 1885), pp. 351–53.

10. Carl Dubitsky, "History of Shiatsu Anma," *Massage Therapy Journal* (fall 1992), p. 110.

11. Ibid.

12. Ibid., p. 112; Toru Namikoshi, *Shiatsu Therapy: Theory and Practice* (Japan Publications, 1974), p. 13.

13. Namikoshi, *Shiatsu Therapy,* p. 16.

14. Dubitsky, "History of Shiatsu Anma," p. 112. I am grateful to Carl Dubitsky for much information in this section on the development of Shiatsu.

15. Ibid.

16. Carl Dubitsky, telephone interview, Aug. 20, 1994.

17. Namikoshi, *Shiatsu Therapy,* p. 13.

18. Shizuto Masunaga, quoted in Susan Moss, "The Ancient Art of Applying Pressure Where It Counts," *Dance Magazine* (May 1982), p. 143.

19. See Michio Kushi and Aveline Tomoyo Kushi, *The Resource Book of Do-In: Exercise for Physical and Spiritual Development* (Japan Publications, 1988).

20. Derived from Ronald Kotzsch, "Hoshino Therapy," *East/West* (Dec. 1988), pp. 54–62.

21. Swami Vishnudevananda quoted in Georg Feuerstein and Stephen Bodian, *Living Yoga: A Comprehensive Guide for Daily Life* (J. P. Tarcher/Perigee, 1993), p. 31.

22. Emma Bragdon, *The Call of Spiritual Emergency: From Personal Crisis to Personal Transformation* (Harper & Row, 1990).

## CH. 13: OTHER ENERGETIC SYSTEMS

1. In the Hawaiian Islands, *lomilomi* refers not only to massage but also to a common dish, lomilomi salmon, in which you tear up the salmon into small pieces and mix them with chopped tomatoes, onions, and seaweed to make a thick salsa.

2. Terry Oleson and William Flacco, "Randomized Controlled Study of Premenstrual Symptoms Treated with Ear, Hand, and Foot Reflexology," *Obstetrics and Gynecology* 82 (Dec. 1993), pp. 906–11.

3. Bill Thompson, "Massage Takes to the Water" *East/West* (July 1990), p. 63.

4. Dolores Krieger, *Accepting Your Power to Heal*, p. 48.

5. Dolores Krieger, "The Relationship of Touch, with Intent to Help or Heal, to Subjects' In-Vivo Human Hemoglobin: A Study in Personalized Interaction," *Proceedings of the Ninth American Nurses Association Nursing Research Conference,* San Antonio, Texas, March 21–23, 1973, pp. 39–58; "Therapeutic Touch During Childbirth Preparation by the Lamaze Method and Its Relation to Marital Satisfaction and State Anxiety of the Married Couple," Department of Health and Human Resources, U.S. Public Health Service, #NU-00833-02, 1983. A host of doctoral dissertations, postdoctoral studies, master's theses, and clinical studies have been written on the use of TT. Check *Medline,* a computer data retrieval program, for dozens of articles on TT, some of which appear in foreign-language health-care publications. The Department of Defense awarded a University of Alabama researcher $355,000 to study the effects of TT on burn patients; the NIH Office of Alternative Medicine has also awarded a grant on the effect of TT on immune response.

6. Janet Quinn, "Therapeutic Touch as Energy Exchange: Testing the Theory," *Advances in Nursing Science* 6:2 (Jan. 1984), pp. 42–49.

7. Becker, *Cross Currents,* p. 108.

8. Jack Bretske, "Letter to the Editor," *Massage Magazine* (Nov./Dec. 1994), p. 14.

## CH.14: EASTERN MOVEMENT ARTS

1. Morihei Ueshiba, *The Art of Peace*, trans. John Stevens (Shambhala, 1992), p. 105.

2. There are many theories about Capoeira's origins: that it developed out of the dynamic dances and music of ancient African kingdoms, that it arose as a self-defense system among African slaves in Brazil, and so on. In the 1800s, *capoeiristas* were fined, threatened with imprisonment, or deported if caught practicing, but by 1928 the Brazilian government formally recognized the art and in 1972 officially designated it a competitive sport. The movements are patterned after animals and elements and follow precise rhythms, especially those of the *berimbau,* a one-string, bow-shaped instrument. They include *ginga* or footwork, kicks, and *esquivas* or evasive techniques. Capoeira is now spreading to the large urban areas of North America. See Bira Almeida, *Capoeira: A Brazilian Art Form: History, Philosophy, and Practice,* 2nd ed. (North Atlantic, 1986), and Nestor Capoeira, *The Little Capoeira Book,* trans. Alex Ladd (North Atlantic, 1995). Almeida also has a video on Capoeira, (800) 445-2454. There is also a United World Capoeira Association, (510) 236-2332.

3. For a comprehensive discussion, see John Donohue and Kimberley Taylor, "The Classification of the Fighting Arts," *Journal of Asian Martial Arts* 3:4 (1994), pp. 10–37.

4. Paul Linden, personal communication, Oct. 17, 1994.

5. Michael A. DeMarco, "The Necessity for Softness in Taijiquan," *Journal of Asian Martial Arts* 3:3 (1994), p. 93.

6. For a collection of women's essays on the transformative role of martial arts in personal growth and healing, self-defense, empowerment, and everyday situations, see Carol A. Wiley, ed., *Women in the Martial Arts* (North Atlantic, 1992). See also Stuart Heller, *The Dance of Becoming: Living Life as a Martial Art* (North Atlantic, 1991).

7. Ueshiba, *The Art of Peace,* p. 95.

8. John Porta and Jack McCabe, "The Karate of Chojun Miyagi," *Journal of Asian Martial Arts* 3:3 (1994), pp. 62–71.

9. Milorad V. Stricevic et al., "Karate: Historical Perspective and Injuries Sustained in National and International Tournament Competitions," *American Journal of Sports Medicine* 11 (Sept.–Oct. 1983), pp. 320–24.

10. Karlfried Graf Durckheim, *Hara: The Vital Center of Man* (Rutledge, Chapman, and Hall, 1988).

11. Alfred Huang, *Complete Tai-Chi: The Definitive Guide to Physical and Emotional Self-Improvement* (Charles E. Tuttle, 1993), p. 25.

12. See "The Roots of Martial Arts," in John Corcoran and Emil Farkas, *Martial Arts: Traditions, History, People* (Gallery, 1983); Donn Draeger and Robert W. Smith, *Comprehensive Asian Fighting Arts* (Kodansha, 1981); and Paul Crompton, *The Complete Martial Arts* (McGraw-Hill, 1989). For historical details on T'ai Chi Chuan, see Master Alfred Huang, *Complete Tai-Chi,* pp. 45–76.

13. According to B. K. Frantzis, the original name was *Nei Gung* (internal power); *Chi Gung* has become a popular term in the last fifty years, and all forms of it are derived from the parent Nei Gung systems. He lays out the difference between them in *Opening the Energy Gates of Your Body: Gain Lifelong Vitality* (North Atlantic, 1993), pp. 27–31.

14. David Eisenberg, *Encounters with Qi,* pp. 199–200.

15. For research on the electromagnetic basis of this practice, see Robert O. Becker, *Cross Currents,* especially pp. 111–14.

16. David Eisenberg, *Encounters With Qi,* p. 200; Craig Reid, "Qi Healing: Can It Be Explained Scientifically?" *Qi: Journal of Traditional Eastern Health and Fitness* (winter 1993), pp. 28–32; Kenneth S. Cohen, "External Qi Healing: Chinese Therapeutic Touch," *Qi* (summer 1993), pp. 10–17. For a computerized English-language Qigong database which documents the application of Chinese Qigong in clinical work and experimental research, contact the Qigong Institute, East West Academy of Healing Arts, 450 Sutter St., Suite 2104, San Francisco, CA 94108. For a summary of research on external and internal Chi Kung, see Chapter 8 in Charles T. McGee, M.D., with Effie Poy Yew Chow, *Miracle Healing from China . . . Qigong* (MediPress, 1994).

17. David Eisenberg, *Encounters with Qi,* p. 211.

18. "Healing with Chi Kung" is adapted from Craig D. Reid, "Qi Healing: Can It Be Explained Scientifically?" *Qi* (winter 1993), pp. 28–32.

19. Michael Province et al., "The Effects of Exercise on Falls in Elderly Patients: A Preplanned Meta-analysis of the FICSIT Trials," *Journal of the American Medical Association* 273:17 (May 3, 1995), pp. 1341–47; Timothy Hain, M.D., at Northwestern University, received a grant from the Office of Alternative Medicine to study the effect of T'ai Chi on mild balance disorders. Zhou Lishang cites Chinese research on T'ai Chi as the "best medical sport" for its health preservation function in "A Panoramic View of the T'ai Chi," *T'ai Chi* (Feb. 1995), pp. 22–24.

20. Jay Dunbar, "Selections from *Let 100 Flowers Bloom:* A Profile of Taijiquan Instruction in America," *Qi* 5:2 (summer 1995), pp. 28–29.

21. Ibid., p. 26.

22. Sophia Delza, *T'ai Chi Ch'uan: Body and Mind in Harmony* (Good News, 1961), pp. 16–19.

23. John Stevens, *Abundant Peace: The Biography of Morihei Ueshiba, Founder of Aikido* (Shambhala, 1987), p. 33.

24. Ibid., pp. 94–95.

25. Wendy Palmer, *The Intuitive Body: Aikido as a Clairsentient Practice* (North Atlantic, 1994). See also William Gleason, *The Spiritual Foundations of Aikido* (Destiny Books/Inner Traditions, 1995).

26. Stevens, *Abundant Peace,* p. 32.

27. Mitsugi Saotome, *The Principles of Aikido* (Shambhala, 1989), p. 1.

28. See Richard Strozzi Heckler, ed., *Aikido and the New Warrior* (North Atlantic, 1985), a collection of essays on how Aikido instructors have applied its principles to different arenas in contemporary life.

29. Gichin Funakoshi, *Karate-do Kyohan* (Kodansha, 1973), pp. 3, 4, 6. For a discussion of Karate-do and the martial arts as peaceful methods of resolving conflict by understanding the roots of violence, see Terence Webster-Doyle, *Karate: The Art of Empty Self* (Atrium, 1989).

30. *The Bhagavad Gita,* trans. Juan Mascaró (Penguin, 1965), verse 1.39.

31. Yehudi Menuhin, "Foreword," in B.K.S. Iyengar, *Light on Yoga* (Schocken, 1975), p. 13.

32. Partially adapted from Anne Cushman, "The ABCs of Yoga," *Yoga Journal, 1994–1995 Yoga Teachers Directory,* pp. 2–12.


## CH. 15: CONVERGENCE SYSTEMS

1. I am grateful to Clyde Ford for a discussion in which he suggested I use the term *convergence* to convey the idea of an approach in which body and emotions are addressed simultaneously.

2. Mirka Knaster, "Ilana Rubenfeld: Our Lady of Synergy," *Massage Therapy Journal* (winter 1991), p. 40.

3. Ilana Rubenfeld, personal communication, Nov. 29, 1994.

4. Barbara Kaplan, interview, Dec. 19, 1994.

5. Joseph LePage, *Integrative Yoga Therapy Manual* (Joseph LePage, 1994).

6. Peter Levine, "Shadows from a Forgotten Past," unpublished manuscript, p. 4.

7. Peter Levine, telephone interview, May 26, 1994.

8. Pat Ogden, interview transcript for *Contact Quarterly,* no date.

9. Pat Ogden and Anne Peters, "Translating the Body's Language," *Massage Therapy Journal* (spring 1990), p. 54.

# INDEX

## A

abuse:
    and body memory, 20
    and disembodiment, 28
acu-points, 278, 280, 289
Acupressure, 282–85
    contraindications, 284
    Process, 375–77
Adler, Janet, 266
aging, 18
Aikido, 339–42
Alexander, F. M., 5, 164, 218–19
Alexander, Gerda, 121, 222–24
Alexander Technique, 218–22, 268
alienation, 23–40
    cultural evolution, 26
    education, 36–38
    family influences, 32–36
    Goddess civilization, 24
    heresy and orthodoxy, 26–27
    industrial revolution, 25–26
    marketplace, 28–32
    mechanical Enlightenment, 25
    religious dualism, 24–25
    self-image and body image, 38–40
    the split, 23–27
alignment, checking, 196, 268
anatomy and physiology, 143
anger, and breathing, 16
anma, 288
Arica School, 119
arm circles, 250–51
Arndt-Schulz Law, 81
aromatherapy, 137–38
arousal, 82–83
asanas, 346, 347
Aston, Judith, 193, 202
Aston-Patterning, 202–204
athletic (sports) massage, 159–61
Authentic Movement, 266–68
Auto-Contractile Pain Response (ACPR), 366
automatic patterns, 95
awareness, 127–30
    mindfulness, 128–29

sensory, 211–13, 226–28
stimulating, 10–12
Ayurveda, 295–97

## B

Baby Elsi's story, 21
baby massage, 156–59
Bainbridge Cohen, Bonnie, 242
balance, and inner ear, 214
ball work, 263–66
Barnes, John, 208
Bartenieff, Irmgard, 248
Bartenieff Fundamentals, 250–52
beauty, cultural ideals of, 31
Becker, Robert O., 280, 323
befriending the body, 42
Being In Movement (BIM), 377–79
Benjamin, Ben E., 164
Benjamin System of Muscular Therapy, 164
Berry, Lauren, 171
Bindegewebsmassage, 165–67
bioenergy, 117
biofeedback, 137
body:
    asking what it wants, 111
    emotions in, 121
    honoring and loving, 43
    how you treat, 32
    intelligence in, 46–48
    mapping of, 108
    in the marketplace, 28–32
    miracle of, 42–48
    mood changes and, 16
    perception of, 52–54
body-centered therapy, growth of, 121–23
body ego, 116–23
body electric, 279–82
body image, 38–40
Body Logic, 186–87
body memory, 20, 83, 123–27
Body-Mind Centering, 242–45
body reading, 120–21
bodyways, 3–22
    access to memories, 20

aging and, 18
avoiding loss, 12
benefits of, 6
deciding on, *see* deciding on a bodyway
embodiment, 20–22
emotional and spiritual development, 13–17
goal of, 40
inner knowledge and freedom, 9–10
overcoming trauma, 20
pleasure, 12–13
psychological dimensions, 113–31
relationships, 7–9
skill improvement, 17–18
touch, 18–20
why people turn to, 3–5
body wisdom journal, xxii–xxiii, 88
Bonnie Prudden Myotherapy, 175–77
boundaries, 68
Bowen, Tom, 173
Bowen Technique, 171–74
breath, observing, 11, 16
breathwork, 138
Breema bodywork, 304–306
Burmeister, Mary, 308–10

### C

categories and models, 103–107
catharsis, 119
cellular memory, 123
central nervous system (CNS), 213
certification and licensing, 76
chakras, 118, 297–99
character armor and orgone, 117–20
Charcot, Jean-Martin, 114
chest, opening, 355–56
chi, 118, 273, 274, 276–78, 280, 282
Chia, Mantak, 285
Chi Kung, 331–35
child massage, 156–59
Chi Nei Tsang (CNT), 285–87
Chinese tradition, 274–87, 330–39
    acu-points, 278
    body electric, 279–82
    chi, 118, 273, 274, 276–78, 280, 282
    Chi Kung, 331–35
    Chi Nei Tsang, 285–87
    contraindications, 284
    five elements, 275–76
    Massage/Acupressure, 282–85
    meridians, 277–78
    self-responsibility, 278–79
    T'ai Chi Chuan, 335–39
    yin and yang, 274–76
chiropractic, 137
Chua Ka, 119
client-therapist psychodynamics, 66–68

Cohen, Bonnie Bainbridge, 242
commitment, 66
communication, 5–7
compression, 185
connectedness, 102
connective tissue massage, 165–67
Conrad Da'oud, Emilie, 260, 261
conscious sensing, 226
Contact Improvisation, 258–60
Continuum, 260–63
convergence systems, 352–79
    Being In Movement, 377–79
    body and psyche in, 352–53
    Hakomi Integrative Somatics, 372–73
    Integrative Yoga Therapy, 362–64
    Jin Shin Do, 374–75
    Phoenix Rising Yoga Therapy, 360–62
    Process Acupressure, 375–77
    Rosen Method, 354–56
    Rubenfeld Synergy Method, 357–60
    SHEN Physio-Emotional Release Therapy,
        366–68
    Somatic Experiencing, 368–71
    Somatosynthesis, 364–66
CORE Bodywork, 207
Craniosacral Therapy, 181–84
Cyriax, James, 164
cultural evolution, 26
cultural ideals, 31
curing and healing, 97, 273, 297, 332, 334

### D

dance, and movement arts, 246–48
dance therapy, 249
Da'oud, Emilie Conrad, 260, 261
Darras, Jean-Claude, 280
deciding on a bodyway, 92–112
    goals, 97–100
    internal sensor, 110–112
    meandering, 109–10
    mixing and matching, 107–109
    models and categories, 103–107
    one vs. many, 92–94
    personality, 94–95
    personal preference, 94
    physical preferences, 96
    scope of practice, 100–103
dermatone map, 165, 166
Dhonden, Yeshi, 104
Diamond Net of Indra, 102
Dicke, Elisabeth, 4–5, 166, 167
disembodiment, causes of, 28
Do-In, 292–93
dream life, in body wisdom journal, xxiii
Dull, Harold, 316–17
dura mater, 142, 181, 182

**E**

Eastern energy, 273–99
   body electric, 279–82
   Chinese tradition, 274–87
   contraindications, 284
   Indian tradition, 295–99
   Japanese tradition, 288–94
   life force, 273–74
Eastern model, 104, 105, 140–41
Eastern movement arts, 326–51
   Chinese tradition, 330–39
   Indian tradition, 344–51
   Japanese tradition, 339–44
   martial arts, 328–30
   meditation in, 326–28
education, 36–38, 98, 211
ego, body, 116–23
embodiment, 20–22
emotional development, 13–17
emotional feelings:
   in body wisdom journal, xxiii
   and physical feelings, 48–50
   in your body, 121
emphasis, 142–43
energetic bodyways, *see* Eastern energy
energetic systems, other, 300–25
   Breema bodywork, 304–306
   Jin Shin Jyutsu, 308–10
   Lomilomi, 306–308
   Polarity Therapy, 313–16
   Reflexology, 310–13
   Reiki, 324–25
   Thai massage, 301–304
   Therapeutic Touch, 319–23
   Watsu, 316–17
   Zero Balancing, 318–19
energy field, assessing, 322
energy level, in body wisdom journal, xxii–xxiii
energy of injury, 125, 182
energy sense, 59–60, 281, 371
Enlightenment, mechanical aspect of, 25
Esalen style massage, 149–51
ethics, 68–70
evaluation of session, 84–90
expectations, reasonable, 79–80
experiences:
   Acupressure, 283
   arm circles, 250–51
   asking body what it wants, 111
   assessing the energy field, 322
   Aston-Patterning, 203
   automatic patterns, 95
   awareness, 212
   body image, 39
   Body-Mind Centering, 244
   body wisdom journal, xxii–xxiii, 88
   Bowen, 173
   breaking the pencil, 343
   checking alignment, 196
   Chi Nei Tsang, 286
   connectedness, 102
   Contact Improvisation, 259
   in Continuum, 262
   cultural ideals, 31
   disembodiment, 28
   Do-In, 292–93
   easy flexibility, 234–35
   emotions in your body, 121
   examining fascia, 190
   family models, 35
   feeling energy, 281
   feelings, 49
   felt sense, 371
   in Gerda Alexander Eutony, 224–25
   going with the grain, 193
   gravity, 192
   guided journey to body wisdom, 51
   in Hakomi Integrative Somatics, 373
   hand massage, 162
   harmonizing energy, 309
   heel squeeze, 160
   honoring and loving your body, 43
   how you treat your body, 32
   infant massage, 157
   intentional projection, 378
   kidney charge, 305
   in Kinetic Awareness, 265
   lie down, 220–21
   mapping your body, 108
   Mentastics, 180
   mindfulness, 128–29
   mood changes, 16
   observing your breath, 11, 16
   opening the chest, 355–56
   physical style, 96
   Polarity Therapy, 314
   posture, 37
   proprioception, 58
   relieving trigger points, 176
   ringing the gong, 332–33
   Shiatsu thumb pressure, 290
   Skinner Releasing Technique, 269–70
   somatics, 217, 240
   standing and walking patterns, 200
   T'ai Chi basic stance, 337
   talking hands, 365
   truth, 56
   unbendable arm, 340
   Yoga asana, 347

**F**

false memories, 126
family influences, 32–36

fascia, 141–42, 188–91
  deep, 142
  examining, 190
  gravity and vertical alignment, 190–91
  superficial, subcutaneous, 142
  and tensegrity, 190–91
feelings:
  in body wisdom journal, xxii–xxiii
  emotional and physical, 48–50
Feldenkrais, Moshe, 5, 232–33, 236, 238
Feldenkrais Method, 232–38
Ferenczi, Sandor, 117
Fitzgerald, William, 310, 311
five elements of yin and yang, 275–76
flexibility, 5–7, 234–35
Ford, Clyde W., 7, 124, 364
freedom and inner knowledge, 9–10
Freud, Sigmund, 113–17
Funakoshi, Gichin, 342
functional approaches, 209–45
  adding sensory information, 213–15
  Alexander Technique, 218–22
  benefits of, 216–17
  Body-Mind Centering, 242–45
  Feldenkrais Method, 232–38
  Gerda Alexander Eutony, 222–26
  Hanna Somatic Education, 238–42
  learning to move, 209–18
  Mensendieck System, 230–32
  proprioception, 214
  Sensory Awareness, 226–28
  see also Western structure and function

G

Gelb, Michael, 17
Gerda Alexander Eutony, 222–26
geriatric massage, 162–63
  contraindications, 163
Gestalt therapy, 121, 226
getting started, 73–74
  obstacles to, 63–64
Gindler, Elsa, 4, 226, 227
Gnosticism, 26–27
goals, 97–100
  curing and healing, 97
  goal and process, 98–99
  short-term and long-term, 99–100
  treatment and education, 98
  triple-lens look, 102–103
Goddess civilization, 24
going with the grain, 193
Goju-Ryu, 329
Goldman, Ellen, 252
gravity, natural center of, 171
gravity and vertical alignment, 190–91
Greene, Anita, 5

Groddeck, Georg, 114
guide, how to use, 135–39
guided journey to body wisdom, 51
guilt, and disembodiment, 28

H

habits, in body wisdom journal, xxiii
Hakomi Integrative Somatics, 372–73
hand massage, 162
Hanna, Thomas, 18, 238
Hanna Somatic Education, 238–42
healing and curing, 97, 273, 297, 332, 334
Healing Tao System, 285–87
heel squeeze, 160
Heller, Joseph, 13, 204
Hellerwork, 204–205
heresy and orthodoxy, cycles of, 26–27
Hippocrates, 143–44
holism, 101–102
homeopathy, 137
honesty, 55–56
Hoshino, Tomezo, 294
Hoshino Therapy, 294
Huang Ti, 274

I

Ichazo, Oscar, 119
Ideokinesis, 256–58
Indian tradition, 295–99, 344–51
  Ayurveda, 295–97
  chakras, 297–99
  contraindications, 284
  kundalini, 297–99
  oil massage, 296
  Yoga, 344–51
industrial revolution, 25–26
infant massage, 156–59
Ingham, Eunice, 310–11
inner ear and balance, 214
inner knowledge and freedom, 9–10
inner voice, 50–52
insight meditation, 130
Integrative Yoga Therapy, 362–64
intelligence in the body, 46–48
Internal Organs Chi Massage, 285
internal sensor, 110–12
intimacy, 69

J

Jack's back, 358–59
Japanese tradition, 288–94, 339–44
  Aikido, 339–42
  anma, 288
  contraindications, 284

Hoshino Therapy, 294
  Karate, 342–44
  Shiatsu, 289–93
Jin Shin Do (JSD), 374–75
Jin Shin Jyutsu (JSJ), 308–10
Johnny's story, 15
Johnson, Don, 193
journal, body wisdom, xxii–xxiii, 88
Juhan, Deane, 3, 20, 213
Jung, Carl Gustav, 122

**K**

Kabat-Zinn, Jon, 127
Karate, 342–44
Kaufman, Raun, 9–10
ki (chi), 118, 273, 274, 276–78, 280, 282
kidney charge, 305
kinesthesia, 57–59, 219, 258
Kinetic Awareness, 263–66
knowledge, inner, 9–10
Kousaleos, George P., 207
Krieger, Dolores, 320–21, 323
kundalini, 297–99
Kunz, Dora, 320
Kurashova Wine, Zhenya, 163–64

**L**

Laban, Rudolf, 248
Laban-Bartenieff, 248–52
Laban Movement Analysis (LMA), 248–50
Lauren Berry method, 171
Lee, Michael, 360
LePage, Joseph, 362–63
Levine, Peter, 124–27, 368, 370
libido, 116
licensing and certification, 76
lie down, 220–22
life force, 273–74
life-to-life communication, 52
Linden, Paul, 125, 377, 379
Ling, Per Henrik, 144, 145
Lomilomi, 306–308
long-term goals, 99–100
loss, avoiding, 12
Louise's "frozen" shoulder, 239
lubricants, 147, 296
lymphatic massage, 167–69

**M**

Machado, Aunty Margaret, 307
mapping your body, 108
marketplace, body in, 28–32
martial arts, 328–30
massage, 143–64

Bindegewebsmassage, 165–67
  Chinese, 282–85
  connective tissue, 165–67
  contraindications for, 149
  Do-In, 292–93
  enhancement of, 148
  Esalen style, 149–51
  geriatric, 162–63
  hand, 162
  infant and child, 156–59
  lubricants for, 147
  lymphatic, 167–69
  oil, 296
  pregnancy, 153–55
  research on, 151
  Russian, 163–64
  seated, 152–53
  sports, 159–61
  Swedish style, 145–48
  Thai, 301–304
massage therapist, 144–45
Masunaga, Shizuto, 289–90, 291
matter over mind, 41–42
meandering, 109–10
medical models, comparing, 140–43
meditation in movement, 326–28
memory, access to, 20, 83, 123–27
Mensendieck, Bess, 229, 230
Mensendieck System, 229–32
Mentastics, 178–81
meridians, 277–78, 280, 290
Mezger, Johan Georg, 144, 145
mindfulness, 128–29
Mindfulness Meditation, 127–31
miracle of the body, 42–48
mixing and matching, 107–109
Miyagi, Chojun, 329
models and categories, 103–107
mood changes, 16
movement bodyways, 272; *see also* Eastern
  movement arts; Western movement arts
movement therapy, 249
Murai, Jiro, 308
Murphy, Michael, 12
muscle groups, 210
muscles, 141–42
muscle spacing, 186
Myofascial Release (MFR), 208
myofascial system, 188–90

**N**

Namikoshi, Tokujiro, 289
Nancy's story, 370
naprapathy, 137
naturopathy, 137
Neuromuscular Therapy (NMT), 176
neuropeptides, 123

**O**

Ogden, Pat, 372
oil massage, 147, 296
on-site massage, 152–53
orgone, 117–20
Ortho-Bionomy (O-B), 184–85
orthodoxy and heresy, cycles of, 26–27
osteopathy, 137, 191

**P**

pain, positive vs. negative, 80–82
Painter, Jack, 205
Palmer, Daniel David, 137
Pandicular Response, 241
participation, 66
PASS (Promoting Achievement in School
    Through Sports), 14–15
patterns:
    automatic, 95
    standing and walking, 200
Pauls, Arthur Lincoln, 184
Pavek, Richard, 366
Paxton, Steve, 258
perception, body, 52–54
peripheral nerve massage, 165
Perls, Fritz, 121, 226
personality, 94–95
Pfrimmer, Thérèse, 169–70
Pfrimmer Deep Muscle Therapy, 169–70
Phipps, Toshiko, 289, 291
Phoenix Rising Yoga Therapy, 360–62
physical and emotional feelings, 48–50
Physical Response Educational Systems
    (P.R.E.S.), 17
physical style, 96
physical therapy, 137
picking up the vibes, 52
Pilates, Joseph, 253, 255
Pilates or Physicalmind Method, 253–56
pleasure, 12–13
Polarity Therapy, 313–16
Postural Integration, 205–206
posture, 17, 37, 188–90, 194
practitioners, 63–91
    arousal and, 82–83
    before session, 79
    boundaries and, 68
    certification, 76
    client-therapist psychodynamics, 66–68
    compatibility, 74
    competence, 74–76
    countertransference and, 67
    differences among, 71–72
    ending relationship with, 90–91
    ethics and, 68–70
    evaluating, 84–90
    expectations, 79–80
    getting your feet wet with, 73–74
    good vs. bad pain, 80–82
    intimacy and, 69
    licensing, 76
    and memories, 83
    misunderstandings, avoiding, 77–78
    obstacles to getting started, 63–64
    projection and, 67
    relationship with, 64–70
    resistance to, 86–90
    self as, 64
    session with, 77–83
    sexual misconduct of, 383–85
    sources of, 72–76
    transference and, 67
prana, 295, 297
pregnancy:
    contraindications, 153, 155, 194, 284
    massage, 153–55
P.R.E.S. (Physical Response Education Systems),
    17
pressure therapy, contraindications, 284
process, 98–99
Process Acupressure (PA), 375–77
projection, intentional, 378
Promoting Achievement in School Through
    Sports (PASS), 14–15
proprioception, 57–59, 214
Prudden, Bonnie, 175–76
psychological dimensions, 113–31
    awareness, 127–31
    body-centered therapy, 121–23
    body ego, 116–23
    body memory, 123–27
    body reading, 120–21
    character armor and orgone, 117–20
    libido, 116
    repression, 115
    seduction theory, 116–17
    therapeutic tradition, 113–15
    unconscious, 114–15
psychotherapies and originators, 122

**Q**

qi (chi), 118, 273, 274, 276–78, 280, 282
Qi Gong, 331

**R**

Raheem, Aminah, 375–76
Rathbone, Jennifer, 271
receptivity, 66
Reflexology (Zone Therapy), 310–13
Reich, Wilhelm, 113, 117–20, 121, 164, 374

Reiki, 324–25
relationships, 7–9, 64–70
relaxation, 100–101
religion, and disembodiment, 28
religious dualism, 24–25
remediation, 101
repression, 115
rescripting, 127
resistance, 86–90
ringing the gong, 332–33
Rolf, Ida, 15, 195, 198–99
Rolfing (Structural Integration), 195–202
Rosen, Marion, 354
Rosen Method, 354–56
Rubenfeld, Ilana, 124, 258–59, 358–59
Rubenfeld Synergy Method, 357–60
Russian massage, 163–64

**S**

scope of practice, 100–103
seated/chair massage, 152–53
seduction theory, 116–17
Self-Breema, 305, 306
self-image, and body image, 38–40
self-responsibility, 278–79
Selver, Charlotte, 226, 228
Selye, Hans, 238
sense, felt, 371
sensitivity, 5–7
sensory awareness, 211–13, 226–28
sensory information, 213–15
sensory-motor amnesia, 241
sensory-motor period, 116
Serizawa, Katsusuke, 289
sessions, 77–83
    after, 87
    avoiding misunderstandings in, 77–78
    before, 79
    cost and time, 78
    evaluation of, 84–90
    getting started, 63–64, 73–74
    good vs. bad pain, 80–82
    not working, 86
    reasonable expectations, 79–80
    resistance in, 86–90
sexual arousal, 82–83
sexual misconduct, how to deal with, 383–85
sexual pleasure, 13
SHEN Physio-Emotional Release Therapy,
    366–68
Shiatsu, 288, 289–93
    contraindications, 284
    thumb pressure, 290
    water, 316–17
    Zen, 289–90
short-term goals, 99–100

skills, improvement of, 17–18
skin, 53, 54, 57
skin detoxification, 287
Skinner, Joan, 268, 270
Skinner Releasing Technique, 268–70
Smith, Fritz Frederick, 318
Smith, Oakley G., 137
social mores, and disembodiment, 28
soft tissues, 141–42
solid knowledge, 59
Soma Neuromuscular Integration, 206–207
Somatic Experiencing, 368–71
somatic memory, 123
somatic perception, 52–54
somatics, 217, 240
Somatosynthesis, 364–66
space-making, 186
spiritual development, 13–17
sports massage, 159–61
standing and walking patterns, 200
stereognosis, 59
Still, Andrew, 137
Stone, Randolph, 313, 315
structural approaches, 188–208
    Aston-Patterning, 202–204
    contraindications, 194
    CORE Bodywork, 207
    gravity and, 190–92
    Hellerwork, 204–205
    Myofascial Release, 208
    myofascial system, 188–90
    Postural Integration, 205–206
    Rolfing, 195–202
    Soma Neuromuscular Integration, 206–207
    standing upright, 188–95
    vertical alignment, 190–91
    see also Western structure and function
Structural Integration (Rolfing), 195–202
Summers, Elaine, 263
Sutherland, William, 181–82
Swedish style massage, 145–48
Sweigard, Lulu E., 256–57
synergy, 357, 359

**T**

T'ai Chi Chuan, 335–39
Takata, Hawayo, 324
talking hands, 365
Taoist teachings, 285, 286, 328, 330–31
Teeguarden, Iona Marsaa, 374
Tempaku, Tamai, 289
tensegrity, 190–91
Thai massage, 301–304
Therapeutic Touch (TT), 319–23
therapeutic tradition, 113–15
therapists, see practitioners

tissue memory, 123
touch, 18–20
  and awareness, 19–20
  and disembodiment, 28
Touch Research Institute, 17, 101, 151
Trager, Milton, 178, 179
Trager Psychophysical Integration, 178–81
Transcendental Meditation (T.M.), 128
trauma, overcoming, 20, 28
treatment, 98
Trigger Point Therapy, 174–77
truth, body of, 55–56
tsubo, 289

**U**

Ueshiba, Morihei, 339–42
unbendable arm, 340
unconscious, 114–15
unwinding, 184
Upledger, John E., 125, 182, 183
Usui, Mikao, 324
Usui System of Natural Healing, 324

**V**

vegetotherapy, 119–20
verbal therapy, 20
Vernejoul, Pierre de, 280
vertical alignment, 190–91
violence, and disembodiment, 28
Vipassana, 129, 130, 131
vivacious perception, 52
Vodder Manual Lymph Drainage (MLD), 167–69
voice, inner, 50–52

**W**

Ward, Robert, 208
Watsu, 316–17
Western model, 104, 105, 140–41
Western movement arts, 246–72
  Authentic Movement, 266–68
  Contact Improvisation, 258–60
  Continuum, 260–63
  dance and, 246–48
  dance therapy, 249
  Ideokinesis, 256–58
  Kinetic Awareness, 263–66
  Laban-Bartenieff, 248–52

Pilates Physicalmind Method, 253–56
  Skinner Releasing Technique, 268–70
  Wetzig Coordination Patterns, 271–72
Western structure and function, 140–87
  Benjamin System of Muscular Therapy, 164
  Bindegewebsmassage, 165–67
  Body Logic, 186–87
  Bowen Technique, 171–74
  comparing medical models, 140–43
  Craniosacral Therapy, 181–84
  Lauren Berry method, 171
  lymphatic massage, 167–69
  massage, 143–64
  Ortho-Bionomy, 184–85
  Pfrimmer Deep Muscle Therapy, 169–70
  Trager Psychophysical Integration, 178–81
  Trigger Point Therapy, 174–77
Wetzig, Betsy, 271
Wetzig Coordination Patterns, 271–72
Whitehouse, Mary Starks, 266
Williams, Bill M. and Ellen Gregory, 206
Wine, Zhenya Kurashova, 163–64
wisdom, 41–60
  befriending the body, 42
  body perception, 52–54
  feelings, 48–50
  guided journey to, 51
  honesty, 55–56
  inner voice, 50–52
  matter over mind, 41–42
  miracle of the body, 42–48
  sources of, 57–60
Woga, 317
Wu Yux-iang, 335

**Y**

yin and yang, 274–76
Yoga, 344–51
  asanas, 346, 347
  styles, 349–50
Yoga Therapy, Integrative, 362–64
Yoga Therapy, Phoenix Rising, 360–62

**Z**

Zake, Yamuna, 186, 187
Zen Shiatsu, 289–90
Zero Balancing, 318–19
Zone Therapy (Reflexology), 310–13

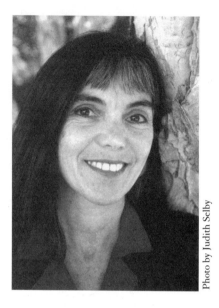

Photo by Judith Selby

# ABOUT THE AUTHOR

Mirka Knaster was born in Europe and raised in New York City. Her life-long experience of living, traveling, and conducting research in different parts of the world have contributed to her cross-cultural perspective on how people view, take care of, and heal their bodies.

A licensed massage therapist who has trained in diverse body methods and disciplines, she has been involved in the alternative health field for more than twenty years. As a contributing editor of *East/West* (now *Natural Health*) and *Massage Therapy Journal,* she has interviewed many of the field's luminaries and reported on the latest trends. Her writing on health and other subjects has appeared in a wide variety of publications, including *The Washington Post, Ladies' Home Journal,* and *Women's Health Care: A Guide to Alternatives.* She was a consultant, writer, and on-screen instructor for the best-selling video "Massage for Health," hosted by Shari Belafonte.

Prior to her work in holistic health, Mirka was a Ford Foundation Fellow at Stanford University's Center for Latin American Studies and taught English in Colombia. She also did research and published academically in the field of women's studies.

For information on Discover the Body's Wisdom™ lectures and bodyways consulting for individuals and corporations, write:

Mirka Knaster
P.O. Box 7464
Asheville, NC 28802
E-mail: Knaster@AOL.com